MCQs in Dental Sciences

National Boards of USA and Canada

- Anatomy and Histology
- Physiology and Biochemistry
- Microbiology and Pathology
- Pharmacology
- Dental Anatomy
- General Medicine
- Oral Pathology
- Periodontics
- Orthodontics, Pedodontics and Endodontics
- Prosthodontics
- Operative Dentistry
- Oral Surgery
- Radiology
- Preventive Medicine Including Microbiology and Biochemistry

Other CBS titles by the same author:

Short Notes for Dental PG Entrance Examinations, Vol I

Short Notes for Dental PG Entrance Examinations, Vol II

Short Notes for Dental PG Entrance Examinations, Vol III

Viva in Orthodontics

MCQs in Dental Sciences

National Boards of USA and Canada

SANDEEP GOYAL MDS (Orthodontics)
Reader, Department of Orthodontics and
Dentofacial Orthopedics, MM College of
Dental Sciences and Research,
Mullana, Ambala, Haryana

Edited by

Sonia Goyal MDS (Oral and Maxillofacial Surgery)
Department Oral and Maxillofacial Surgery,
M. M. College of Dental Sciences and Research,
Mullana, Ambala, Haryana

CBS

CBS PUBLISHERS & DISTRIBUTORS
NEW DELHI • BANGALORE

First Edition : 2004
Reprint : 2005

ISBN : 81-239-1094-0

Production Director : Vinod K. Jain

Published by :
Satish Kumar Jain for CBS Publishers & Distributors,
4596/1-A, 11 Darya Ganj, New Delhi - 110 002 (India)
E-mail : cbspubs@del3.vsnl.net.in
Website : http://www.cbspd.com

Branch Office :
Seema House, 2975, 17th Cross, K.R. Road,
Bansankari 2nd Stage, Bangalore - 560070
Fax : 080-6771680 • E-mail : cbsbng@vsnl.net

Typeset at CBS P&D Typesetting unit and printed at
Asia Printograph, Shahdara, Delhi - 110032 (India)

dedicated

to

Late Sh. Kanhaiya Lal,

Late Sh. Ram Kishan

and

Late Sh. Jaiveer Parkash

Preface

Keeping in view the modern style of the examinations, it is necessary that the students should have a vast knowledge of the subjects to deal with any difficult situation and the questions asked in the examination. Their quiver should be full of all the arrows and instruments so that they are not dependent on any other person during the examination. My other series ***Short Notes For Dental PG Entrance Examinations*** has been compiled keeping in view the requirements of the students during the time of preparation so as to put together all the required information for the special topics under one heading and to compensate the shortcomings present in all the other books available in the market which are totally based on the MCQs.

Since the multiple choice questions help in testing the knowledge of the students by churning the mind and making it exercise on a broad front, the study of the MCQ-based books is necessary. It gives an opportunity to correlate all the choices given with a question and to discuss and omit the wrong choices. Also, they help in finding out the logical statement correlated with the not-required statements.

It has been observed that the books flooding the market at present are based on the MCQs in which many of the answers have been marked wrong, enough to confuse the students. This compilation, which is totally based on the standards set by the national boards of America, has taken care in removing even the smallest possible mistake to avoid confusion. It is suggested that the students should try to get to the depth of the statements and the choices supplied to get a clear knowledge of the question asked. This exercise will help in sharpening the mind and improve the selection power of the brain. This book contains all the subjects of the basic and clinical dentistry. It can prove a boon for the students preparing for the entrance examinations. It can also help the undergraduate dental students to prepare for their *viva-voce* and to clear their ideas. The basic subjects and the questions included can also act as an exercise and help the MBBS students preparing for PG entrance examinations.

I will again suggest the students to keep themselves abreast of the correct and proven scientific statements for the questions, and not get misguided by the wrong choices placed in many MCQ-books. For this, they should be thorough with their theoretical knowledge and remove their confusions after studying standard textbooks.I request the readers to evaluate the volume critically and send me their invaluable suggestions for the improvement of the contents, because only criticism leads to progress and improvements. These suggestions will be solicited in future editions/ volumes of this book. My e–mail address is **goyalsandeep2000@sify.com**

Dr Sandeep Goyal

Acknowledgement

I bow my head to Almighty God for giving my strength to complete this book, as without His wishes, nothing can be done. I can never forget my parents and family members, whose constant encouragement and words of advice keep me working in this field for the benefit of the students.

Words are lacking with me, as it will not be an exaggeration to say that without the blessings of my teachers and guides who taught me during my graduation and postgraduation courses, I would not have been able to reach this level of academics, and I will always have deep respect for all of them at the core of my heart. **Dr D N Kapoor, Dr V P Sharma; Dr Pradeep Tandon and Dr Sanjay Tiwari** have helped me a lot during and after my studies and encouraged me at every stage of my life and took me out of the troubled moments.

My wife, **Dr Sonia Goyal**, who is currently senior lecturer at M M College of Dental Sciences and Research, Mullana, Ambala, Haryana, has always been a constant and unending source of inspiration for this project. It is her editorial and compilation skills which have enabled me to present this project in this form.

I wish to thank **Mr S K Jain**, managing director, and **Mr Y N Arjuna**, publishing director, of CBS Publishers and Distributors, and their team of experts for giving the final touches to the contents of the book.

Last but not the least, I wish to thank all my near and dear ones who have silently helped me during the entire project.

Dr Sandeep Goyal

Contents

Suggested Readings

Since the author does not claim this book to be complete in all respects, the students are advised to further supplement their information by going through other standard textbooks on particular topics. The following table lists some selected books which the student must study thoroughly for gaining the theoretical knowledge.

Author	*Textbook*
Ananthanarayan	Microbiology
Arora/Arora	TB of Microbiology for Dental Students
Boucher	Prosthodontics: Basics of CD
Burkitt's	Oral Medicine
Chatterjee	Physiology
Chaurasia	Human Anatomy, Vols 1, 2 & 3
Cohen's	Endodontics: Pathways to the Pulp
Dixit	Human Embryology
Dykema	Prosthodontics: Basics of FPD
Faruqi	Osteology for Dental Students
Fenn	Clinical Dental Prosthetics, 4/e
Fenn	Prosthodontics: Basics of CD
Finn	Pedodontics
Garg/Bahl/Kaul	Textbook Of Histology
Glickermann	Periodontics
Goaz And White	Radiology
Graber	Orthodontics – An Art or Science
Grossman	Endodontics
Ingle	Endodontics
Joseph	TB of Preventive and Community Dentistry
Khosla/Khosla	Medicine for Dental Students
Killey	Oral Surgery
Kruger	Oral Surgery
Malamed	Local Anesthesia
Marya	TB of Physiology for Dental Students
Marzouk	Operative Dentistry
McCracken	Prosthodontics: Basics of RPD
Mcdonald	Pedodontics

Author	*Textbook*
Monheim	Local Anesthesia
Orban	Dental and Oral Histology
Profitt	Orthodontics
Robins	Pathology
Shafer's	Oral Pathology
Sharma	Essentials of Pharmacology, 2/E
Shenoy	Manipal Manual of Surgery
Shillinburg	Prosthodontics: Basics of FPD
Sikri	TB of Operative Dentistry
Singh	Embryology
Singh	Histology
Singh	Textbook of Dental Biochemistry
Skinners	Dental Materials
Steward	Prosthodontics: Basics of RPD
Stone's	Oral Pathology
Sturdevant	Operative Dentistry
Ten Cate's	Oral Histology
Tiagi	Dental Materials
Tripathi	Pharmacology
Weine	Endodontics
Wheeler's	Dental Anatomy
Wieurmann's	Radiology
Winkler	Prosthodontics: Basics of CD

Standard books of MCQs which should be read definitely:

- ❑ Series of NDBs, i.e. national dental board papers, available upto L – series in I & II volumes.
- ❑ Rudman's
- ❑ Cawson's
- ❑ Boucher's
- ❑ Reed's vols. I & II
- ❑ Steele's
- ❑ Arco's vols. I & II
- ❑ Gardiner's

MCQs in Dental Sciences

- Anatomy and Histology
- Physiology and Biochemistry
- Microbiology and Pathology
- Pharmacology
- Dental Anatomy
- General Medicine
- Oral Pathology
- Periodontics
- Orthodontics, Pedodontics and Endodontics
- Prosthodontics
- Operative Dentistry
- Oral Surgery
- Radiology
- Preventive Medicine including Microbiology and Biochemistry

MCQs

included in this volume
are based on the examinations of

National Boards of
USA and Canada

1

Anatomy and Histology

1. **The Golgi apparatus functions to**
   A. Give form to the cell and control passage of materials in and out of the cell
   B. Serve as a matrix substance in which chemical reactions occur
   C. Synthesize complex carbohydrate molecules which combine with protein produced by rough endoplasmic reticulum to form secretory products such as lipoproteins
   D. Release energy from food molecules and transform energy into usable ATP

2. **All of the following statements concerning the sphenoid bone are true except:**
   A. The greater wing of the sphenoid bone forms the lateral wall of the orbit and the roof of the infratemporal fossa
   B. The lesser wing of the sphenoid bone contains the optic canal (optic foramen) and helps from the superior orbital fissure and roof of the orbit
   C. The medial pterygoid plates of the sphenoid bone provide attachment sites for two muscles of mastication
   D. Foramina within the greater wing of the sphenoid bone provide access to both the pterygopalatine and infratemporal fossa
   E. The body of the sphenoid bone contains the sella turcica and the sphenoid sinus

3. The os coxa or hipbone is formed by the fusion of the three structures listed below except?

A. Ilium
B. Ischium
C. Acetabulum
D. Pubis

4. Which part of the face listed below is the first to form in the embryo?

A. The maxilla
B. The mandible
C. Both of the above
D. None of the above

5. All of the following are functions of the skeletal system, except:

A. Support
B. Protection
C. Body movement
D. Hemopoiesis
E. Fat storage
F. Mineral storage

6. The auxiliary vein begins at the border of the teres major muscle as the continuation of the basilic vein. As it ascends to the inferior margin of the first rib it becomes which vein listed below?

A. Brachial vein
B. Brachiocephalic vein
C. Cephalic vein
D. Subclavian vein

7. Mitosis results in:

A. One daughter cell
B. Two daughter cells
C. Three daughter cells
D. Four daughter cells

8. Which type of tissue listed below supports or binds other tissues and provides metabolic needs to all body organs?

A. Epithelial tissue
B. Connective tissue
C. Muscle tissue
D. Nervous tissue

9. All of the following structures empty into the cavernous sinus, excepts the

A. Superior ophthalmic vein
B. Inferior ophthalmic vein
C. Maxillary artery
D. The cerebral veins
E. Sphenoparietal sinus
F. Central vein of the retina

10. The greater petrosal nerve originates from which ganglion listed below?

A. Otic ganglion
B. Pterygopalatine ganglion
C. Geniculate ganglion
D. Celiac ganglion

11. Which structures listed below form the root of the lung?

A. Bronchi
B. Pulmonary artery
C. Pulmonary vein
D. Lymph vessels
E. Bronchial vessels
F. Nerves
G. All of the above

12. Which cranial nerve provides preganglionic parasympathetic fibers through the otic ganglion to the parotid gland?

A. Trigeminal nerve (CN V)
B. Facial nerve (CN VII)
C. Glossopharyngeal nerve (CN IX)
D. Vagus nerve (CN X)

13. Which of the following has the most extensive distribution of all the cranial nerves?

A. Facial nerve (CN VII)
B. Trigeminal nerve (CN V)
C. Hypoglossal nerve (CN XII)
D. Vagus nerve (CN X)

14. Which nerve listed below is the largest of the 12 cranial nerves and is the principal general sensory nerve to the head, particularly the face?
A. Vagus (CN X)
B. Glossopharyngeal (CN IX)
C. Facial (CN VII)
D. Trigeminal (CN V)

15. Which organ listed below extends from the pyloric opening to the ileocecal junction and is that where digestion and food absorption mainly takes place?
A. Stomach
B. Liver
C. Small intestine
D. Large intestine

16. The thymus gland produces which hormone listed below?
A. Glucagon
B. Thymopoietin
C. Calcitonin
D. Insulin

17. In relationship to the occlusal plane of the mandibular molars, the mandibular foramen is:
A. Below the occlusal plane and posterior to the molars
B. Above the occlusal plane and posterior to the molars
C. Above the occlusal plane and anterior to the molars
D. Below the occlusal plane and anterior to the molars

18. All of the following statements concerning neurons are true except:
A. They are unipolar, bipolar, or multipolar in shape
B. They are specialized for the reception, integration, and transmission of information
C. They are the basic structural and functional component of the nervous system
D. Their axons carry impulses toward the cell body
E. They consist of cell bodies, axons and dendrites

19. Wharton's duct is associated with which salivary grand listed below?

A. Parotid gland
B. Submandibular gland
C. Sublingual gland
D. von Ebner's glands

20. Specialized structures, which are found periodically along lymph vessels, are

A. Thrombocytes
B. Lacteals
C. Lymph nodes
D. Gap junctions

21. Which of the following is the hardest substance in the body?

A. Enamel
B. Dentin
C. Cementum
D. Bone

22. All of the following structures are found in the superior mediastinum, except:

A. The arch of the aorta
B. The branchio-cephalic veins
C. Trachea
D. Lungs
E. Thymus gland

23. In which type of muscle fiber listed below, would you expect to find fusiform cells?

A. Skeletal muscle fibers
B. Smooth muscle fibers
C. Cardiac muscle fibres
D. Neither of the above

24. Which type of epithelium listed below would be found lining the stomach?

A. Simple squamous epithelium
B. Simple columnar epithelium
C. Stratified cuboidal epithelium
D. Pseudostratified columnar epithelium

25. All muscles listed below are considered to be the circular muscles of the pharynx except?
A. Superior constrictor
B. Middle constrictor
C. Inferior constrictor
D. Stylopharyngeus

26. Which group of gingival fibers listed below connects all teeth and maintains the integrity of the dental arches?
A. Alveolo-gingival fibers
B. Transseptal fibers
C. Dentoperiosteal fibers
D. Dentogingival fibers

27. Muscle fiber contraction results from the interaction of contractile proteins in which the length of the sarcomeres is reduced. Which two proteins listed below are responsible for this muscle contraction?
A. Elastin
B. Myosin
C. Collagen
D. Actin

28. The exchange of nutrients and wastes between blood and tissue takes place across the walls of:
A. Veins
B. Arteries
C. Capillaries
D. Venules
E. Arterioles

29. Thrombosis in the coronary sinus might cause dilation of all of the following veins except:
A. Small cardiac veins
B. Great cardiac vein
C. Middle cardiac vein
D. Anterior cardiac veins

30. Which structure listed below gives rise to cementoblasts?
A. Dental papilla
B. Enamel organ
C. Dental sac
D. Inner enamel epithelium

31. Which of the following are the two terminal branches of the internal thoracic artery?

A. Superior epigastric and musculophrenic arteries
B. Anterior and posterior intercostal arteries
C. Subclavian and inferior epigastric arteries
D. None of the above

32. Compared to companion arteries, veins show all of the following except:

A. Less muscles
B. Lower blood pressure within them
C. Less elastic tissues
D. Same general tissues
E. Smaller diameter

33. Which two structures listed below join to form Hertwig's epithelial root sheath?

A. Stratum intermedium
B. Inner enamel epithelium
C. Stellate reticulum
D. Outer enamel epithelium

34. All of the following statements concerning the nasal cavity are true, except

A. The roof is formed by the nasal, frontal, sphenoid (the body) and ethmoid (the cribriform plate of. bones)
B. The floor is formed by the palatine process of the maxilla and the horizontal plate of the palatine bone.
C. The lateral walls are formed by the superior, middle, and inferior conchae.
D. The medial wall or nasal septum is formed entirely by the vomer bone
E. The bridge of the nose is formed by the two nasal bones

35. The middle ear cavity and the sphenoid sinus are separated by a thin layer of bone from which part of the cranial fossa listed below?

A. Anterior cranial fossa
B. Middle cranial fossa
C. Posterior cranial fossa
D. None of the above

36. The common carotid artery divides into its external and internal branches at the level of the superior border of the:
A. Jugular notch
B. First cervical vertebra
C. Cricoid cartilage
D. Thyroid cartilage
E. Hyoid bone

37. Which of the following is the principle artery to the nasal cavity, supplying the conchae, meatus, and paranasal sinuses?
A. Anterior tympanic artery
B. Sphenopalatine artery
C. Middle meningeal artery
D. Lingual artery

38. Which cell listed below is considered to be a phagocytic cell and is concerned with defense against bacterial invasion?
A. Plasma cell
B. Mast cell
C. Macrophage
D. Schwann cell

39. The cell cycle consists of all of the following except:
A. Growth
B. Synthesis
C. Fusion
D. Mitosis

40. Which of the following is the best way to palpate the posterior aspect of the mandibular condyle?
A. Intraorally
B. Through the external auditory meatus
C. Lateral to the external auditory meatus
D. Any of the above

41. Which structure listed below is a band or cord of dense, regular fibrous connective tissue that attaches muscle to bone?
A. Ligament
B. Tendon
C. Joint
D. Disc

42. The external laryngeal branch of the superior laryngeal nerve innervates which muscle listed below?
A. Thyrohyoid muscle
B. Middle pharyngeal constrictor muscle
C. Cricothyroid muscle
D. Superior pharyngeal constrictor muscle

43. Anatomically the dental pulp is divided into two portions, the coronal and radicular pulp. Which portion is located in the pulp chamber and pulp horns?
A. Coronal pulp
B. Radicular pulp
C. Both of the above
D. None of the above

44. Which nerve listed below innervates the facial muscles with motor fibers, the lacrimal gland and salivary glands with parasympathetic fibers, and the anterior tongue with sensory fibers?
A. Trigeminal
B. Vagus
C. Facial
D. Glossopharyngeal

45. Which of the following is the main function of cementum?
A. Compensation for tooth wear
B. Reparative
C. To attach the principle fibers of the periodontal ligament to the tooth
D. Protection

46. The splanchnic nerves (greater, lesser and least) arise from which region of the sympathetic trunks listed below?
A. Cervical region
B. Thoracic region
C. Lumbar region
D. Sacral region

47. Which nerve listed below carries general sensation from the anterior two-thirds of the tongue?
A. Hypoglossal nerve
B. Chorda tympani

C. Lingual nerve
D. Recurrent laryngeal nerve
E. Glossopharyngeal nerve

48. Non-neuronal tissue of the CNS that performs supportive and other ancillary functions is called:
A. Dermatome
B. Neuroglia
C. Bursa
D. Synapse

49. All structures listed below make up the brainstem except?
A. Diencephalon
B. Pons
C. Medulla oblongata
D. Mesencephalon

50. Which part of the adrenal gland listed below behaves more like neural tissue as opposed to a typical endocrine gland?
A. Adrenal cortex
B. Adrenal medulla
C. None of the above
D. Both of the above

51. Which salivary gland listed below is the smallest and contains both serous and mucous acini?
A. Submandibular gland
B. Parotid gland
C. Sublingual gland
D. None of the above

52. Which pharyngeal pouch listed below gives rise to the inferior parathyroid gland and the thymus gland?
A. First
B. Second
C. Third
D. Fourth
E. Fifth

53. Which endocrine gland listed below plays a vital role in the regulation of calcium and phosphorus metabolism?
A. Adrenal gland

B. Parathyroid gland
C. Pancreas
D. Pineal gland

54. The soft plate ends posteriorly in the midline as a conical projection called the:
A. Palatine aponeuroses
B. Uvula
C. Piriform fossa
D. Pharyngeal isthmus

55. Which longitudinal muscle of the pharynx listed below is innervated by the glossopharyngeal nerve?
A. Stylopharyngeus
B. Palatopharyngeus
C. Salpingopharyngeus
D. None of the above

56. Most of the joints of the body are:
A. Fibrous joints
B. Cartilaginous joints
C. Synovial joints
D. Fibrocartilaginous joints

57. Bruner's glands are found in which area listed below?
A. Submucosa of the stomach
B. Submucosa of the duodenum
C. Submucosa of the jejunum
D. Submucosa of the ileum

58. Which type of oral mucosa listed below covers the dorsum of the tongue and the taste buds?
A. Masticatory mucosa
B. Lining or reflective mucosa
C. Specialized mucosa
D. None of the above

59. All of the following statements concerning the periodontal ligament are true except:
A. It is a specialized connective tissue that is soft, fibrous, cellular and vascular
B. Its average width is 2.0 mm

C. Its principle function is to support the tooth, in its socket
D. It occupies the space between the cementum and the alveolar bone

60. Which muscle of the soft palate listed below draws the soft palate down to the tongue closing the oropharyngeal isthmus
A. Tensor veli palatini
B. Levator veli palatini
C. Palatoglossus
D. Palatophyarynngeus
E. Muscularis uvulae

61. Which muscle of the larynx listed below is the only one innervated by the external laryngeal branch of the vagus nerve?
A. Cricothyroid
B. Posterior cricoarytenoid
C. Lateral cricoarytenoid
D. Oblique arytenoid
E. Thyroarytenoid

62. The arterial blood supply of the heart is provided by
A. The right and left pulmonary arteries
B. The right and left coronary arteries
C. The right & left subclavian arteries
D. The right and left innominate arteries

63. Which heart valve listed below guards the opening between the right atrium and right ventricle?
A. Mitral (bicuspid) valve
B. Tricuspid valve
C. Pulmonary semilunar valve
D. Aortic semilunar valve

64. Which branch of the external carotid artery listed below supplies the submandibular gland?
A. Posterior auricular artery
B. Ascending pharyngeal artery
C. Maxillary artery
D. Facial artery

65. The maxillary artery divides into three parts. Which one of the following is not one of those parts?
A. Pterygopalatine part
B. Pterygoid part
C. Infratemporal part
D. Mandibular part

66. Histologically, the dentin of the root is distinguished readily from the dentin of the crown by the presence of which structure listed below?
A. Incremental lines of Retzius
B. Rete pegs
C. Tomes granular layer
D. Sharpey's fibers

67. Epithelia with two or more layers of cells, with only the deepest layer in contact with the basal lamina, are classified as:
A. Simple epithelia
B. Stratified epithelia
C. Pseudostratified epithelia
D. Columnar epithelium

68. The oral epithelium is covered by a layer of
A. Stratified cuboidal epithelium
B. Stratified squamous epithelium
C. Stratified columnar epithelium
D. Pseudostratified columnar epithelium

69. The pterygoid processes are part of which bone listed below?
A. Palatine bone
B. Temporal bone
C. Sphenoid bone
D. Occipital bone

70. The portal vein is formed by the union of splenic vein and:
A. Superior mesenteric vein
B. Inferior phrenic vein
C. Paraumbilical vein
D. None of the above

71. Under the microscope, erythrocytes (red blood cells) appear as:
A. Oval discs with multilobed nuclei
B. Circular discs with centrally located nuclei

C. Biconcave discs without nuclei
D. Circular discs with several nuclei

72. Which fossa listed below is an irregular-shaped space lying posterior to the maxilla, between the pharynx and the ramus of the mandible?
A. Pterygopalatine fossa
B. Mandibular fossa
C. Infratemporal fossa
D. Coronoid fossa

73. Which cell listed below is considered to be the most versatile in the body?
A. Macrophage
B. Hepatocyte
C. Kupffer cell
D. Erythrocyte

74. Platelets are best described as
A. Giant multinucleated cells
B. Cytoplasmic fragments of cells
C. Immature leukocytes
D. Lymphoid cells

75. The articular surfaces of the TMJ are covered by:
A. Elastic cartilage
B. Hyaline cartilage
C. Fibrocartilage
D. Periosteum

76. The basophils in the circulating blood are similar to which cell listed below?
A. Platelets
B. Mast cell
C. Macrophage
D. Kupffer cell

77. Which cranial nerve listed below supplies motor function to the trapezius and sternocleidomastoid muscles?
A. Vagus nerve
B. Glossopharyngeal nerve
C. Accessory nerve
D. Hypoglossal nerve

78. Which of the following ligaments normally is found in the inguinal canal of the female?

A. Ovarian ligament
B. Broad ligament
C. Round ligament of the uterus
D. Suspensory ligament of the ovary

79. Apical abscesses of which teeth listed below have a marked tendency to produce cervical spread of infection most rapidly?

A. Mandibular central and lateral incisors
B. Mandibular canine and first premolar
C. Maxillary first and second molars
D. Mandibular second and third molars

80. Which of the following statements concerning urine are true?

A. Adults pass about a quart and a half of urine each day depending on the fluids and foods consumed.
B. The volume of urine formed at night is about half that formed in the daytime.
C. Normal urine is sterile. It contains fluids, salts and waste products but is free of bacteria, viruses and fungi.
D. The tissues of the bladder are isolated from urine and toxic substance by a coating that discourages bacteria from attaching and growing on the bladder wall.
E. All of the above statements concerning urine are true.

81. Most skull joints found between the flat bones of the skull are

A. Fibrous joints
B. Cartilaginous joints
C. Synovial joints
D. Ligamentous joints

82. All of the following statements concerning the temporalis muscle are true, except:

A. It is fan-shaped and originates from the bony floor of the temporal fossa and from the deep surface of the temporal fascia.
B. The anterior and superior fibers elevate the mandible; the posterior fibers retract the mandible.

C. It inserts on the coronoid process of the mandible and the posterior fibers retract the mandible.
D. It is innervated by the maxillary division of the trigeminal nerve (V-2).
E. It is considered to be one of the muscles of mastication.

83. Which of the following can classify exocrine glands?
A. Type of secretion
B. Mode of secretion
C. Structure of duct system
D. Shape of secretory unit
E. All of the above

84. Metabolically active follicular colloid in the usual thyroid follicle stains
A. Acidophilic
B. Basophilic
C. Mixed
D. None of the above

85. Which of the following is the function of hyaline cartilage during endochondral ossification in a long bone of an extremity?
A. Provides a region where a long bone grow in length.
B. Provides a region where a long bone çan grow in width.
C. Hyaline cartilage has no function during endochondral ossification in a long bone.
D. All of the above

86. The cardiac notch is a deep indentation on the
A. Superior lobe of the left lung.
B. Inferior lobe of the left lung
C. Inferior lobe of the right lung
D. Middle lobe of the right lung
E. Superior lobe of the right lung

87. Which space listed below is entered when performing a spinal tap?
A. Arachnoid space
B. Central canal
C. Subarachnoid space.
D. Conus medullaris

88. Which division of the trigeminal nerve listed below passes through the foramen ovale and supplies motor innervation to the tensor veli palatini, tensor tympani, muscles of mastication (Temporalis, masseter and lateral and medial pterygoid and the anterior belly of digastric and myhyoid muscles?

A. Ophthalmic division
B. Maxillary division
C. Mandibular division
D. None of the above

89. Resting lines as seen in a histologic section of cortical bone of the mandible are the result of which of the following?

A. Growth of the mandible by the interstitial growth
B. Growth of the mandibular by appositional growth.
C. Growth of the mandible by both interstitial and appositional growth
D. None of the above

90. Which of the following statements concerning the breast and mammary gland are true?

A. The mammary glands lie in the superficial fascia
B. The mammary gland is actually a modified sweat gland.
C. The breast receives arterial blood through branches of the lateral thoracic (branch of the axillary artery) and internal thoracic arteries
D. Fibrous Copper's ligaments support the breasts
E. All of the above statements are true.

91. Which of the following characteristics are true concerning veins?

A. Thin tunica media with few muscle fibers
B. Thick tunica adventitia with little elastic tissue
C. Larger lumen and thinner walls than the arteries they accompany
D. Some contain valves and vasa vasorum
E. They receive blood from the venules and carry it from the body (except the lungs) to the right atrium of the heart.
F. All of the above are true.

92. Which cell listed below is the most common type found in the epidermis of the skin?
A. Melanocytes
B. Keratinocytes
C. Langerhans cells
D. None of the above

93. The primary purpose of cilia in mammalian cells is to
A. Move solids over their surfaces
B. Move fluid, mucous, or cells over their surfaces
C. Absorb fluid, mucous of cells over their surfaces
D. Absorb solids and liquids over their surfaces

94. Which of the following is the distinctive array of microtubules in the core of cilia and flagella composed of a central pair surrounded by a sheath of nine doublet microtubules (Characteristic ("9+2" pattern)?
A. Tubulin
B. Centriole
C. Axoneme
D. Malleolus

95. The mandibular fossa is a part of which bone listed below:?
A. Ethmoid bone
B. Sphenoid bone
C. Temporal bone
D. Parietal bone

96. Which method of bone development or formation involves a cartilaginous model being laid around it?
A. Intramembranous ossification
B. Endochondral ossification
C. Both of the above
D. None of the above

97. Which structure below gives the first indication of tongue development in the embryo?
A. The stomodeum
B. The tuberculum impar
C. The copula
D. The hypobranchial eminence

98. Calcitonin and thyroxine are produced and stored in which gland listed below?
A. Parathyroid glands
B. Adrenal glands
C. Thyroid gland
D. Thymus

99. The veins of the brain are direct tributaries of the
A. Internal jugular vein
B. Dural sinuses
C. Diploic veins
D. Emissary veins
E. Pterygoid venous plexus

100. The ductus venosus present in the fetus becomes what in the newborn?
A. Ligamentum arteriosum
B. Ligamentum teres
C. Fossa ovalis
D. Ligament venosum

101. Which type of epithelium listed below lines the mucous membranes of the nasopharynx?
A. Simple squamous epithelium
B. Stratified squamous epithelium
C. Pseudostratified ciliated columnar epithelium
D. Transitional epithelium

102. Which of the following cells form cementum?
A. Cementoblasts
B. Odontoblasts
C. Cementoblasts.
D. Ameloblasts

103. Which area of the oral cavity has mucosa that is lined with keratinized epithelium?
A. Soft palate
B. Gingiva
C. Sublingual regions
D. Buccal regions

104. Which of the following is the region where the optic nerve exits the eye?

A. Lens
B. Iris
C. Cornea
D. Optic disc.

105. The two optic nerves unite in the floor of the diencephalon to form which of the following?

A. Optic tract
B. Lateral geniculate body
C. Optic chiasma.
D. Lateral geniculate nuclei

106. Which parasympathetic ganglion listed below lies in the infratemporal fossa just below the foremen ovale between the mandibular nerve and the tensor veli palatini muscle?

A. Ciliary ganglion
B. Pterygopalatine ganglion
C. Submandibular ganglion
D. Otic ganglion.

107. Which of the following nerves innervate the TMJ?

A. Auriculotemporal nerve
B. Masseteric nerve
C. Deep temporal nerve
D. All of these

108. A lesion occurring in the jugular foramen may damage all of the following structures except:

A. Spinal accessory nerve
B. Vagus nerve
C. Glossopharyngal nerve
D. Internal jugular vein
E. Facial nerve

109. Which of the following is a pear-shaped muscular sac lying on the undersurface of the liver

A. Pancreas
B. Gall bladder
C. Stomach
D. Esophagus

110. Which gland listed below is the major gland of immune system?

A. Thyroid gland
B. Adrenal gland
C. Thymus glands
D. Pineal gland

111. Which of the following contains mucous- secreting cells?

A. Submandibular gland
B. Sublingual gland
C. Buccal glands
D. Glands of the esophagus
E. Mucosa of the trachea
F. All of the above

112. The nervous system can be divided into which two main parts listed below?

A. Central nervous system (CNS)
B. Somatic nervous system (SNS)
C. Peripheral nervous system (PNS)
D. Autonomic nervous system

113. Myelin is the fat-like substance forming a sheath around certain nerve fibers in the PNS (peripheral nervous system) which type of cell listed below form myelin?

A. Oligodendrocytes
B. Schwann cells
C. Astrocytes
D. Micoglia

114. The middle ear (tympanic cavity) communicates anteriorly with the nasopharynx via the

A. Acoustic apparatus
B. Vestibular apparatus
C. Eustachian (auditory) tube
D. External acoustic (auditory meatus)

115. Which of the following statements concerning the thoracic duct are true?

A. Begins below in the abdomen as a dilated sac, the cisterna chyli

B. Ascends through the aortic opening in the right side of the descending aorta
C. Empties into the junction of the left internal jugular vein and the left subclavian vein (which is the beginning the left brachiocephalic vein)
D. Contains valves and ascend between the aorta and azygos vein in the thorax
E. Conveys to the blood all lymph from the lower limbs, pelvic cavity, abdominal cavity, left side of the thorax and left side of the head and left arm
F. All of the statements concerning the thoracic duct are true

116. Which of the following explains how the epidermis of the skin obtains nourishment?
A. By diffusion of tissue fluid from capillary beds in the hypodermis
B. By diffusion of tissue fluid from capillary beds in the dermis
C. By diffusion of tissue fluid from capillary beds in the subcutaneous tissue
D. By diffusion of tissue fluid from capillary beds in the stratum corneum

117. Which of the following is the fundamental morphologic unit of enamel?
A. Enamel tuft
B. Enamel spindle
C. Enamel rod
D. Enamel lamellae

118. The epithelium of the oral mucous membrane may be
A. Keratinized
B. Parakeratinized
C. Nonkeratinized
D. All of the above

119. Which of the following refers to the sarcoplasmic reticulum present in skeletal muscle?
A. Releases and stores phosphate ions during muscle contraction and relaxation
B. Releases and stores glucose during muscle contraction and relaxation

C. Releases and stores calcium ions during muscle contraction and relaxation
D. None of the above

120. Which muscle listed below can flex the thigh and extend the leg?
A. Biceps femoris
B. Sartorius
C. Rectus femoris
D. Semimembranosus

121. All of the following statements concerning skeletal muscles are true, except:
A. Are considered voluntary in that they may be consciously contracted
B. Are usually long and narrow, span a joint, and are attached at either end by a tendon
C. Their origin is the more movable attachment and their insertion is the more stationary attachment
D. They may be classified according to their fiber arrangement as parallel, convergent, circular or pinnate
E. Each individual muscle fiber is innervated by a motor neuron terminal at a motor end plate
F. They are enclosed by epimysium, perimysium, and endomysium
G. They comprise approximately 40% of a person's body weight

122. All of the following statements concerning cardiac muscle are true, except:
A. It makes up the muscular component of the heart known as the myocardium
B. Cardiac muscle cells are faintly striated, branching cells which connect by means of intercalated disks to form a functional network
C. It contracts voluntarily
D. Its fibers are separate cellular units which (unlike other striated muscle fibers) don't contain many nuclei
E. It responds to increased demands by increasing the size of its; this is known as compensatory hypertrophy

123. The fossa ovalis and the anulis ovalis lie on the:
A. SA node
B. Atrial (interatrial) septum
C. Interventricular (ventricular) septum
D. AV node

124. The liver is one of the organs, along with lungs to receive a dual blood supply. Which two structures listed below are responsible for that dual blood supply to the liver?
A. Common carotid artery
B. Hepatic artery
C. Splanchnic vein
D. Hepatic portal vein

125. Which of the following is the first layer of dentin formed?
A. Mantle dentin
B. Peritubular dentin
C. Intertubular dentin
D. Interglobular dentin

126. Which muscle listed below has fibers that insert into neck of the mandibular condyle and into the capsule and articular disc of the TMJ?
A. Temporalis muscle
B. Buccinator muscle
C. Medial pterygoid muscle
D. Lateral pterygoid muscle

127. Which of the following is the main function of the dental pulp?
A. Nutritive
B. Sensory
C. Protective
D. Formative

128. All of the following statements concerning the left vagus nerve are true except?
A. It can be cut on the lower part of the esophagus to reduce gastric secretion (termed a vagotomy)
B. It forms the anterior vagal trunk at the lower part of the oesophagus.
C. It passes in front of the left subclavian artery as it enters the thorax

D. It contains parasympathetic postganglionic fibers
E. It contributes to the anterior esophageal plexus

129. All of the following are the four distinct layers of the enamel organ except?
A. Outer enamel epithelium
B. Inner enamel epithelium
C. Stratum granulosum
D. Stratum intermedium
E. Stellate reticulum

130. Listed below are the usual events in the histogenesis of a tooth. Place them in their correct sequence (from what happens first to what happens last)
1. Deposition of the first layer of dentin
2. Differentiation of odontoblasts
3. Deposition of the first layer of enamel
4. Elongation of inner enamel epithelial cells
   A. 4,2,1,3
   B. 1,2,3,4
   C. 2,3,4,1
   D. 3,2,1,4

131. The first sign of human tooth development is seen during the:
A. First week
B. Third week
C. Sixth week
D. Ninth week

132. The ground substance of hyaline cartilage is basophilic because it contains which substance listed below?
A. Muramic acid
B. Glycogen granules
C. Sulfated proteoglycans
D. Polysaccharides

133. Which organelle listed below contains centrioles which are short cylinders adjacent to the nucleus that take part in cell division?
A. Mitochondria
B. Peroxisomes

C. Ribosomes
D. Centrosomes

134. What is the collective name given to lifeless substances, such as yolk, fat and starch - that may be stored in various parts of the cytoplasm?
A. Ectoplasm
B. Metaplasm
C. Protoplasm
D. Nucleoplasm

135. Which artery listed below gives rise to the right subclavian and the right common carotid arteries?
A. Maxillary artery
B. Coronary artery
C. External iliac artery
D. Brachiocephalic artery

136. Which one of the meninges that cover the spinal cord and brain is a dense, strong fibrous sheet?
A. Dura mater
B. Arachnoid mater
C. Pia mater
D. All of the above

137. Which cranial nerve listed below sends motor fibers to levator palpebrae superioris and all extrinsic eye muscles except superior oblique and lateral rectus?
A. Trochlear nerve
B. Abducens nerve
C. Oculomotor nerve
D. Optic nerve

138. Which structures listed below makes up the forebrain?
A. Cerebrum
B. Pons
C. Medulla oblongata
D. Diencephalon

139. Which hormones listed below are released from the posterior pituitary?
A. Prolactin
B. Growth hormone (GH)

C. Antidiuretic hormone (ADH)
D. Luteinizing hormone (LH)
E. Oxytocin

140. Which of the following determines whether gigantism or acromegaly will occur when there is over-secretion of growth hormone by the pituitary gland?
A. Whether or not the epiphyses of the short bone have fused with the shaft
B. Whether or not there is enough calcium present to cause fusion of the epiphyses
C. Whether or not the epiphyses of the long bones have fused with the shaft
D. None of the above

141. Which structure listed below divides the anterior body cavity into an upper thoracic cavity and a lower abdomino-pelvic cavity?
A. Liver
B. Diaphragm
C. Stomach
D. Lungs

142. During the fourth week of embryonic development, the first branchial arch divides to form
A. The two lateral nasal processes
B. The mandibular and maxillary process
C. The two medial nasal processes
D. The lateral and medial nasal process

143. All of the following comparisons between the large intestine and small intestine are true, except:
A. The large intestine is about one-fourth the size of the small intestine
B. The lumen of the large intestine is of a greater diameter than that of the small intestine
C. The smooth muscle coat of the large intestine consists of three bands called teniae coli that cause the colon to form pouches (called Haustra). The small intestine lacks this characteristic.
D. The walls (or tunics) of the large intestine have more villi then the small intestine.

E. The external surface of the large intestine has small areas of fat-filled peritoneum called epiploic appendages. The small intestine lacks this characteristic.

144. Which two muscles listed below form a sling around the angle of the mandible?

A. Buccinator muscle
B. Masseter muscle
C. Medial pterygoid muscle
D. Lateral pterygoid muscle

145. Gingival fibers are found

A. In the free gingiva
B. At the DEJ
C. In the attached gingiva
D. At the muco-gingval junction

146. The point of exit from the stomach, where the stomach joins with the small intestine is guarded by a:

A. Greater omentum
B. Pyloric sphincter
C. Lesser omentum
D. Cardiac orifice

147. Which type of smooth muscle listed below has numerous gap junctions?

A. Single-unit smooth muscle
B. Multiunit smooth muscle
C. Both of the above
D. None of the above

148. The periodontal ligament is composed primarily of:

A. Elastic fibers
B. Reticulin fibers
C. Collagen fibers
D. Spindle fibers

149. Which heart valve is best heard over the apex of the heart?

A. Tricuspid valve
B. Mitral valve
C. Pulmonary valve
D. Aortic valve

150. Which muscle of the neck listed below separates the anterior and posterior triangles of the neck?
A. Digastric
B. Mylohyoid
C. Sternocleidomastoid
D. Omohyoid

151. Which artery listed below supplies the tongue?
A. Palatine artery
B. Inferior alveolar artery
C. Lingual artery
D. Vertebral artery

152. The thick middle muscular layer of the heart wall is called the:
A. Epicardium
B. Myocardium
C. Endocardium
D. Pericardium

153. Which chamber of the heart listed below is associated with the apex of the heart?
A. Right atrium
B. Left atrium
C. Right ventricle
D. Left ventricle

154. Of the following blood vessels, which one plays a significant role in peripheral vascular resistance and in the regulation of pressure?
A. Capillaries
B. Arterioles
C. Veins
D. Venules

155. Which one of the five layers of epidermis listed below contains the pigment producing melanocytes?
A. Stratum basale (basal layer)
B. Stratum spinosum (spiny layer)
C. Stratum granulosum (grainy layer)
D. Stratum lucidum (clear layer)
E. Stratum corneum (horny layer)

156. Which structure listed below is considered to be remnants of Hertwig's epithelial root sheath?
A. Accessory root canals
B. The epithelial rests of Malassez
C. Dentino-enamel junction (DEJ)
D. Cemento-enamel junction (CEJ)

157. Which vein listed below drains venous blood from structures of the posterior abdominal and thoracic body wall
A. External jugular vein
B. Internal jugular vein
C. Azygos vein
D. Femoral vein

158. Which type of tissue below can be classified according to the shape of the cell and the number and arrangement of cell layers?
A. Nervous tissue
B. Muscle tissue
C. Connective tissue
D. Epithelial tissue

159. Which of the following is the basic structural unit of adult compact bone?
A. Lamellae
B. The osteon
C. Volkmann's canals
D. Osteocytes

160. Which of the following is known as the sex chromatin body?
A. Golgi body
B. Barr body
C. Pineal body
D. Lateral body

161. Which of the following is a bone-forming cell that is derived from mesenchyme?
A. Osteoclast
B. Osteoblast
C. Osteoid
D. Osteocyte

162. Which structure listed below is a sieve-like bone at the base of the skull, behind the root of the nose that runs through the mid - sagittal plane and aids to connect the cranial skeleton to the facial skeleton?

A. Temporal bone
B. Maxilla
C. Ethmoid bone
D. Vomer bone

163. Mitosis includes all of the following stages except:

A. Prophase
B. Metaphase
C. Hypophase
D. Anaphase
E. Telophase

164. Which of the following is the cartilaginous bar of the first branchial arch?

A. Meckel's cartilage
B. Reichert's cartilage
C. John's cartilage
D. Smith's cartilage

165. At each intervertebral foramen the spinal nerves are formed by the union of which of the following?

A. Fibers originating in the cranial nerves
B. Anterior and posterior roots
C. Fibers originating in the cervical plexus
D. Mediolateral roots

166. Which veins listed below unite in the superior mediastinum to form the superior vena cava?

A. Right and left external jugular veins
B. Right and left subclavian veins
C. Right and left brachiocephalic veins
D. Right and left gastric veins

167. The gonads are the:

A. The uterus in females and the epididymis in males
B. The vagina in females and the ductus deferens in males
C. The ovaries in females and the testis in males
D. The uterine tubes in females and the ejaculatory ducts in males

168. Which of the following is formed very rapidly in response to irritants

A. Primary dentin
B. Secondary dentin
C. Reparative dentin
D. Sclerotic dentin

169. Which of the following are the last bronchioles of the bronchial tree?

A. Terminal bronchioles
B. Respiratory bronchioles
C. Primary bronchioles
D. Tertiary bronchioles

170. Which form of connective tissue listed below can be described as cells and fibers embedded in a gel-like matrix (amorphous ground substance)?

A. Bone
B. Cartilage
C. Adipose tissue
D. Vascular tissue

171. Which types of nerves listed below are the principle types found in the dental pulp?

A. Parasympathetic and efferent fibers
B. Sympathetic and afferent fibers
C. Parasympathetic and afferent fibers
D. Sympathetic and efferent fibers

172. Which nerve listed below innervates the posterior belly of the digastric muscle?

A. Oculomotor nerve
B. Facial nerve
C. Abducens nerve
D. Trochlear (CN IV)

173. Which ganglia listed below is located at the level of the cricoid cartilage?

A. The superior cervical ganglia
B. The middle cervical ganglia
C. The inferior cervical ganglia
D. All of the above

174. Which of the following causes the folding of the embryo during the fourth week of development?
A. Growth of the epithelial tissues
B. Growth of the connective tissues
C. Growth of the muscle tissues
D. Growth of the neural tissues

175. The internal acoustic meatus transmits which two of the following structures?
A. Vestibulocochlear nerve
B. Trigeminal nerve
C. Facial nerve
D. Vagus nerve

176. All of the following nerves pass through the superior orbital fissure, except:
A. Ophthalmic nerve
B. Abducens nerve
C. Optic nerve
D. Oculomotor nerve
E. Trochlear nerve

177. Which duct listed below is the main excretory duct of the pancreas?
A. Wharton's duct
B. Duct of Wirsung
C. Bartholin duct
D. Wolffian duct

178. Which gland listed below is both an exocrine and endocrine gland?
A. Thyroid gland
B. Thymus
C. Pancreas
D. Parathyroid glands

179. Which spinal cord tracts listed below convey impulses concerned with touch and pressure?
A. Anterior spinothalamic tracts
B. Lateral spinothalamic tracts
C. Lateral corticospinal tracts
D. Anterior corticospinal tracts

180. Which lobe of the cerebrum listed below is responsible for hearing?

A. Temporal lobe
B. Occipital lobe
C. Frontal lobe
D. Parietal lobe

181. In the head and neck, all the lymph ultimately drains into the:

A. Submental lymph nodes
B. Submandibular lymph nodes
C. Deep cervical lymph nodes
D. Retropharyngeal lymph nodes

182. What percentage of dentin is organic?

A. 5-10 %
B. 20 %
C. 30 %
D. 60 %

183. Which of the following statements concerning enamel are true?

A. The DEJ is the interface between in dentin and enamel, it is also the remnant of the formation of the tooth.
B. Enamel forms more evenly before birth than after birth Deciduous teeth, therefore are almost always uniform in appearance, while permanent teeth show variations in color and degree of calcifications.
C. Ameloblasts enter their first formative state after the first layer of dentin is formed. They secrete enamel matrix as they retreat away from the DEJ, which then mineralizes.
D. Enamel is produced in a rhythmical fashion
E. All of the above statements are true

184. Surrounding each tooth is specialized epithelium known as a

A. Connective tissue attachment
B. Periodontal ligament attachment
C. Junctional epithelium
D. Nasmyth's membrane

185. Which papillae of the tongue listed below are characterized by the absence of taste buds and increased keratinization?
A. Circumvallate papillae
B. Fungiform papillae
C. Filiform papillae
D. Foliate papillae

186. The intrinsic muscles of the thorax are involved in which process listed below ?
A. Laughing
B. Swallowing
C. Breathing
D. Digestion

187. Which muscle of the anterior abdominal wall listed below helps form the cremaster muscle?
A. External oblique
B. Internal oblique
C. Transversus
D. Rectus abdominis

188. The nerve to the mylohyoid muscle is a branch of which nerve listed below?
A. Ophthalmic nerve
B. Maxillary nerve
C. Mandibular nerve
D. Facial nerve

189. Which cells listed below secrete mucus and are abundant in the ileum of the small intestine?
A. Paneth cells
B. Absorptive cells
C. Entero-endocrine cells
D. Goblet cells

190. Which structure listed below is located in the wall of the right atrium near the superior vena cava and acts as a "pacemaker" for the heart?
A. Atrioventricular (AV) node
B. Atrial septum
C. Sinoatrial (SA) node
D. Tricuspid valve

191. Which artery listed below supplies the mucosa of the palate posterior to the maxillary canine?
A. Sphenopalatine artery
B. Greater palatine artery
C. Posterior superior artery
D. Nasopalatine artery

192. Which of the following is the most prominent functional component in the tunica media of small arteries
A. Collagen fibers
B. Elastic fibers
C. Smooth muscle cells
D. Skeletal muscle cells

193. When a tooth first erupts into the oral cavity, where the attachment epithelium derived from?
A. Dental papilla
B. Dental sac
C. Reduced enamel epithelium
D. Dental pulp

194. All of the following are components of a junctional complex, except:
A. Tight junctions
B. Gap junctions
C. Intermediate junctions
D. Desmosomes

195. A tubercle is:
A. A large, rounded roughened process
B. A sharp slender projecting process
C. A small rounded process
D. A prominent elevated ridge or border of a bone

196. Which bone listed below forms the prominence of the cheek and part of the lateral wall and floor to the orbital cavity
A. Sphenoid bone
B. Ethmoid bone
C. Zygomatic bone
D. Occipital bone

197. In the adult, hematopoiesis occurs in which two types of tissue listed below?
A. Nervous tissue
B. Lymphoid tissue
C. Muscle tissue
D. Myeloid tissue

198. The inferior mesenteric artery supplies all of the following organs except the:
A. Sigmoid colon
B. Descending colon
C. Transverse colon
D. Rectum
E. Ascending colon

199. Which of the following cells are found in the seminiferous tubules of the testis?
A. Endothelial cells
B. Interstitial cells
C. Sertoli cells
D. Clara cells

200. Which basic component of a typical cell listed below serves as the cell's external boundary separating it from other cells and from the external environment?
A. Protoplasm
B. Cell membrane
C. Nucleus
D. Golgi bodies

201. The first sign of human tooth development is seen during the:
A. first week
B. third week
C. sixth week
D. ninth week

202. Dislocation of the TMJ is almost always
A. Posteriorly bilateral, and occurs while sleeping.
B. Anteriorly bilateral, and occurs while laughing or yawning
C. Anteriorly unilateral and occurs while chewing food
D. Posteriorly unilateral and occurs while laughing or yawning

203. The sphenomandibular ligament of the TMJ attaches to the spine of the sphenoid bone and
A. The neck of the mandibular condyle
B. The lingula of the mandible
C. The ramus of the mandible
D. The angle of the mandible

204. Which ganglion listed below is located within the facial canal and contains sensory neurons that innervate taste buds on the anterior two-thirds of the tongue?
A. Otic ganglion
B. Ciliary ganglion
C. Semilunar ganglion
D. Geniculate ganglion

205. Which structure listed below is the first formed by the tooth germ and remains in evidence in the formed tooth?
A. Cementoenamel junction CEJ)
B. Dentinoenamel junction (DEJ)
C. Cementodentinal junction (CDJ)
D. Mucogingival junction (MGJ)

206. The ovaries are:
A. Heart-shaped organs located on either side of the adrenal glands
B. Almond shaped organs located on either side of the uterus
C. Pear- shaped organs situated between the bladder and the rectum
D. Muscular tubes located between the urethra and the rectum

207. Where would you expect to see incremental lines of Retzius?
A. In dentin
B. In cementum
C. In enamel
D. In the pulp

208. Which recurrent laryngeal nerve listed below crossed the arch of the aorta, hooks around the ligamentum arteriosum and ascends in the groove between the trachea and esophagus?
A. Right recurrent laryngeal nerve
B. Left recurrent laryngeal nerve

C. None of the above
D. Both of the above

209. Which muscle listed below is a landmark for locating the glossopharyngeal nerve (CN IX) in the neck?
A. Posterior belly of the digastric muscle
B. Inferior pharyngeal constrictor muscle
C. Stylopharyngeal muscle
D. Anterior scalene muscle

210. All preganglionic and postganglionic neurons of the parasympathetic nervous system release:
A. Dopamine
B. Norepinephrine
C. Acetylcholine
D. Epinephrine

211. Which of the following folds of cranial dura separate the lateral lobes of the cerebellum?
A. Tentorium cerebelli
B. Falx cerebri
C. Falx cerebelli
D. Diaphragma sellae

212. The body contains two types of glands exocrine and endocrine. Which type secrets its products into ducts, where the secretions are then carried to the target site?
A. Exocrine glands
B. Endocrine glands
C. Both of the above
D. None of the above

213. All portions of the pituitary gland listed below are derived from oral ectoderm except
A. Pars distalis
B. Pars tuberalis
C. Pars intermedia
D. Pars nervosa
E. Infundibulum

214. Which gland listed below is often called the "master endocrine gland"
A. Pancreas

B. Thymus gland
C. Pituitary gland
D. Parathyroid glands

215. Which hormone listed below is the most plentiful anterior pituitary hormone?
A. Thyroid stimulating hormone (TSH)
B. Adrenocorticotropic hormone (ACTH)
C. Growth hormone (GH)
D. Follicle stimulating hormone (FSH)
E. Luteinizing hormone (LH)

216. Which muscle listed below flexes, adducts, and medially rotates the arm?
A. Pectoralis major
B. Latissimus dorsi
C. Deltoids
D. Teres major

217. The myofibrils of a skeletal muscle fiber are arranged into the compartments called:
A. Z lines
B. Sarcomeres
C. H bands
D. A bands

218. Which type of joint listed below is characterized by a joint cavity?
A. Fibrous joint
B. Cartilaginous joint
C. Synovial joint
D. All of the above

219. Which of the following is a muscular tube that extends from the pharynx through the mediastinum to the stomach?
A. Pancreas
B. Duodenum
C. Esophagus
D. Large intestine

220. Which of the following cells may be found in the periodontal ligament?
A. Fibroblasts

B. Osteoblasts
C. Cementoblasts
D. Macrophages
E. All of the above

221. Approximately one - third of all principal fibers of the periodontal ligament are:
A. Alveolar crest fibers
B. Horizontal fibers
C. Oblique fibers
D. Apical fibers
E. Inter-radicular fibers

222. All of the following statements concerning cardiac muscle fibers are true except.
A. Make up the thick, middle layer of the heart known as the myocardium
B. Have larger t-tubules and less developed sarcoplasmic reticulums as compared to skeletal muscle fibers
C. In contrast to skeletal muscle fibers, cardiac muscle fibers are short branched, and single or binucleated
D. Their characteristic feature is the presence of intercalated discs
E. Cardiac muscle fibers have less mitochondria between myofibrils and are poorer in myoglobin than most skeletal muscle fibers

223. The lateral wall of the axilla (armpit) is formed by:
A. The clavicle
B. The scapula
C. Serratus anterior muscle
D. The humerus

224. Which chamber of the heart listed below receives blood from the superior and inferior venae cavae and also from the anterior cardiac vein?
A. Right atrium
B. Left atrium
C. Right ventricle
D. Left ventricle

225. The pectinate muscles are located within the heart
A. On the interatrial septum
B. In the right ventricle
C. On the inner surfaces of the right atrium
D. On the sinus venosum
E. On the right side of the interventricular septum

226. Which of the following arteries does not accompany the corresponding nerve through out its course?
A. Infraorbital artery
B. Inferior alveolar artery
C. Lingual artery
D. Posterior superior alveolar artery

227. Which of the following arteries supply the stomach?
A. Right and left gastric arteries
B. Right and left gastroepiploic arteries
C. Short gastric arteries
D. All of the above

228. The tooth germ is composed of all the structures listed below except
A. Enamel organ
B. Dental sac
C. Dental papilla
D. Hertwig's epithelial root sheath

229. Which stage in the life cycle of a tooth listed below includes final shaping of the tooth?
A. Initiation (Bud stage)
B. Proliferation (Cap stage)
C. Differentiation (Bell stage)
D. Apposition

230. Branches of which artery listed below supply the maxillary and mandibular teeth?
A. Vertebral
B. Occipital
C. Maxillary
D. Subclavian.

231. In a young child, which area of the maxilla listed below grows in height and length to accommodate the developing dentition?

A. Frontal process
B. Zygomatic process
C. Alveolar process
D. Orbital plate

232. Which structure listed below covers the surface of bone and consists of dense regular connective tissue?

A. Diaphysis
B. Endosteum
C. Epiphysis
D. Periosteum

233. The pterygoid plexus of veins surrounds which artery listed below?

A. Maxillary artery
B. Subclavian artery
C. Facial artery
D. Internal carotid artery

234. Which of the following statements concerning the hypoglossal nerve (CN XII) are true?

A. It is a motor nerve supplying all of the intrinsic and extrinsic muscles of the tongue except the palatoglossus, which is supplied by the vagus nerve
B. It leaves the skull through the hypoglossal canal which lie medial to the carotid canal and jugular foramen
C. It passes above the hyoid bone on the lateral surfaces of the hyoglossus muscle deep to the mylohyoid muscle
D. It loops around the occipital artery and passes between the external carotid artery and internal jugular vein
E. In the upper part of its course, it is joined by C1 fibers from the cervical plexus
F. All of the above are true concerning the hypoglossal nerve

235. Which cranial nerve listed below supplies the derivatives of the first branchial arch?

A. Facial nerve (CN VII)
B. Glossopharyngeal nerve (CN IX)

C. Trigeminal nerve (CN V)
D. Vagus nerve (CN X)

236. Which type of cartilage listed below is the most abundant in the body?
A. Hyaline cartilage
B. Fibrocartilage
C. Elastic cartilage
D. All of the above

237. Which structure listed below is a noncellular, protein - polysaccharide layer that anchors an epithelium to the underlying connective tissue
A. Plasma membrane
B. Basement membrane
C. Dermis
D. Tight junction

238. The inferior nasal concha is a part of which bone listed below?
A. Nasal bone
B. Sphenoid bone
C. Ethmoid bone
D. None of the above

239. Which vein listed below is formed by the union of the superficial temporal and maxillary veins within the parotid gland?
A. Hemiazygos vein
B. Left superior intercostal vein
C. Retromandibular vein
D. Subclavian vein

240. What is the function of neutrophils?
A. Transport oxygen
B. Involved in the processes of hemostasis and blood coagulation
C. Involved in the specific immune response
D. Ingest bacterial and other foreign substances

241. Which of the following can be defined as a small pit or depression in bone?
A. Fossa

B. Fissure
C. Fovea
D. Meatus

242. Which cell listed below is committed to differentiate into antibody producing plasma cells?
A. Stem cell
B. Macrophage
C. T cell
D. B cell

243. The liquid portion of the blood is called what?
A. Formed elements
B. Saline
C. Plasma
D. Lymph

244. Which structure listed below associated with the TMJ is fibrous, saddle - shaped and separates the condyle and the temporal bone?
A. Articular fossa
B. Articular disc (meniscus)
C. Articular eminence
D. None of the above

245. Which cell listed below is present in mesenchyme and capable of differentiating into of the special types of connective tissue or supporting tissues, smooth muscle vascular endothelium or blood cells?
A. Alpha cells
B. B cells
C. Mesenchymal cells
D. Leydig cells

246. If a tooth is being tilted mesially during orthodontics, which two of the following four statements are true?
A. The coronal half of the distal wall will show resorption as a result of osteoclastic activity
B. The coronal half of the mesial wall will show resorption as a result of osteoclastic activity
C. The coronal half of the distal wall will show deposition as a result of osteoblastic activity

D. The coronal half of the mesial wall will show deposition as a result of osteoblastic activity

247. Which part of the urinary system listed below transports urine from the renal pelvis to the urinary bladder?

A. Kidney
B. Ureters
C. Urethra
D. Bowmann's capsule

248. Which of the following is a delicate membrane covering the crown of a newly erupted tooth?

A. Perikymata
B. Primary enamel cuticle
C. Hertwig's root sheath
D. Plasmalemma

249. Which structure listed below is lined with stereocilia?

A. Ovaries
B. Urethra
C. Epididymis
D. Uterus

250. Which cranial nerve listed below passes through the cribriform plate of the ethmoid bone to enter the olfactory bulb where synapses are made?

A. Optic nerve (CN II)
B. Olfactory nerve (CN I)
C. Oculomotor nerve (CN III)
D. Trochlear nerve (CN IV)

251. The urethra is longer in

A. Males
B. Females
C. Is of equal length

252. Which areas of the brain listed below are filled with cerebrospinal fluid?

A. Gray matter
B. Ventricles
C. White matter
D. Pons

253. Which of the following statements concerning the cervical plexus and its branches are true?

A. The motor nerve for most of the infrahyoid muscles are branches of the ansa cervicalis (loop formed by C1, C2 and C3)

B. Cervical nerves C 1- C4 contribute motor fibers to the cervical plexus

C. It is positioned deep on the side of the neck, lateral to the first four cervical vertebrae.

D. An important branch of each cervical plexus is the phrenic nerve which supplies the diaphragm.

E. The supraclavicular nerve innervates the skin over the shoulder

F. The transverse cervical nerves provide sensory innervation to the anterior and lateral parts of the neck

G. All of the above statement concerning the cervical plexus and its branches are true

254. The posterior lobe of the pituitary gland consists of which type of nerve fibers listed below?

A. Unmyelinated nerve fibers

B. Myelinated nerve fibers

C. Both myelinated and unmyelinated nerve fibers

255. The peripheral nervous system can be divided into which two divisions listed below?

A. Afferent (sensory) division

B. Afferent (motor) division

C. Efferent (motor) division

D. Efferent (sensory) division

256. All hormones listed below are made in anterior pituitary except —

A. Antidiuretic hormone (ADH)

B. Follicle stimulating hormone (FSH)

C. Luteinizing hormone (LH)

D. Growth hormone (GH)

E. Adrenocorticotropic hormone (ACTH)

F. Thyroid-stimulating hormone (TSH)

257. Which structure listed below can be seen in histologic examination of the submandibular and sublingual glands but not in the adult parotid gland?
A. Myoepithelial cells
B. Serous cells
C. Intercalated ducts
D. Serous demilunes
E. Striated ducts

258. All of the following statements concerning the buccinator muscle are true except:
A. It originates from the outer surface of the alveolar margins of the maxilla and mandible opposite the molar teeth and from the pterygomandibular raphe
B. It is innervated by the buccal branch of the hypoglossal nerve (CN XIII)
C. It compresses the cheeks and lips against the teeth
D. It inserts at the orbicularis oris muscle and skin at the angle of the mouth
E. It is pierced by the parotid duct

259. The facial nerve, the retromandibular vein, and the external carotid artery lie within which salivary gland below?
A. Submandibular
B. Parotid gland
C. Sublingual gland

260. Synarthroses are:
A. Immovable joints
B. Slightly movable joints
C. Freely movable joints

261. Which muscle listed below is not one of the muscles of mastication?
A. Temporalis muscle
B. Masseter muscle
C. Buccinator muscle
D. Medial pterygoid muscle
E. Lateral pterygoid muscle

262. All of the following statements concerning the respiratory system are true, except:

A. It has two major parts - a branching tree- like set of hollow tubes (the conducting airways) and very thin- walled pouches (the alveoli) at the ends of these tubes
B. The lungs lie in the mediastinum
C. Cartilaginous rings are found in the main bronchi
D. The left lung has a smaller volume than the right lung
E. Alveolar sacs form the functional unit of the lung

263. Lymph leaves the lymph node through the

A. Afferent lymphatic vessels
B. Efferent lymphatic vessels
C. Both of the above

264. All of the following statements concerning the intrinsic muscles of the tongue are true except:

A. They are continued to the tongue and are not attached to bone
B. They are innervated by the pharyngeal plexus
C. They alter the shape of the tongue
D. They are named according to the three spatial planes in which they run

265. Which space listed below should be entered when performing an emergency tracheotomy?

A. Epidural space
B. Medullary space
C. Cricothyroid space
D. Pleural space

266. Which of the following abdominal organs (or viscera) is not located retroperitoneally?

A. Kidneys
B. Aorta
C. Adrenal glands (suprarenal glands)
D. Liver
E. Pancreas

267. Of the muscles listed below that move the forearm, which one is not involved in flexing the forearm?

A. Biceps brachii

B. Brachialis
C. Brachioradialis
D. Triceps brachii

268. All of the following statements concerning the liver are true except:
A. It is the body's largest and most active gland
B. It receives blood from the hepatic artery and portal vein
C. It receives autonomic nerve fibers from the celiac plexus
D. Its function is to store and concentrate bile
E. It is divided into a large right lobe and a small left by the attachment of the peritoneum of the falciform ligament
F. The right lobe is further divided into a quadrate lobe and a caudate lobe by the presence of gall bladder, the fissure for the ligamentum teres, the inferior vena cava and the fissure for the ligamentum venosum

269. All of the following statements concerning the heart are true except:
A. It is hollow muscular organ that is somewhat pyramidal in shape and lies within the pericardium in the middle mediastinum.
B. It is connected at its base to the great vessels but otherwise lies free within the pericardium
C. It contains four hollow chambers: the two upper atria and the two lower ventricles. The atria are separated by the interatrial septum and the ventricles are separated by the interventricular septum.
D. It contains five valves: two atrio-ventrivcular (AV) valves and three semilunar valves.
E. The wall of the heart consists of three layers: the epicardium, myocardium, and endocardium

270. All of the following statements concerning the kidneys are true, except
A. They are located retroperitoneally, the right kidney lies slightly lower than the left kidney due to the large size of the right lobe of the liver.
B. Each kidney is surrounded by a fibrous renal capsule and is supported by the adipose capsule.

C. Each kidney is divided into an outer dark- brown renal medulla and an inner light- brown renal cortex.
D. The renal medulla is composed of renal pyramid separated by renal columns.
E. Each kidney has an indentation, the hilus, on its medial border, through which the ureters, renal vessels and nerves enter or leave.
F. Each kidney receives its blood supply form a renal artery, a branch of the aorta.

271. Which type of connective tissue listed below provides strong, flexible support and is found in tendons and ligaments?
A. Loose (areolar) connective tissue
B. Dense connective tissue
C. Adipose connective tissue
D. Bone tissue

272. Which of the following statements concerning the carotid sinus is true?
A. It is innervated by the facial nerve
B. It is located at the terminal end of the external carotid artery
C. It communicates freely with the cavernous sinus
D. It is stimulated by changes in blood pressure
E. It functions as a chemoreceptor

273. Which vein listed below communicates with the superior ophthalmic vein and thus with the cavernous sinus allowing a route of infection from the face to the cranial dural sinus?
A. Suprascapular vein
B. Facial vein
C. Subclavian vein
D. Transverse cervical vein

274. Hyaline cartilage differs from bone in that hyaline cartilage may grow by which process listed below?
A. Appositional growth
B. Interstitial growth
C. Both of the above
D. None of the above

275. Which of the following is a precursor cell found in the red bone marrow that gives rise to all of the formed elements of the blood?
A. Monoblast
B. Myeloblast
C. Hemocytoblast
D. Lymphoblast

276. Which leukocytes (white blood cells) listed below are the least abundant?
A. Neutrophils
B. Monocytes
C. Eosinophils
D. Basophils
E. Lymphocytes

277. Chromosomes are composed of:
A. RNA and DNA
B. DNA and protein
C. Protein and RNA
D. Lipids and phospholipids

278. The nucleolus of a cell functions to:
A. Synthesize t-RNA
B. Synthesize r-RNA
C. Synthesize m-RNA
D. Synthesize DNA

279. The pterygoid processes or plates are a part of which bone?
A. Temporal
B. Sphenoid
C. Palatine
D. Zygoma

280. Which of the following statements concerning the portal vein is true?
A. It carries half as much blood as the hepatic artery
B. It has also no tributaries superior to its beginning
C. It is formed posterior to the neck of the pancreas by the union of the splenic and renal veins.
D. It ascends anterior to the bile duct and the proper hepatic artery.

E. It passes anterior to the epiploic foramen in the free edge of the lesser omentum.

281. Which of the following are the anatomical and functional units of the kidney
A. Axonemes
B. Nephrons
C. Myofibrils
D. Lobules

282. Which layer of the dermis listed below is a thick, fibrous layer?
A. Papillary layer
B. Reticular layer
C. Both of the above
D. None of the above

283. Which cell junction listed below seems to allow for the passage of ions and small molecules?
A. Tight junctions
B. Hemidesmosomes
C. Gap junctions
D. Intermediate junctions

284. Which of the following substitute for capillaries in the liver, spleen, pituitary gland, adrenal gland, carotid body, pancreas and parathyroid glands?
A. Lymph nodes
B. Venules
C. Sinusoids
D. Lacteals

285. Which artery listed below supplies the brain through its terminal branches - the anterior and middle cerebral arteries?
A. Vertebral artery
B. Coronary artery
C. Internal carotid artery
D. Superior mesenteric artery

286. The primary palate develops as a result of the merger of:
A. The two maxillary processes
B. The two lateral nasal processes

C. The two mandibular processes
D. The two medial nasal processes

287. Teniae coli are characteristic of which organ listed below
A. Stomach
B. Pancreas
C. Large intestine
D. Small intestine

288. Which structure listed below is called the adenoid when enlarged?
A. Lingual tonsil
B. Palatine tonsil
C. Pharyngeal tonsil
D. None of the above

289. Which opening of the diaphragm listed below transmits the aorta, thoracic duct, and azygos vein?
A. Aortic opening
B. Esophageal opening
C. Caval opening
D. None of the above

290. All of the following statements concerning the inguinal canal are true, except:
A. It transmits the spermatic cord in males and the round ligament of the uterus in females; as well as the ilioinguinal nerve in both sexes.
B. It begins at the deep inguinal ring and extends to the superficial inguinal ring .
C. It is much larger in females than in males
D. The interior wall is formed by aponeuroses of the external oblique and internal oblique muscles.

291. Which part of the alveolar process listed below immediately surrounds the root of the tooth and serves as an attachment for the fibers of the PDL?
A. Alveolar bone proper
B. Supporting alveolar bone
C. Lamina dura
D. None of the above

292. Which organ of the male reproductive system listed below produces spermatozoa and secretes sex hormones?
A. Prostate gland
B. Ductus deferens
C. Testis
D. Epididymis

293. Each odontoblast of dentin gives rise to a long slender cytoplasmic extension called
A. Triacetate fibers
B. Tomes fibers
C. Tag fibers
D. Korff's fibers

294. When a patient attempts protrusion, the mandible deviates markedly to the left. Which muscle listed below is unable to contract?
A. Buccinator muscle
B. Temporalis muscle
C. Right lateral pterygoid muscle
D. Left lateral pterygoid muscle

295. During an inferior alveolar nerve block injection, the needle passes through the mucous membrane and the buccinator muscle and lies lateral to which muscle listed below?
A. Masseter
B. Temporlais
C. Medial pterygoid
D. Lateral pterygoid

296. The trachea is a tube that begins below the cricoid cartilage (C6 of larynx) and ends at the level of the sternal angle T5 where it divides into:
A. terminal bronchi
B. respiratory bronchi
C. primary bronchi
D. tertiary bronchi

297. Which cranial nerve listed below passes through the cavernous sinus, enters the orbit through the superior orbital fissure and supplies the motor functions to the lateral rectus muscle?
A. Trigeminal nerve

B. Facial nerve
C. Abducens nerve
D. Vestibulocochlear nerve

298. The pterygopalatine fossa communicates laterally with the infratemporal fossa by way of which of the following?
A. Sphenopalatine foramen
B. Pterygoid canal
C. Foramen rotundum
D. Petrotympanic fissure
E. Pterygomaxillary fissure

299. Which bones listed below form the floor of the nasal cavity?
A. Ethmoid and palatine bones
B. Nasal bone and maxilla
C. Palatine bone and maxilla
D. Nasal and vomer bones

300. Which two of the following decrease with age in the dental pulp?
A. Number of collagen fibers
B. Number of reticulin fibers
C. The size of the pulp
D. Calcifications within the pulp

301. Which subdivision of the pharynx listed below contains the pharyngeal tonsils in its posterior wall?
A. Nasopharynx
B. Oropharynx
C. Laryngopharynx
D. None of the above

302. Which of the following act to integrate sensory stimuli that give rise to the sensations of heat and pain
A. Substantia nigra
B. Substantia gelatinosa
C. Substantia adamantina
D. Substantia grisea

303. Which of the following statements concerning the spinal cord are true?
A. It is cylindrical, occupies approximately the upper two-third of the vertebral canal, and is enveloped by the meninges.

B. In contrast to the cerebral hemispheres (brain) it has centrally located gray matter and peripherally located white matter.
C. It ends at about the level of L1 in the adult and at the level of L3 in the young child.
D. All of the above statements are true concerning the spinal cord

304. Which structure listed below houses the pituitary gland (hypophysis)?
A. Cribriform plate
B. Crista galli
C. Sella turcica
D. Lacrimal fossa
E. Diaphragma sellae

305. The epiploic foramen (Winslow's foramen) permits free communication between which two structures listed below?
A. The large and small intestine
B. The middle and inner ear
C. The lesser and greater omentum
D. The esophagus and stomach

306. Which structure listed below secretes hormones that are not essential to life?
A. Adrenal cortex
B. Anterior pituitary
C. Adrenal medulla
D. Pancreatic islets of Langerhans

307. Which anterior pituitary hormone listed below controls the production and secretion of hormones called glucocorticoids by the cortex of the adrenal gland?
A. Follicle-stimulating hormone (FSH)
B. Luteinizing hormone (LH)
C. Adrenocorticotropic hormone (ACTH)
D. Thyroid -stimulating hormone (TSH)

308. The area of skin supplied by a single spinal nerve is called a;
A. Fasciculus
B. Dermatome
C. spindle
D. Bundle

309. Which muscle of the pectoral girdle listed below is innervated by the accessory nerve (CN XI)?
A. Serratus anterior
B. Pectoralis minor
C. Subclavius
D. Trapezius
E. Levator scapulae

310. Which component of the lymphatic system listed below has the following functions: important blood reservoir, phagocytosis of undesirable particles of blood, and manufacturer of mononuclear leukocytes?
A. Thymus
B. Spleen
C. Bone marrow
D. Lymph nodes

311. Which joint listed below allows movement of the head about its vertical axis (rotation to the right or left)?
A. Atlanto-occipital joint
B. Intervertebral joint
C. Atlanto- axial joint
D. Costovertebral joint

312. The nasal cavities are lined by:
A. Stratified squamous epithelium
B. Stratified cuboidal epithelium
C. Pseudostratified ciliated columnar epithelium
D. Pseudostratified cuboidal epithelium

313. All of the following statements concerning the lymphatic system are true except:
A. The main function is to collect and transport tissue fluids from the intercellular spaces in all the tissues of the body back to the veins in the blood system
B. Lymph is a transparent, usually slightly yellow, often opalescent liquid found in the lymphatic vessels
C. It consist of the bone marrow spleen thymus gland lymph nodes tonsils, appendix. Peyer's patches, lymph, and lymphatic vessels

D. Just like the circulatory system, the lymphatic system has a central heart-like organ to pump lymph throughout the lymph vessels
E. The chief characteristic common to all lymphatic organs is the presence of lymphocytes

314. Which of the following statements is true concerning the triangle of auscultation?
A. It is bounded by the upper border of the latissimus dorsi, the lower border of the trapezius, and the medial margin of the scapula
B. It is the site where breathing sounds can be heard most clearly
C. Its floor is formed by the rhomboid major
D. All of the above statements are true

315. Which tooth tissue listed below has the highest mineral content?
A. Enamel
B. Dentin
C. Cementum
D. Pulp

316. The pharyngeal plexus does not innervate which muscle of the soft palate listed below?
A. Tensor veli palatini
B. Levator veli palatini
C. Palatoglossus
D. Palatopharyngeus
E. Muscularis uvulae

317. Which muscle listed below opens and protrudes the mandible?
A. Temporalis muscle
B. Masseter muscle
C. Medial pterygoid muscle
D. Lateral pterygoid muscle

318. All of the following comparisons between the ileum and the jejunum are correct except:
A. They are both suspended by mesentery
B. The ileum has more plicae circulares (valves of Kerckring) and more villi

C. Less digestion and absorption nutrients occur in the ileum
D. The mesentery of the ileum contains more fat

319. The Spleen:
A. Lies in the lower right inguinal region of the abdominal cavity
B. Lies in the upper right hypochondrium of the abdominal cavity between the stomach and the diaphragm
C. Lies in the upper left hypochondrium of the abdominal cavity between the stomach and the diaphragm
D. Lies in the hypogastrium of the abdominal cavity just below the river

320. The external carotid artery:
A. Extends from the upper border of the thyroid cartilage to the base of the skull
B. Contributes to form the basilar artery
C. Supplies the occipital lobe of the cerebral hemisphere
D. Gives off the inferior thyroid artery
E. Lies within the substance of the parotid gland

321. The mouth or oral cavity initially appears as a slight depression of the surface ectoderm called the:
A. Medial tongue bud
B. Frontal nasal process
C. Stomodeum
D. Pyramidal lobe

322. Which of the following are found between the basal cells of epithelium and the underlying basal lamina?
A. Focal contacts
B. Hemidesmosomes
C. Desmosomes
D. Gap junctions

323. The small deep penetrating arteries of the basal ganglia known as the lenticulostriate arteries are branches of which of the following?
A. Middle cerebral artery
B. Internal carotid artery
C. Anterior choroidal artery
D. All of the above

324. Three pair of veins return most of the venous blood from the head and neck regions to the heart. Which pair listed below does not?

A. Right and left internal jugular veins
B. Right and left external jugular veins
C. Right and left vertebral veins
D. Right and left gastric veins

325. What bones form the floor of the nasal cavity?

A. Nasal and vomer bones
B. Ethmoid and palatine bones
C. Maxilla and nasal bones
D. Palatine and maxilla bones

326. A patient was in a bad car accident and received a severe blow to the head that fractured his her optic canal. Which of the following pairs of structures are most likely to be injured?

A. Ophthalmic artery and ophthalmic vein
B. Optic nerve (CN II) and ophthalmic vein
C. Optic nerve (CN II) and ophthalmic artery
D. Ophthalmic nerve (CN V-1) and ophthalmic artery

327. Parasympathetic effects

A. Prepare the body to resist stress
B. Lead to acceleration of body activity
C. Cause rage and emotional reactions
D. Maintain normality of body functions
E. All of the above

328. Which extrinsic tongue muscle listed below depresses the tongue?

A. Genioglossus muscle
B. Hyoglossus muscle
C. Styloglossus muscle
D. Palatoglossus muscle

329. Which structure listed below is the functional unit in salivary gland?

A. Nephron
B. Microfilament
C. Adenomere
D. Lobule

330. Which of the following arteries does not accompany the corresponding nerve throughout its course?

A. Lingual
B. Infraorbital
C. Inferior alveolar
D. Posterior superior alveolar

331. What muscles are elevators of the mandible?

A. Medial pterygoid, digastric-both anterior and posterior belly and lateral pterygoid
B. Digastric-both anterior and posterior belly-and lateral ptrerygoid
C. Medial pterygoid, temporalis, and masseter
D. Digastric- both anterior and posterior belly, temporalis, and masseter

332. All of the following structures are found in dentin except:

A. Globular dentin
B. The neonatal line
C. Contour lines of Owen
D. Tome's granular layer
E. Intertubular matrix

333. What of the following may cause "dead tracts" in dentin.

A. Caries
B. Erosion
C. Cavity preparation
D. Odontoblastic crowding
E. All of the above

334. What group of periodontal ligament fibers has a cementum-to - cementum attachment?

A. Oblique
B. Horizontal
C. Trans-septal
D. Apical
E. Alveolar crest

335. Where are circular fibers found?

A. Free gingiva
B. Attached gingiva

C. Mucogingival junction
D. Epithelial attachment

336. Which of the following structures transmits the internal carotid artery and the greater petrosal nerve?
A. Petrotympanic fissure
B. Sphenopalatine foramen
C. Foramen lacerum
D. Mandibular foramen

337. Permanent teeth move in what direction when erupting?
A. Occlusally and buccally
B. Occlusally and lingually
C. Occlusally and mesially
D. Occlusally and distally

338. Apical abscesses of which teeth listed below have a marked tendency to produce cervical spread of infection most rapidly?
A. Mandibular central and lateral incisors
B. Mandibular canine and first premolar
C. Maxillary first and second molars
D. Mandibular second and third molars

339. The oculomotor nerve (III) enters the orbit through what opening?
A. Sphenomaxillary fissure
B. Superior orbital fissure
C. Pterygomaxillary fissure
D. Optic canal

340. Tropocollagen is a protein molecule found in which fibers?
A. Collagen
B. Elastic
C. Reticular
D. A and C, only

341. What connective tissue cell is most concerned with defense against bacterial invasion?
A. Macrophage
B. Basophil
C. Plasma cells
D. Mast cells

342. Which blood element is a fragment of megakaryocytic cytoplasm?

A. Erythrocytes
B. Platelets
C. Leukocytes
D. Plasma

343. Cyclic DNA is associated with what organelle within a cell?

A. Smooth endoplasmic reticulum
B. Nucleus
C. Mitochondrion
D. Vacuole

344. Which of the following cells is most likely to have an abundant amount of rough surfaced endoplasmic reticulum?

A. Osteocyte
B. Macrophages
C. Osteoblast
D. Mesothelial cell
E. Small lymphocyte

345. What muscle divides the maxillary artery into three parts?

A. Buccinator
B. Lateral Pterygoid
C. Masseter
D. Superior constrictor m of pharynx.

346. Which of the following structures is formed from the first branchial arch?

A. Hyoid bone
B. Buccinator muscle
C. Stylopharyngeus muscle
D. Lateral pterygoid muscle
E. Superior parathyroid gland

347. Which branchial arches are concerned with the development of the tongue?

A. First and second
B. First, third and fourth
C. Second and third
D. First, second, and third

348. What is the first part of the face to form in the embryo?
A. Maxilla
B. Mandible
C. Nasal prominence
D. None of the above

349. Which of the following has no lymph sinuses or crypts and is surrounded partly by connective tissue and partly by epithelium?
A. Thymus
B. Peyer's patch
C. Lingual tonsil
D. Palatine tonsil
E. Pharyngeal tonsil

350. Where would you find valves of Kerckring?
A. Duodenum
B. Jejunum
C. Ileum
D. Appendix

351. Metabolically active follicular colloid in the usual thyroid follicle stains how?
A. Basophilic
B. Acidophilic
C. Variable
D. None of the above

352. What is the average capacity of a stomach?
A. 0.5 liters
B. 0.7 liters
C. 1.0 liters
D. 1.4 liters

353. In what band on transmission electron microscopic preparations of skeletal muscle, would thick myofilaments be observed?
A. I - band
B. Z - band
C. A – band
D. None of the above

354. Alveolar bone proper consists of what type of bone?
A. Woven bone
B. Cortical bone
C. Bundle bone
D. Lamellar bone

355. The splanchnic nerve arise from which region?
A. Pelvis region
B. Lumbar region
C. Thoracic region
D. Sacral region

356. Which of the following structures can be seen in histologic examination of the submandibular and sublingual glands but not in the adult parotid?
A. Striated ducts
B. Serous demilunes
C. Intercalated ducts
D. Myoepithelial cells
E. Grandular serous cells

357. What muscle inserts on the mastoid process of the temporal bone?
A. Digastric (posterior belly)
B. Sternocleidomastoid
C. Longus capitis
D. Geniohyoid

358. Which fissure divides the mandibular fossa into two parts?
A. Petrotympanic fissure
B. Sphenomaxillary fissure
C. Tympanomastoid fissure
D. Pterygomaxillary fissure

359. What two muscles form a sling around the angle of the mandible?
A. Medial pterygoid and lateral pterygoid
B. Posterior belly of digastric and lateral pterygoid
C. Masseter and medial pterygoid
D. Buccinator and anterior belly of digastric

360. The eustachian canal, salpingopharyngeal fold, pharyngeal recess, and pharyngeal tonsils (adenoids) are located in which of the following?
A. Nasopharynx
B. Palatopharynx
C. Oropharynx
D. None of the above

361. The middle nasal concha is part of which bone?
A. Sphenoid
B. Ethmoid
C. Maxilla
D. Nasal

362. The nasolacrimal duct drains into what?
A. Inferior meatus
B. Middle meatus
C. Superior meatus
D. Lacrimal meatus

363. Which nerve supplies motor innervation to the mylohyoid muscle?
A. Nerve to mylohyoid (branch of V-3)
B. Hypoglossal
C. Glossopharyngeal
D. Phrenic

364. Which nerve provides major sensory innervation to TMJ?
A. Masseteric nerve
B. Auriculotemporal nerve
C. Facial nerve
D. Maxillary nerve

365. What is the only direction in which the TMJ can be dislocated?
A. Laterally
B. Medially
C. Anteriorly
D. Posteriorly

Answer key to anatomy and histology

1	C	2	C	3	C	4	B
5	E	6	D	7	B	8	B
9	C	10	C	11	G	12	C
13	D	14	D	15	C	16	B
17	B	18	D	19	B	20	C
21	A	22	D	23	B	24	B
25	D	26	B	27	B, D	28	C
29	D	30	C	31	A	32	E
33	B, D	34	D	35	B	36	D
37	B	38	C	39	C	40	B
41	B	42	C	43	A	44	C
45	C	46	B	47	C	48	B
49	A	50	B	51	C	52	C
53	B	54	B	55	A	56	C
57	B	58	C	59	B	60	C
61	A	62	B	63	B	64	D
65	C	66	C	67	B	68	B
69	C	70	A	71	C	72	C
73	B	74	B	75	C	76	B
77	C	78	C	79	D	80	E
81	A	82	D	83	E	84	B
85	A	86	A	87	C	88	C
89	B	90	E	91	F	92	B
93	B	94	C	95	C	96	B
97	B	98	C	99	B	100	D
101	C	102	C	103	B	104	D
105	C	106	D	107	D	108	E
109	B	110	C	111	F	112	A, C
113	B	114	C	115	F	116	B
117	C	118	D	119	C	120	C
121	C	122	C	123	B	124	B, D
125	A	126	D	127	D	128	D
129	C	130	A	131	C	132	C
133	D	134	B	135	D	136	A
137	C	138	A, D	139	C, E	140	C
141	B	142	B	143	D	144	B, C
145	A	146	B	147	A	148	C

149	B	150	C	151	C	152	B
153	D	154	B	155	A	156	B
157	C	158	D	159	B	160	B
161	B	162	C	163	C	164	A
165	B	166	C	167	C	168	C
169	B	170	B	171	B	172	B
173	B	174	D	175	A, C	176	C
177	B	178	C	179	A	180	A
181	C	182	B	183	E	184	C
185	C	186	C	187	B	188	C
189	D	190	C	191	B	192	C
193	C	194	B	195	C	196	C
197	B, D	198	E	199	C	200	B
201	C	202	B	203	B	204	D
205	B	206	B	207	C	208	B
209	C	210	C	211	C	212	A
213	D, E	214	C	215	C	216	A
217	B	218	C	219	C	220	E
221	C	222	E	223	D	224	A
225	C	226	C	227	D	228	D
229	C	230	C	231	C	232	D
233	A	234	F	235	C	236	A
237	B	238	D	239	C	240	D
241	C	242	D	243	C	244	B
245	C	246	B, C	247	B	248	B
249	C	250	B	251	A	252	B
253	G	254	A	255	A, C	256	A
257	D	258	B	259	B	260	A
261	C	262	B	263	B	264	B
265	C	266	D	267	D	268	D
269	D	270	C	271	B	272	D
273	B	274	B	275	C	276	D
277	B	278	B	279	B	280	E
281	B	282	B	283	C	284	C
285	C	286	D	287	C	288	C
289	A	290	C	291	A	292	C
293	B	294	D	295	C	296	C
297	C	298	E	299	C	300	B, C
301	A	302	B	303	D	304	C

305 C	306 C	307 C	308 B
309 D	310 B	311 C	312 C
313 D	314 D	315 A	316 A
317 D	318 B	319 C	320 E
321 C	322 B	323 A	324 D
325 D	326 C	327 D	328 B
329 C	330 A	331 C	332 D
333 E	334 C	335 A	336 C
337 A	338 D	339 B	340 D
341 A	342 B	343 C	344 C
345 B	346 D	347 D	348 B
349 E	350 B	351 A	352 C
353 C	354 C, D	355 C	356 B
357 B	358 A	359 C	360 A
361 B	362 A	363 A	364 B
365 C			

Reader's Notes

2

Physiology and Biochemistry

1. The neurotransmitter of the preganglionic sympathetic neurons is:
A. Norepinephrine
B. Acetylcholine
C. Dopamine
D. Serotonin

2. The isoelectric point (p) is the pH at which:
A. The number of positive charges outnumbers the negative charges
B. The number of positive charges equals the number of negative charges
C. The number of negative charges outnumbers the number of positive charges
D. None of the above

3. All of the following are factors that decrease insulin secretion EXCEPT:
A. Decrease in blood glucose level
B. Secretion of somatostatin
C. Secretion of glucagon
D. Secretion of either epinephrine or norepinephrine

4. The primary purine bases in both RNA and DNA are:
A. Thymine (T) and Guanine (G)
B. Adenine (A) and Guanine (G)
C. Cytosine (C) and Thymine (T)
D. Guanine (G) and Cytosine (C)

5. Which major type of protein present in the plasma functions to provide colloid osmotic pressure in the plasma?
A. Globulin
B. Albumin
C. Fibrinogen
D. None of the above

6. The largest number of chemoreceptors which are important for detecting changes in oxygen in the blood and help regulate respiratory activity are located in the:
A. Basal bodies
B. Carotid bodies
C. Residual bodies
D. Nissl bodies

7. The processes which take place in the nephrons, ultimately leading to urine formation include:
A. Glomerular filtration
B. Tubular reabsorption
C. Tubular secretion
D. All of the above

8. Proteins that make up the cell membrane serve as:
A. Transporters
B. Enzymes
C. Receptors
D. Mediators
E. All of the above

9. The four structural and functional portions of the cardiac conduction system are listed below. Which portion is called the "pacemaker" of the heart?
A. Sinoatrial node
B. Atrioventricular node
C. Atrioventricular bundle
D. Purkinje fibers

10. Which of the following statements concerning the Frank-Starling law of the heart are true?

A. It is the mechanism that allows the heart to adjust intrinsically to changing demands
B. It is the mechanism that matches cardiac output to venous return
C. The basis for this law is the intrinsic ability of the heart to adapt itself to changing loads of in-flowing blood
D. It is the mechanism that normally allows the heart to pump automatically whatever amount of blood flows into the right atrium from the veins
E. All of the above

11. The major hormone responsible for lactogenesis is:

A. Growth hormone
B. Adrenocorticotropic hormone (ACTH)
C. Prolactin
D. Thyroid-stimulating hormone (TSH)

12. Cortisol (hydrocortisone) has a direct inhibitory effect on which two structures listed below:

A. Adrenal cortex
B. Hypothalamus
C. Anterior pituitary gland
D. Posterior pituitary gland

13. Which of the following is the best known stimuli for increasing the rate of thyroid-stimulating hormone (TSH) secretion by the anterior pituitary gland?

A. Exposure to heat
B. Exposure to cold
C. Exposure to stress
D. All of the above

14. Which of the following is the major regulatory enzyme of cholesterol synthesis?

A. Squalene synthetase
B. Mevalonate kinase
C. HMG CoA reductase
D. HMG CoA synthetase

15. The globin (protein) portion of a hemoglobin molecule consists of:
A. One alpha chain and one beta chain
B. Two alpha chains and two beta chains
C. Three alpha chains and three beta chains
D. Four alpha chains and four beta chains

16. The thick ascending loop of Henle reabsorbs:
A. Potassium ions and water
B. Water only
C. Sodium and chloride ions
D. Potassium and chloride ions

17. Genetic recombination experiments depend heavily upon the action of which two enzymes listed below?
A. Restriction endonucleases
B. Alkaline phosphatase
C. DNA ligases
D. Creatine kinase

18. 84% of the entire blood volume of the body is in the:
A. Pulmonary circulation
B. Systemic circulation
C. Heart
D. Pulmonary vessels

19. Folic acid:
A. Is a coenzyme in carboxylation reaction, in which it serves as a carrier of activated carbon dioxide
B. Is a component of coenzyme A
C. Plays a key role in one-carbon metabolism, and is essential for the biosynthesis of the purines and the pyrimidine, thymine
D. Is a component of the visual pigments of rod and cone cells

20. Inhibitors of enzymes decrease the rate of enzymatic reactions. Which type of inhibitor listed below binds to the enzyme or the enzyme-substrate complex at a site different from the active site?
A. Competitive inhibitors
B. Noncompetitive inhibitors
C. Irreversible inhibitors
D. None of the above

21. Which intraocular structure listed below controls the amount of light that enters the eye by opening and closing like the aperture of a camera lens?

A. Sclera
B. Cornea
C. Iris
D. Pupil
E. Lens

22. All of the following are synthesized from the amino acid tyrosine EXCEPT:

A. Dopamine
B. Serotonin
C. Norepinephrine
D. Epinephrine

23. All of the following statements concerning niacin are true EXCEPT:

A. It is also called nicotinic acid
B. It is a component of NAD and NADP
C. It can be formed from the amino acid arginine
D. High supplemental doses are effective in treating hyperlipidemia
E A deficiency leads to pellagra

24. The Michaelis constant, Km, is:

A. Independent of pH
B. Numerically equal to -½ V_{max}
C. Dependent on the enzyme concentration
D. Numerically equal to the substrate concentration that gives half-maximal velocity

25. Which of the following ions has a higher concentration in the intracellular fluid (ICF) than in the extracellular fluid (ECF)?

A. Chloride (Cl)
B. Potassium (K)
C. Sodium (Na)
D. Bicarbonate (HCO)

26. Spatial summation occurs when:

A. Two inhibitory inputs arrive at a postsynaptic neuron within one minute of each other

B. Two excitatory inputs arrive at a postsynaptic neuron simultaneously

C. Two inhibitory inputs arrive at a postsynaptic neuron 10 seconds apart

D. Two excitatory inputs arrive at a postsynaptic neuron in rapid succession

27. All of the following statements are true EXCEPT:

A. Peripheral nerve fibers can sometimes regenerate if the some (cell body) is not damaged and some of the neurilemma remains intact

B. The neurilemma forms a regeneration tube through which the growing axon reestablishes its original connection

C. If the nerve originally led to a skeletal muscle, the muscle atrophies in the absence of innervation but regrows when the connection is reestablished

D. Nerve fibers of the CNS (brain and spinal cord) possess the thickest neurilemma

28. Which of the following affect bone mass, structural integrity, and bone loss?

A. Age

B. Race

C. Gender

D. All of the above

29. Which two amino acids listed below, have sulfur containing side chains (R-groups)?

A. Lysine

B. Cysteine

C. Arginine

D. Glutamate

E. Methionine

30. Which of the following serves as a principal source of carbon for nonessential amino - acids?

A. Fats

B. Water

C. Carbohydrates
D. Urea

31. A synapse consists of:
A. An axon terminal
B. A synaptic cleft
C. Postsynaptic membrane
D. All of the above

32. Buffers:
A. Prevent a change in pH when Cl ions are added to or removed from a solution
B. Prevent a change in pH when H ions are added to or removed from a solution
C. Prevent a change in pH when K ions are added to or removed from a solution
D. Prevent a change in pH when Na ions are added to or removed from a solution

33. Which of the following causes the secretion of secretin?
A. High pH in the duodenum
B. Neutral pH in the duodenum
C. Low pH in the duodenum
D. None of the above

34. The most important aspect of the DNA double helix is:
A. The randomness of the pairing of bases
B. The specificity of the pairing of bases
C. The phosphodiester linkages
D. That it forms a double spiral coil

35. Serum contains which of the following?
A. Blood cells
B. Platelets
C. Fibrinogen
D. None of the above

36. Which structure listed below controls or affects body temperature, appetite, water balance, pituitary secretions, emotions, and autonomic functions, (including sleep and wakeful cycles)?
A. Basal ganglia

B. Thalamus
C. Hypothalamus
D. None of the above

37. All of the following will cause a decrease in the glomerular filtration rate (GFR) EXCEPT:
A. Constriction of the afferent arteriole
B. Constriction of the efferent arteriole
C. Increased plasma protein concentration of glomerular capillary blood
D. Ureteral stone

38. Molecules that can easily penetrate a biologic membrane are usually:
A. Large and nonpolar
B. Small and polar
C. Large and polar
D. Small and nonpolar

39. Which of the following represents the standard bipolar limb lead I of the ECG?
A. Right arm (-) and left arm (+)
B. Right arm (-) and left leg (+)
C. Left arm (-) and left leg (+)
D. All of the above

40. The three factors that affect the magnitude of the resistance the blood encounters as it flows through vessels are listed below. Which factor has the most powerful relationship?
A. Blood viscosity
B. Vessel length
C. Vessel radius
D. Thickness of the intimal wall

41. All of the following statements concerning calcitonin are true EXCEPT:
A. It is synthesized and secreted by the parafollicular cells of the thyroid gland
B. Its secretion is stimulated by a decrease in serum calcium
C. It acts primarily to inhibit bone resorption
D. Along with parathyroid hormone and 1.25-DHC, it is a major regulator of calcium metabolism

42. Secretion of growth hormone is increased by all of the following EXCEPT:
A. Sleep
B. Stress
C. Obesity
D. Starvation
E. Exercise
F. Hypoglycemia
G. Hormones related to puberty

43. Which hormone listed below is secreted in response to dilation of the cervix?
A. Parathyroid hormone (PTH)
B. Follicle-stimulating hormone (FSH)
C. Oxytocin
D. Estradiol

44. The cell (plasma) membrane is a fluid mosaic of:
A. Lipids
B. Proteins
C. Lipids and proteins
D. Carbohydrates

45. Erythropoietin:
A. Raises the blood sugar level
B. Controls blood pressure
C. Promotes protein production
D. Stimulates red blood cell production

46. Which mechanism below is essential to the production of an osmotically concentrated urine?
A. Proprioceptive mechanism
B. Association mechanism
C. Countercurrent mechanism
D. Investing mechanism

47. The Nucleic acids (DNA) are complex molecules composed of all of the following EXCEPT:
A. Nitrogenous bases
B. Five-carbon sugars
C. Glycans
D. Phosphate groups

48. Which two forces listed below tend to move fluid out of a capillary membrane?
A. Capillary pressure
B. Interstitial fluid pressure
C. Colloid osmotic pressure of the plasma
D. Colloid osmotic pressure of the interstitial fluid

49. The pH of saliva is:
A. Between 1.0 and 3.0
B. Between 2.5 and 4.5
C. Between 6.0 and 7.0
D. Between 9.0 and 10.0

50. All of the following characterized saliva EXCEPT:
A. High potassium and bicarbonate ion concentrations
B. Low sodium and chloride concentrations
C. It is hypertonic
D. Its production is inhibited by vagotomy

51. Coenzyme A contains:
A. Riboflavin
B. Niacin
C. Pantothenic acid
D. Biotin

52. Enteropeptidase (enterokinase) which is produced by intestinal cells converts:
A. Chymotrypsinogen to chymotrypsin
B. Trypsinogen to trypsin
C. Pepsinogen to pepsin
D. Proelastase to elastase

53. All of the following are water-soluble vitamins EXCEPT:
A. Vitamin B-complex
B. Vitamin C
C. Vitamin E
D. Vitamin H

54. Gastric secretion is regulated by which two mechanism listed below?
A. Counter-current mechanism
B. Neural mechanism

C. Hormonal mechanism
D. Immunological mechanism

55. Action potentials in the skeletal muscle cell membrane initiate depolarization of the T tubules, which opens calcium ion release channels in the sarcoplasmic calcium. The calcium ions that are released from the sarcoplasmic calcium bind to which of the following?
A. ATP
B. Acetylcholine
C. Troponin
D. Tropomyosin

56. The descending (motor) spinal tracts carry impulses from the brain to lower motor neurons that regulate the activity of skeletal muscles. Upper motor neurons originate in the brain and form which two major systems listed below?
A. Pyramidal system (corticospinal tract)
B. Spinothalamic system
C. Extrapyramidal system
D. Reticulospinal system

57. Excitatory neurotransmitters in the CNS include all of the following EXCEPT:
A. Acetylcholine (ACH)
B. Glycine
C. Epinephrine
D. Dopamine
E. Serotonin

58. Which of the following solutions has an osmotic pressure different from the other two solutions?
A. 1 M glucose
B. 1 M sodium chloride
C. 1 M potassium nitrate
D. None of the above

59. Ovulation occurs as a result of:
A. The progesterone-induced LH surge
B. The estrogen-induced FSH surge
C. The progesterone-induced FSH surge
D. The estrogen-induced LH surge

60. All of the following are actions of estrogen EXCEPT:

A. Causes of development of female secondary sex characteristics at puberty
B. Causes of development of the breasts
C. Maintains pregnancy
D. Promotes secretory changes in the uterine endometrium during the latter half of the monthly female sexual cycle, thus preparing the uterus for implantation of the fertilized ovum.

61. All of the following statements are true EXCEPT:

A. Blood is normally slightly acidic, with a pH range of 6.45 to 6.55
B. The blood's acid-base balance is controlled precisely because even a minor deviation from the normal range can severely affect many organs
C. The body uses three mechanisms to control the blood's acid-base balance
D. An abnormality in one or more of these pH control mechanisms can cause one of two major disturbances in acid-base balance acidosis or alkalosis

62. Histones are small proteins that are positively charged at physiological pH due to their high content of which two amino acids listed below?

A. Cysteine
B. Arginine
C. Lysine
D. Glutamine

63. Which of the following would cause the release of norepinephrine and epinephrine from storage vesicles in the adrenal medulla?

A. Response to fright
B. Exercise
C. Cold
D. Low levels of blood glucose
E. All of the above

64. Which enzyme listed below is abundant in the liver?

A. Creatine kinase (CK)
B. Lactate dehydrogenase (LDH)

C. Glutamate - pyruvate transaminase (GPT)
D. Glutamate-oxaloacetate transaminase (GOT)

65. Glycogen, starch, and glycosaminoglycans are classified as:
A. Monosaccharides
B. Disaccharides
C. Oligosaccharides
D. Polysaccharides

66. Jaundice refers to yellow discoloration of the skin, sclera, and tissues caused by:
A. Hyperlipidemia
B. Hyperglycemia
C. Hyperbilirubinemia
D. Hypercalcemia

67. Which fatty acids listed below are essential fatty acids?
A. Lauric and myristic acids
B. Palmitic and stearic acids
C. Linoleic and linolenic acids
D. Butyric and caproic acids

68. During intense exercise, which of the following accumulates in muscle?
A. Glucose
B. Ethanol
C. Lactate
D. Glycogen

69. Which of the following parameters is decreased during exercise?
A. Heart rate (HR)
B. Cardiac output (CO)
C. Total peripheral resistance (TPR)
D. Stroke volume (SV)

70. Which valve below is composed of two cusps that prevent a backflow of blood from the left ventricle to the left atrium during ventricular contraction?
A. Tricuspid valve
B. Mitral valve
C. Pulmonary valve
D. Aortic valve

71. **Which GI hormone listed below has the ability to enhance the release of insulin in response to infusions of glucose?**
A. Gastrin
B. Gastric inhibitory peptide (GIP)
C. Cholecystokinin (CCK)
D. Secretin

72. **End-organ resistance to which hormone listed below results in polyuria and elevated serum osmolarity?**
A. Oxytocin
B. Antidiuretic hormone (ADH)
C. Parathyroid hormone (PTH)
D. Aldosterone

73. **Aldosterone's primary effect is on the:**
A. Liver
B. Heart
C. Kidneys
D. Lungs

74. **Which electron-carrier complex of the respiratory chain listed below contains NADH as the electron donor?**
A. Complex I
B. Complex II
C. Complex III
D. Complex IV

75. **Which of the following glycosaminoglycans is also known as the cement substance of tissues?**
A. Chondroitin sulfate
B. Dermatan sulfate
C. Hyaluronic acid
D. Keratan sulfate
E. Heparin sulfate

76. **Which of the following are steroids with detergent properties and are used to emulsify lipids in foodstuff passing through the intestine to enable fat digestion and absorption through the intestinal wall?**
A. Phospholipids
B. Proteins
C. Bile salts
D. Carbohydrates

77. All of the following statements concerning the backbone of DNA are true EXCEPT:

A. It is constant throughout the molecule
B. It consists of deoxyriboses linked by "phosphodiester bridges" or "phosphodiester linkages"
C. It is hydrophobic
D. It is highly polar

78. The cerebellum functions to:

A. Maintain muscle tone
B. Coordinate muscle movement
C. Control balance
D. All of the above

79. All of the following statements concerning the pentose phosphate pathway are true EXCEPT:

A. It produces carbon dioxide (CO_2)
B. It can produce NADPH
C. It requires ATP for phosphorylation
D. It can produce five-carbon sugars (used for DNA and RNA)
E. It is controlled by inhibition of glucose 6-phosphate dehydrogenase by NADPH

80. Carbonic anhydrase catalyzes the reaction between:

A. Carbon dioxide and oxygen
B. Oxygen and water
C. Carbon dioxide and bicarbonate
D. Carbon dioxide and water

81. All of the following statements concerning vitamin C are true EXCEPT:

A. It is also called biotin
B. It is an antioxidant
C. Diets high in vitamin C reduce the risk of certain types of cancer
D. It is a cofactor required for the hydroxylation of proline and lysine

82. The proteolytic enzyme that dissolves fibrin is:

A. Prothromobin
B. Thrombin
C. Fibrinogen
D. Plasmin

83. All of the following conditions increase the likelihood of edema formation EXCEPT:
A. Inflammation
B. Standing
C. Venous constriction
D. Arteriolar constriction

84. Which of the following are functions of the stretch reflex?
A. To maintain muscle tone for posture
B. To increase efficiency for locomotion
C. To smooth out movements
D. Acts as site of coordination for higher order inputs
E. All of the above

85. A motor neuron and all of the muscle fibers that it innervates is called a:
A. Map unit
B. Svedberg unit
C. Motor unit
D. Kind unit

86. FAD and FMN contain:
A. Folic acid
B. Riboflavin
C. Ascorbic acid
D. Thiamine

87. Alveolar ventilation is expressed as:
A. Respiratory rate x (Tidal volume + Dead space)
B. Respiratory rate + (Tidal volume + Dead space)
C. Respiratory rate x (Tidal volume - Dead space)
D. Respiratory rate + (Tidal volume - Dead space)

88. Which of the following factors influence pulmonary ventilation?
A. Arterial PO_2
B. Arterial PCO_2
C. Arterial pH
D. All of the above

89. In protein, amino acids are joined covalently by:
A. Hydrogen bonds
B. Peptide bonds

C. Ionic bonds
D. Van der Waals interactions

90. Which of the following can be defined as electron or protein-transfer proteins having one or several heme groups?
A. Aminotransferases
B. Cytochromes
C. Isomerases
D. Vitamin B complex

91. The two main types of adrenergic receptors in the autonomic nervous system are:
A. Nicotinic and muscarinic
B. Alpha and gamma
C. Gamma and beta
D. Alpha and beta

92. Rods and cones of the retina are examples of:
A. Mechanoreceptors
B. Photoreceptors
C. Chemoreceptors
D. Thermoreceptors

93. Which enzyme below is an RNA-directed DNA polymerase?
A. RNA ligase
B. DNA polymerase
C. Reverse transcriptase
D. DNA ligase

94. Under normal conditions, oxygen is carried to the tissues almost entirely by:
A. Albumin
B. Hemoglobin
C. Insulin
D. Cytochrome C

95. Which structures listed below are the last small branches of the arterial system and act as control valves through which blood is released into the capillaries?
A. Venules
B. Arteries
C. Arterioles
D. Veins

96. Which of the following are complex lipids similar to fats, but with a phosphorus and nitrogen-containing compound replacing one of the fatty acid molecules?
A. Carbohydrates
B. Phospholipids
C. Steroids
D. Proteins

97. The liver releases glucose back into the circulating blood during exercise. Besides the skeletal muscle, what other organ takes up this extra glucose?
A. Kidneys
B. Heart
C. Brain
D. Lungs

98. The P wave of the normal electrocardiogram (ECG or EKG) represents:
A. ventricular repolarization
B. Atrial repolarization
C. Ventricular depolarization
D. Atrial depolarization

99. The cardiac cycle is the period from the beginning of one heartbeat to the beginning of the next. How many phases does this cycle have?
A. One
B. Two
C. Three
D. Four

100. After food has become mixed with stomach (gastric) secretions, the resulting mixture that is passed from the stomach to the duodenum is called"
A. Bile
B. Chyme
C. Mucin
D. glycerol

101. Which compound listed below is important in fat metabolism?
A. Heparin

B. Choline
C. Thrombin
D. Serotonin

102. The complex process by which platelets, plasma, and coagulation factors interact to control bleeding is called?
A. Homeostasis
B. Hemostasis
C. Hermotherapy
D. Hemopoiesis

103. All of the following statements concerning chylomicrons are true EXCEPT:
A. They are the smallest of the lipoproteins
B. They are the least dense of the lipoproteins
C. They contain a high proportion of triacylglycerols
D. They are assembled in the intestinal mucosa as a means to transport dietary cholesterol and triacylglycerols to the rest of the body
E. They function to deliver dietary triacylglycerols to adipose tissue and muscle and dietary cholesterol to the liver

104. Black urine is a common finding in people with:
A. Phenylketonuria
B. Alkaptonuria
C. Cystinuria
D. Albinism

105. Which of the following is the most abundant glycosaminoglycan in the body?
A. Keratan sulfate
B. Hyaluronic acid
C. Dermatan sulfate
D. Chondroitin sulfate
E. Heparin sulfate
F. Heparin

106. A severe thiamine deficiency syndrome found in areas where polished rice is the major component of the diet is called"
A. Pellagra
B. Beri-beri
C. Scurvy
D. Megaloblastic anemia

107. The enzyme glucose 6-phosphatase is found most abundantly in which organ listed below?

A. Brain
B. Lungs
C. Liver
D. Pancreas

108. Vitamin B is a collective term for:

A. Pyridoxine
B. Pyridoxal
C. Pyridoxamine
D. All of the above

109. The key regulatory enzyme for glycogen synthesis is:

A. Glycogen phosphorylase
B. Phosphoglucomutase
C. glycogen synthase
D. Phosphofructokinase

110. The pitch of a sound is related mainly to which of the following characteristics of sound wave?

A. Amplitude of waves
B. Frequency of waves
C. Superimposed wave
D. Secondary waves
E. Length of waves

111. Sensory impulses travel via sensory (afferent, or ascending) neural pathways to the sensory cortex in the parietal lobe of the brain where they are interpreted. Which pathway in the somatosensory system listed below processes sensations of temperature, pain and light touch?

A. The fasciculus gracilis and fasciculus coneatus tracts
B. Spinothalamic tract

112. The action potential is an explosion of electrical activity that is created by a:

A. Polarizing current
B. Depolarizing current
C. Repolarizing current
D. All of the above

113. Which intraocular structure listed below contains the nerves that sense light and the blood supply that nourishes them?

A. Iris
B. Pupil
C. Choroid
D. Retina

114. Hyperopia (far sighted ness) is corrected with which type of lens?

A. Convex lens
B. Concave lens
C. Cylindric lens
D. Toric lens

115. Which GI hormone listed below is secreted form the G cells (enteroendocrine cells) of the stomach in response to a meal?

A. Gastrin
B. Cholecystokinin (CCK)
C. Secretin
D. Gastric inhibitory peptide (GIP)

116. All of the following are actions of glucocorticoids (cortisol) EXCEPT:

A. Stimulation of gluconeogenesis
B. Anti-inflammatory effects
C. Stimulation of fat deposition and inhibition of lipolysis
D. Suppression of the immune response
E. Maintenance of vascular responsiveness to catecholamines

117. All of the following statements concerning heparin are true EXCEPT:

A. Unlike other glycosaminologycans that are extracellular compounds, heparin is an intracellular component of mast cells that the arteries, especially in the liver, lungs, and skin
B. It serves as a powerful anticoagulant
C. It is used in the treatment of certain types of lung, blood vessel, and heart disorders, and during or after certain types of surgery (open heart or bypass surgeries)
D. Small quantities are produced by basophil cells of the blood
E. It is usually found in large quantities in the blood

118. The most calcified of the dental tissues is:
A. Dentin
B. Enamel
C. Cementum
D. Pulp

119. Elastin is composed of all of the following amino acids EXCEPT:
A. Glycine
B. Hydroxylysine
C. Proline
D. Lysine
E. Hydroxyproline

120. Collagen contains approximately 1000 amino acids, one-third of which are:
A. Arginine
B. Glycine
C. Cysteine
D. Histidine

121. The synapse between axons of motor neurons and skeletal muscle is called a:
A. Gap junction
B. Costochondral junction
C. Neuromuscular junction
D. Mucocutaneous junction

122. Glucagon has all of the following actions EXCEPT:
A. Increases the blood glucose concentration
B. Increases blood fatty acid and ketoacid concentration
C. Decreases blood amino acid concentration
D. Increases urea production

123. The degenerate nature of the genetic code implies what?
A. That many amino acids are designated by more than one codon (triplet)
B. That only one amino acid is designated by one codon (triplet)
C. Neither of the above
D. Both of the above

124. The normal plasma concentration of calcium varies between:

A. 3.0 and 5.0 mg/dl
B. 5.5 and 7.5 mg/dl
C. 8.5 and 10.5 mg/dl
D. 15.0 and 20.0 mg/dl

125. Within the spinal cord, the H-shaped mass of gray matter is divided into horns, which consist mainly of neuron cell bodies. Cell bodies in the posterior (dorsal) horn relay:

A. Voluntary motor impulses
B. Reflex motor impulses
C. Sensory impulses
D. All of the above

126. Ammonia is produced from the metabolism of a variety of compounds. Which compound listed below is quantitatively the most important source of ammonia?

A. Glutamine
B. Amino acids
C. Amines
D. Purines and pyrimidines

127. The ventricles are completely depolarized during which isoelectric portion of the electrocardiogram (ECG)?

A. QRS complex
B. Q-T interval
C. S-T segment
D. T wave

128. Blood flow is directly proportional to the pressure difference between the two ends of the vessel but is inversely proportional to the fractional resistance to the blood flow through a vessel. This relationship can be expressed as:

A. Flow = pressure × resistance
B. $\text{Flow} = \frac{\text{resistance}}{\text{pressure}}$
C. $\text{Flow} = \frac{\text{pressure}}{\text{resistance}}$
D. None of the above

129. Steroid hormones include all of the following EXCEPT:
A. Cortisol
B. Progesterone
C. Insulin
D. Testosterone
E. Estrogen
F. Aldosterone

130. The granulose cells in the corpus luteum produce which two hormones listed below?
A. Prolactin
B. Progesterone
C. Estrogen
D. Oxytocin

131. Almost all secretions by the pituitary gland are controlled by signals transmitted from which of the following:
A. The Cerebrum
B. The Medulla
C. The Hypothalamus
D. The Pons

132. Caries activity is directly proportional to all of the following EXCEPT:
A. The consistency of fermentable carbohydrates ingested
B. The quantity of fermentable carbohydrates ingested
C. The frequency of ingesting fermentable carbohydrates
D. The oral retention of fermentable carbohydrates ingested

133. Which of the following is considered to be the normal hemoglobin?
A. Hemoglobin A
B. Hemoglobin C
C. Hemoglobin H
D. Hemoglobin S
E. Hemoglobin M

134. The kidneys regulate acid-base balance by the:
A. Secretion of bicarbonate ions (HCO_3) into the renal tubules and the reabsorption of hydrogen ions (H)
B. Secretion of hydrogen ions (H) into the renal tubules and the reabsorption of bicarbonate ions (HCO_3)

C. Secretion of both hydrogen (H) and bicarbonate ions (HCO_3) into the renal tubules
D. Reabsorption of both hydrogen (H) and bicarbonate ions (HCO_3)

135. Hydrolysis of DNA will yield all of the following EXCEPT:
A. Ribose
B. Phosphoric acid
C. Deoxyribose
D. Nitrogenous bases (adenine, guanine, thymine, and cytosine)

136. Changes in blood pressure are due mainly to alterations in resistance by the:
A. Veins
B. Venules
C. Capillaries
D. Arterioles

137. Biotin is :
A. The precursor of FAD
B. Required for the carboxylation of acetyl CoA, an intermediate in fatty acid synthesis
C. A cofactor required for the hydroxylation of proline and lysine
D. A fat-soluble vitamin

138. Osteoblasts that are actively depositing bone matrix secrete large quantities of which enzyme listed below?
A. Creatinine phosphate
B. Hyaluronidase
C. Alkaline phosphatase
D. Acid phosphatase

139. All of the following statements concerning vitamin D are true EXCEPT :
A. It is involved in calcium metabolism
B. 25-hydroxycholecalciferol is the active form
C. Vitamin D and parathyroid hormone both increase serum calcium
D. A deficiency causes a net demineralization of bone resulting in rickets in children and osteomalacia in adults

140. The normal pH of pancreatic juice is :
A. 1.0 to 2.0
B. 4.0 to 6.0
C. 8.0 to 8.3
D. 9 to 10.5

141. Which of the following are sources of high-energy phosphate that keep the ATP pool filled for muscle contraction?
A. Creatine phosphate
B. Glycolysis of glycogen
C. Cellular respiration in the mitochondria of the muscle fibers
D. All of the above

142. All of the following statements are true EXCEPT.
A. Preganglionic neurons have their cell bodies in the CNS and synapse in autonomic ganglia
B. Sympathetic ganglia are located in the paravertebral chain
C. Cholinergic neurons, whether in the sympathetic or parasympathetic nervous system, release norepinephrine as the neurotransmitter
D. The majority of sympathetic postganglionic neurons are adrenergic

143. All of the major anterior pituitary hormones except one exert their effects by stimulating "target glands". Which of the following does not affect a "target gland"?
A. Prolactin
B. Thyroid-stimulating hormone (TSH)
C. Luteinizing hormone (LH)
D. Growth hormone (GH)
E. Follicle-stimulating hormone (FSH)
F. Adrenocorticotropic hormone (ACTH)

144. All of the following are the cardinal symptoms of diabetes EXCEPT:
A. Polydipsia
B. Polyuria
C. High blood pressure
D. Polyphagia
E. Weight loss
F. Loss of strength

145. The basal ganglia consists of :
A. Caudate nucleus
B. Putamen
C. Globus pallidus
D. Substantia nigra
E. Subthalamic nucleus
F. All of the above

146. Which of the following statements concerning the two principal laws of thermodynamics are true?
A. They apply only to closed systems, that is entities with which there can be no exchange of energy
B. The first law says that the total quantity of energy in the universe remains constant (this is the principle of the conservation of energy)
C. The second law states that the quality of this energy is degraded irreversibly (this is the principle of the degradation of energy)
D. The second law, known as Carnot's principle, is controlled by the concept of entropy
E. All of the above statements are true

147. All of the following statements concerning prostaglandins are true EXCEPT:
A. They have a very short half-life
B. They generally act locally on or near the tissue that produced them
C. They are synthesized only in the liver and the adrenal cortex
D. The common precursor of the prostaglandins is arachidonic acid (an unsaturated fatty acid)
E. Their synthesis can be inhibited by a number of unrelated compounds including aspirin and cortisol

148. All of the following statements concerning enamel hypoplasia are true EXCEPT :
A. It is a defect in the mineralization of the formed enamel matrix
B. The enamel of primary and permanent teeth appear pitted
C. Radiographically the enamel is either absent or very thin over tips of cusps and interproximal areas
D. It can be caused by nutritional deficiencies

149. Ovulation occurs :

A. 7 days before menses, regardless of cycle length
B. 14 days before menses, regardless of cycle length
C. 18 days before menses, regardless of cycle length
D. 21 days before menses, regardless of cycle length

150. When the lungs are in the resting position, the pressure within them, which is called the intrapulmonary pressure, is equivalent to which of the following?

A. Blood pressure
B. Critical pressure
C. Atmospheric pressure
D. Transmural pressure

151. All of the following are causes of metabolic alkalosis EXCEPT :

A. Use of diuretics (thiazides, furosemide, ethacrynic acid)
B. Vomiting
C. Chronic renal failure
D. Overactive adrenal gland (Cushing's syndrome or use of corticosteroids)

152. All of the following are signs indicative of a deficiency of proteins EXCEPT :

A. Lack of vigor and stamina
B. Weakness
C. Mental depression
D. Xerostomia
E. Poor resistance to infection
F. Impaired wound healing
G. Slow recovery from disease

153. Epinephrine and norepinephrine are secreted from the

A. Thyroid gland
B. Adrenal medulla
C. Pineal gland
D. Adrenal cortex

154. All of the following statements concerning transamination reactions are true EXCEPT:

A. These reactions involve the transfer of an amino group from one amino acid to an o-keto acid

B. The enzymes that catalyze these reactions are known as transaminases or aminotransferases

C. Glutamate and a-ketoglutarate are often involved in these reactions, serving as one of the amino acid/-keto acid pairs

D. Pyridoxal phosphate (PLP) which is derived from vitamin B, serves as the cofactor for these reactions

E. All amino acids participate in these reactions at some point in their catabolism

155. Glycosaminoglycans are :

A. Disaccharides

B. Homopolysaccharides

C. Heteropolysaccharides

D. Monosaccharides

156. All of the following statements concerning addison's disease (adrenocortical insufficiency) are true EXCEPT:

A. It results when underactive adrenal glands produce insufficient amounts of corticosteroids

B. It usually occurs in young adults and affects males more often than females

C. In 30% of people with Addison's the adrenal glands are destroyed by a cancer, amyloidosis, an infection such as tuberculosis, or another identifiable disease

D. In the other 70% of people with Addison's disease, the cause isn't known for certain, but is suspected that the adrenal glands are destroyed by an autoimmune reaction

E. It is characterized by hypotensed pigmentation of the skin; low levels of serum sodium chloride and dicarbonate with an elevation of serum potassium

157. Fatty acid breakdown (catabolism) occurs where?

A. In the cytosol

B. In the mitochondria

C. In the nucleus

D. None of the above

158. The branch point molecule of glycolysis is :

A. Glucose 6-phosphate

B. Glyceraldehyde 3-phosphate

C. Phosphoenolpyruvate

D. Pyruvate

159. Which of the following contribute adrenergic fibers to the heart and affect the heart's irritability?

A. First four thoracic spinal nerves (accessory nerves)
B. Left vagus nerve
C. Right vagus nerve
D. Trigeminal nerve

160. Which of the following substances is filtered but not reabsorbed by the kidney tubules?

A. Sodium chloride
B. Inulin
C. Para-aminohippurate (PAH)
D. Glucose

161. Somatostatin inhibits are secretion of all of the following hormones EXCEPT:

A. Insulin
B. Glucagons
C. Antidiuretic hormone (ADH)
D. Gastrin

162. Oral contraceptives inhibit:

A. Follicle growth
B. Ovulation
C. Follicle formation
D. Puberty

163. All of the following statements concerning the citric acid cycle (Krebs' cycle) are true EXCEPT:

A. the cycle starts with the 4-carbon compound oxaloacetate, adds 2 carbons from acetyl CoA, loses 2 carbons as CO, and regenerates the 4-carbon compound oxaloacetate
B. The pyruvate that enters this cycle is generated by the glycolysis of glucose or protein catabolism
C. This cycle is controlled by regulation of several enzyme activities. The most important of these regulated enzymes are citrate synthtase, isocitrate dehydrogenase, and "α-ketoglutarate dehydrogenase complex
D. The enzymes involved in the citric acid cycle are found in the cytosol

E. Aspartic acid and oxaloacetic acid are interconvertible (G) For each molecule of glucose metabolized 2 molecules of ATP are formed.

164. Sucrose, lactose, and maltose are common:
A. Monosaccharides
B. Disaccharides
C. Oligosaccharides
D. Polysaccharides

165. The use of fat instead of glucose for energy leads to an excess of ketone bodies. This condition disturbs normal acid-base balance and homeostatic mechanisms, leading to:
A. Glomerulonephritis
B. Megaloblastic anemia
C. Ketosis
D. Scurvy

166. There are three separate types of RNA, each of which plays an independent and entirely different role in protein synthesis. Which type transports activated amino acids to the ribosomes to be used in assembling the protein molecule?
A. Messenger RNA
B. Transfer RNA
C. Ribosomal RNA
D. None of the above

167. Which type of shock listed below is most often associated with severe trauma and reactive peripheral vasodilation?
A. Hypovolemic shock
B. Cardiogenic shock
C. Septic shock
D. Neurogenic shock
E. Anaphylactic shock

168. Which enzyme listed below catalyzes the oxidative deamination of glutamate?
A. Histidase
B. Aspartate aminotransferase (AST)
C. Glutamate dehydrogenase
D. Alanine aminotransferase (ALT)

169. The aerobic breakdown of a single molecule of glucose produces a net profit of how many ATP?

A. 20-24 ATP
B. 30-32 ATP
C. 36-38 ATP
D. 44-48 ATP

170. A major role of proteins is to serve as:

A. Bile salts
B. Enzymes
C. Fatty acids
D. Ketone bodies

171. All of the following are functions of zinc EXCEPT:

A. It stabilizes cell membranes
B. It functions in taste acuity
C. It is needed in collagen formation / healing
D. It is involved in vitamin B_{12} formation
E. It is essential in cell-mediated immunity

172. All of the following statements concerning muscle spindles are true EXCEPT:

A. They are found within the belly of muscles
B. They consists of small, encapsulated intrafusal fibers and run in parallel with the main muscle fibers (extrafusal fibers)
C. The finer the movement required, the lesser the number of muscle spindles in a muscle
D. They detect both static and dynamic changes in muscle length

173. Muscle cells use which of the following to store energy?

A. Creatine phosphate
B. FADH2
C. NADH
D. Phosphoneolpyruvate

174. Which of the following is the active form of vitamin D?

A. Cholecalciferol
B. 25-hydroxycholecalciferol
C. 1,25-dihydroxycholecalciferol
D. 24,25-dihydroxycholecalciferol

175. The factors that determine how rapidly a gas will pass through the respiratory membrane include:

A. The thickness of the membrane
B. The surface area of the membrane
C. The solubility of the gas in the substance of the membrane
D. The pressure difference between the two sides of the membrane
E. All of the above

176. The volume of air remaining in the lungs after a maximal expiration is called the:

A. Vital capacity (VC)
B. Tidal volume (TV)
C. Residual volume (RV)
D. Functional residual capacity (FRC)

177. The plasma protein of the highest concentration in plasma is:

A. Globulins (alpha, beta, and gamma)
B. Fibrinogen
C. Albumin
D. None of the above

178. All amino acids found in proteins are of the:

A. D-configuration
B. L-configuration
C. F-configuration
D. C-configuration

179. Which of the following is the cause of the "positive" afterpotential which occurs for a few milliseconds after the action potential is over?

A. Many sodium channels remain open for several milliseconds after repolarization of the membrane is complete
B. All potassium channels remain closed for several milliseconds after repolarization of the membrane is complete
C. Many potassium channels remain open for several milliseconds after repolarization of the membrane is complete
D. All sodium and potassium channels remain closed for several milliseconds after repolarization of the membrane is complete

180. Which receptors listed below are sensitive to pressure, pain, and chemical changes in the internal environment of the body?

A. Exteroceptors
B. Interoceptors
C. Both of the above
D. None of the above

181. Which blood group listed below has neither antigen A or B?

A. A
B. B
C. O
D. AB

182. The function of arteries is to:

A. Act as control valves through which blood is released into the capillaries
B. Exchange fluid, nutrients, electrolytes, hormones, and other substances
C. Transport blood under high pressure to the tissues
D. Act as conduit for the transport of blood from the tissues back to the heart

183. All of the following statements concerning fatty acid synthesis are true EXCEPT:

A. Fatty acid synthesis involves two carbon additions from acetyl-CoA and an acyl protein (ACP)
B. The important step in fatty acid synthesis is the first one in which acetyl-CoA, carbon dioxide, and bicarbonate form malonyl-CoA
C. Fatty acid synthesis is not a simple reversal of " β-oxidation used for the catabolism of fatty acids
D. Fatty acid synthesis takes place in the mitochondria while fatty acid breakdown (catabolism) occurs in the cytosol (cytoplasm)

184. Gluconeogenesis, which occurs mainly in the liver, is the synthesis of glucose from compounds that are not carbohydrates. Which organ below is a minor contributor of newly synthesized glucose molecules?

A. Appendix

B. gallbladder
C. Kidneys
D. Pancreas

185. Which valve below is composed of three cusps that prevent a backflow of blood from the aorta into the left ventricle during ventricular relaxation?
A. Pulmonary valve
B. Tricuspid valve
C. Mitral valve
D. Aortic valve

186. The stretch receptors of the atria that elicit the Bainbridge reflex transmit their afferent signals through the:
A. Trigeminal nerves to the medulla of the brain
B. Vagus nerves to the medulla of the brain
C. Facial nerves to the medulla of the brain
D. glossopharyngeal nerves to the medulla of the brain

187. Deficiency of which hormone listed below causes hypocalcemia and hyperphosphatemia?
A. Aldosterone
B. Testosterone
C. Follicle-stimulating hormone (FSH)
D. Parathyroid hormone (PTH)

188. Hemoglobin:
A. Carries carbon dioxide to the cells from the lungs and oxygen away from the cells to the lungs
B. Carries carbon monoxide to the cells from the lungs and carbon dioxide away from the cells to the lungs
C. Carries oxygen to the cells from the lungs and carbon dioxide away from the cells to the lungs
D. Carries carbon monoxide to the cells from the lungs and oxygen away from the cells to the lungs

189. Most of the glomerular filtrate is reabsorbed in the:
A. Descending (thin) loop of Henle
B. Distal convoluted tubule
C. Proximal convoluted tubule
D. Ascending (thick) loop of Henle

190. All of the following are clinical features of hyperthyroidism EXCEPT:

A. Restlessness, irritability, and fatigability
B. Heat intolerance (sweating)
C. Tachycardia (a rapid heat rate)
D. Weight gain
E Fine hair
F Diarrhea
G. Tremor (shakiness)

191. The majority of glycosaminoglycans in the body are linked to core proteins, forming:

A. Glycoproteins
B. Glycolipids
C. Proteoglycans
D. None of the above

192. Which cardiac muscle listed below has a longer refractory period?

A. Ventricular muscle
B. Atrial muscle
C. Bundle of his
D. Purkinje fibers

193. All of the following statements concerning thyroid hormone are true EXCEPT:

A. Collectively referred to as thyroid hormone, T3 and T4 are the body's major metabolic hormones
B. It regulates metabolism by speeding cellular respiration
C. T_3 (tri-iodothyronine) has several times the biologic activity of T4 (thyroxine)
D. It stimulates bone maturation as a result of ossification and fusion of the growth plates
E. It decreases glycogenolysis, gluconeogenesis, and lipolysis

194. Which of the following vitamins is required for blood clotting?

A. Vitamin A
B. Vitamin K
C. Vitamin E
D. Vitamin D

195. A Competitive inhibitor of an enzyme;
A. Increases Km without affecting Vmax
B. Decreases Km without affecting Vmax
C. Increases Vmax without affecting Km
D. Decreases both Vmax and Km

196. Vitamin A (retinol) is:
A. Required for blood clotting
B. Required for the hydroxylation of proline and lysine residues in the precursor of collagen
C. Required for formation of the visual pigments of rod and cone cells
D. Required for synthesis of cofactor required for reactions in the oxidation of pyruvate to carbon dioxide and water

197. Gastric secretions include all of them except
A. Mucus
B. Hydrochloric acid (HCL)
C. Pepsinogen
D. Ptyalin
E. Intrinsic factor

198. Isotopes of an element:
A. Have different chemical properties but the same weights
B. Have the same chemical properties but different weights
C. Have different chemical properties and weights
D. Have the same chemical properties and weights

199. The two types of cholinergic receptors in the autonomic nervous system are:
A. Nicotinic and alpha
B. Alpha and beta
C. Nicotinic and muscarinic
D. Muscarinic and beta

200. Saltatory conduction serves to:
A. Increase the velocity of nerve transmission along myelinated fibers
B. Conserve energy since the sodium and potassium pumps have to reestablish concentration differences only at the nodes of Ranvier
C. Allow repolarization to occur with little transfer of ions
D. All of the above

201. Which of the following are heat-generating mechanisms?
A. Increased metabolism
B. Shivering
C. Vasoconstriction of cutaneous blood vessels
D. All of the above

202. Histamine causes all of the following responses EXCEPT:
A. Bronchoconstriction
B. Increased blood pressure
C. Increased vascular permeability (particularly in capillaries and venules)
D. Secretion of HCl
E. Vasodilation (particularly the arterioles)

203. All of the following are formed via the cyclo-oxygenase pathway EXCEPT:
A. Prostaglandins
B. Prostacyclin
C. Leukotrienes
D. Thromboxanes

204. Tyrosine is produced by hydroxylation of the essential amino acid:
A. Histidine
B. Lysine
C. Valine
D. Phenylalanine

205. All of the following statements are true EXCEPT:
A. During early childhood, a boy does not secrete gonadotropins, and thus has little circulating testosterone
B. Secretion of gonadotropins from the adrenal gland, which usually occurs between the ages 16 and 20, marks the onset of puberty
C. These pituitary gonadotropins stimulate testes functioning as well as testosterone secretion
D. During puberty the penis and testes enlarge and the male reaches full adult sexual and reproductive capability
E. Puberty also marks the development of male secondary sexual characteristics

206. Which of the following is a glycoprotein hormone (10% carbohydrate) that is synthesized by the thyroid follicular cell and iodinated once it has been synthesized?
A. Glucagon
B. Cortisol
C. Thyroglobulin
D. Aldosterone

207. The activity level of which enzyme listed below controls the rate of glycolysis?
A. Aldolase
B. Phosphoglucose isomerase
C. Phosphofructokinase
D. Triose phosphate isomerase

208. The quantitative relation between the concentration of a week acid (HA) and its conjugate base (A) is described by the:
A. Arrhenius equation
B. Henderson-Hasselbalch equation
C. Bohr equation
D. Einthoven equation

209. Of the 20 amino acids commonly found in proteins, how many are not essential in the adult diet because they can be synthesized in the body?
A. 5
B. 9
C. 11
D. 18

210. Simple sugars are also called:
A. Monosaccharides
B. Disaccharides
C. Oligosaccharides
D. Polysaccharides

211. Gaucher's disease is a disorder of lipid metabolism caused by a deficiency of:
A. Hexosaminidase A
B. Sphingomyelinase

C. Glucocerebrosidase
D. α-L- iduronidase

212. Which of the following is the major source of Acetyl CoA for fatty acid synthesis?
A. Creatinine
B. Paraaminohippuric acid (PAH)
C. Glucose
D. Cholesterol

213. All of the following enzymes participate in what anaerobic process? Hint: it occurs in the cytosol of all cells of the body:
- Hexokinase
- Phosphoglucose isomerase
- Phosphofructokinase
- Aldolase
- Triose phosphate isomerase
- Glyceraldehyde 3-phosphate dehydrogenase
- Phosphoglycerate kinase
- Phosphoglyceromutase
- Enolase
- Pyruvate kinase

A. Glycolysis
B. Kreb's cycle
C. Respiratory chain
D. TCA cycle

214. Venous return is the blood returning to the heart via the inferior and superior vena cavae. Which of the following assists venous return?
A. The contraction of skeletal muscles
B. The pressure changes in the thorax and abdomen during breathing
C. The presence of valves
D. All of the above

215. The bundle of His arises in the:
A. SA node
B. AV node
C. Right ventricle
D. Left ventricle

216. The peptide hormone principally involved in the digestion of lipids is:
A. Serotonin
B. Enterogastrone
C. Enkephalins
D. Somatostatin

217. The oxidation of one NADH by the electron transport chain leads to the formation of how many ATP?
A. 1
B. 2
C. 3
D. 4

218. All of the following are reducing sugars EXCEPT:
A. Lactose
B. Maltose
C. Sucrose
D. Glucose

219. The kidneys normally excrete:
A. 1 to 2 L of urine per day
B. 10 to 20 L of urine per day
C. 50 to 75 L of urine per day
D. 100 to 150 L of urine per day

220. A complete DNA molecule consists of two polynucleotide chains or strands that:
A. Are parallel
B. Are perpendicular
C. Are antiparallel
D. Are antiperpendicular

221. Which part of the brainstem listed below serves as an autonomic reflex center to maintain homeostasis, regulating respiratory, vasomotor, and cardiac functions?
A. Midbrain
B. Pons
C. Medulla oblongata
D. None of the above

222. Which two situations listed below will excite the respiratory neurons and increase respiration/

A. A decrease in hydrogen ion concentration in the arterial blood

B. A decrease in the PCO_2 of arterial blood

C. An increase in hydrogen ion concentration in the arterial blood

D. An increase in the PCO_2 of arterial blood

223. Which receptors below are stimulated by distension of the lungs?

A. Irritant receptors

B. J receptors

C. Joint and muscle receptors

D. Lung stretch receptors

224. All of the following statements concerning muscle fibers are true EXCEPT:

A. Fast-twitch fibers are about twice as large in diameter

B. Slow-twitch fibers are mainly organized for endurance, especially for the generation of aerobic energy

C. The enzymes of the aerobic metabolic system are considerably more active in slow-twitch fibers than in fast-twitch fibers

D. Fast-twitch fibers contain more mitochondria and myoglobin

E. Fast-twitch fibers can deliver extreme amounts of power for a few seconds to a minute or so, whereas, slow-twitch fibers deliver a prolonged strength of contraction over many minutes or hours

225. Fluoride (fluorine) is found primarily in:

A. Milk

B. Drinking water

C. Seafood

D. Eggs

226. An isotonic solution is:

A. A solution that when placed on the outside of a cell will cause osmosis out of the cell

B. A solution that when placed on the outside of a cell will cause osmosis into the cell

C. A solution that when placed on the outside of a cell will not cause osmosis
D. None of the above

227. A reflex is:
A. A delayed response to a stimulus
B. An automatic response to a stimulus
C. None of the above
D. Both of the above

228. All of the following are major minerals EXCEPT:
A. Calcium
B. Chloride
C. Copper
D. Phosphorous
E. Magnesium

229. Many of the digestive proteases are produced and secreted as inactive:
A. carbohydrates
B. Lipids
C. Zymogens
D. Ketone bodies

230. ATP is produced via:
A. Substrate-level phosphorylation
B. Electron-transport phosphorylation
C. Photophosphorylation
D. All of the above

231. Which member of the electron transport chain listed below is also called Coenzyme Q?
A. Flavin mononucleotide (FMN)
B. Ubiquinone
C. Cytochromes b and c
D. Cytochromes a + b

232. All of the following statements concerning myoglobin are true EXCEPT:
A. It is a heme-protein present in heart and skeletal muscle
B. It functions both as a reservoir for oxygen and as an oxygen carrier

C. It decreases the rate of transport of oxygen within the muscle cell
D. It consists of a single polypeptide chain that is structurally similar to the individual polypeptide chains of the hemoglobin molecule

233. The difference in electrical charge between the inside and the outside of the cell membrane of an unstimulated (nonconducting) neuron is called the:
A. Relative refractory potential
B. Action potential
C. Resting membrane potential
D. Absolute refractory potential

234. The autonomic nervous system (ANS) is a set of efferent pathways from the central nervous system that innervates and regulates all of the following EXCEPT:
A. Glands (both exocrine and endocrine)
B. Cardiac muscle
C. Skeletal muscle
D. Smooth muscle
E. Visceral organs

235. Glutamate is derived form a-ketoglutarate. All of the following amino acids can be derived from glutamate EXCEPT:
A. Asparagine
B. Glutamine
C. Proline
D. Arginine

236. The sequence of amino acids in a protein is called the:
A. Primary structure
B. Secondary structure
C. Tertiary structure
D. Quaternary structure

237. The cyclic nucleotides cGMP and cAMP are called:
A. Neurotransmitters
B. Second messengers
C. Third messengers
D. Hormones

238. Which cellular structure listed below is composed of rRNA and protein?
A. Mitochondria
B. Golgi apparatus
C. Ribosomes
D. Lysosomes

239. The unpleasant sensation of difficulty in breathing is called:
A. Hypercapnea
B. Dyspnea
C. Apnea
D. Orthopnea

240. Which part of the ear is also called the tympanic cavity?
A. Inner ear
B. Middle ear
C. External ear
D. None of the above

241. Which of the following are the two main types of intrafusal fibers that are encapsulated in sheaths to form muscle spindles?
A. Nuclear bag fibers
B. Nuclear pipe fibers
C. Nuclear chain fibers
D. Nuclear rope fibers

242. The method of measuring heat loss or energy loss is called:
A. Enthalpy
B. Hydropathy index
C. Calorimetry
D. Entropy

243. All of the following will promote the release of oxygen from oxyhemoglobin (the hemoglobin dissociation curve will shift to the right) EXCEPT:
A. Increased carbon dioxide concentration (PCO)
B. Increased body temperature
C. Decrease in the pH
D. Increase in the pH

244. The pulmonary circuit is characterized by:
A. High pressure and low resistance
B. Low pressure and high resistance
C. Low pressure and low resistance
D. High pressure and high resistance

245. All of the following bonds are considered to be weak bonds EXCEPT:
A. Hydrogen bonds
B. Ionic bonds
C. Covalent bonds
D. van der Walls interactions

246. How do local anesthetics effect the nerve membrane?
A. They increase potassium flux
B. They increase the membrane excitability by increasing the membrane's permeability to sodium ions
C. They decrease the membrane's permeability to sodium ions and reduce the membrane excitability
D. They increase the calcium and chloride flux

247. Which vitamin below is synthesized only by microorganisms and is not present in plants?
A. Vitamin A
B. Cobalamin (vitamin B_{12})
C. Vitamin C
D. Vitamin E

248. All of the following statements concerning allosteric enzymes are true EXCEPT:
A They frequently catalyze a committed step early in a metabolic pathway
B They often have two or more subunits each with substrate binding sites that exhibit cooperativity
C. Allosteric activators cause the enzyme to bind substrate more readily
D. Allosteric inhibitors cause the enzyme to bind substrate less readily
E. They follow the Michaelis-Mention kinetics

249. The volume of blood pumped per minute by each ventricle is the:
A. Total peripheral resistance (TPR)
B. Cardiac output (CO)
C. Stroke volume (SV)
D. Heart rate (HR)

250. The first heart sound corresponds to the closure of the:
A. Semilunar valves
B. Pulmonary valve
C. Aortic valve
D. Atrioventricular valves

251. Which blood lipoprotein listed below is the most dense?
A. Chylomicrons
B. VLDLs
C. LDLs
D. HDLs

252. All of the following statements concerning the urea cycle are true EXCEPT:
A. The two nitrogen atoms that are incorporated into urea enter the cycle as ammonia and aspartate
B. Urea is produced by the hydrolysis of ornithine
C. The first two reactions leading to the synthesis of urea occur in the mitochondria, whereas the remaining cycle enzymes are located in the cytosol.
D. The urea that is formed in the urea cycle is passed via the blood stream to the kidneys and is excreted into the urine

253. Which mineral listed below is important in the formation of hemoglobin?
A. Sodium
B. Potassium
C. Iron
D. Magnesium

254. Acetyl CoA is used by the liver for the synthesis of:
A. Cholesterol
B. Bile salts
C. Ketone bodies
D. Hormones

255. All of the following statements concerning vitamin E are true EXCEPT:
A. It is also called tocopherol
B. It serves as an antioxidant
C. It prevents free radicals from oxidizing compounds such as polyunsaturated fatty acids
D. It is the most toxic of the fat-soluble vitamins

256. Which amylase listed below converts starch to maltose and dextrins?
A. Alpha-amylase
B. Beta-amylase
C. Glucamylase
D. All of the above

257. Diabetes insipidus:
A. Results from the decreased production of glucagons
B. Results from the decreased production of antidiuretic hormone (vasopressin)
C. Results from the decreased production of growth hormone
D. Results from the decreased production of thyroid hormone

258. Dextrans are:
A. Polysaccharides of fructose obtained from yeast and bacteria
B. Polysaccharides of galactose obtained from yeast and bacteria
C. Polysaccharides of glucose obtained from yeast and bacteria
D. Polysaccharides of ribose obtained from ycast and bacteria

259. Gastric secretion is said to occur in three phases. Which of the following is not one of those phases?
A. Cephalic phase
B. Caudal phase
C. Gastric phase
D. Intestinal phase

260. Important functions of the liver in protein metabolism include:
A. Deamination of amino acids
B. Formation of urea for removal of ammonia from the body fluids
C. Formation of plasma proteins

D. The ability to synthesize certain amino acids and other important chemical compounds from amino acids
E. All of the above

261. Which hormone listed below is often called the "stress hormone?
A. Growth hormone (GH)
B. Thyroid-stimulating hormone (TSH)
C. Adrenocorticotropic hormone (ACTH)
D. Follicle-stimulating hormone (FSH)

262. The volume of blood expelled by the ventricles of the heart is called what?
A. Stroke volume
B. Cardiac output
C. Residual capacity
D. Reserve volume

263. Cardiac output, blood viscosity, blood volume, and peripheral resistance are all factors involved in the maintenance of what?
A. Diastolic arterial blood pressure
B. Aortic blood pressure
C. Systolic arterial blood pressure
D. Pulse pressure

264. Which circulation is most of the blood volume of the body found in?
A. Systemic
B. Pulmonary
C. No difference in blood volume between the two circulations
D. Brain

265. Which structures below act as control valves through which blood is released into the capillaries?
A. Venules
B. Arterioles
C. Veins
D. Arteries
E. Capillaries

266. Where is the resistance the greatest of any part of the systemic circulation?
A. Aorta
B. Arterioles
C. Veins
D. Capillaries

267. Standard limb lead 1 of the ECG represents cardiac potential differences as they occur between which two limbs?
A. Left arm and left leg
B. Right arm and right leg
C. Right arm and left arm
D. Right arm and left leg

268. Under normal circumstances, what is the major factor determining the cardiac output?
A. Stroke volume
B. Heart rate
C. Rate of venous return

269. Which enzyme affects the intermolecular transfer of amino groups within the myocardium and may increase as a result of myocardial infarction and liver damage?
A. Serum glutamic-pyruvic transaminase (SGPT)
B. Serum glutamate decarboxylase
C. Serum glutamic-oxaloacetic transaminase (SGOT)
D. None of the above

270. Diastole begins with the onset of which heart sound?
A. First
B. Second
C. Third
D. Fourth

271. What is the neurotransmitter at the motor end plates (neuromuscular junctions) between nerve and striated muscle?
A. Norepinephrine
B. Acetylcholine
C. Neostigmine
D. Physiostigmine

272. Calcium ions trigger contraction of muscles by binding to what?
A. Actin
B. Tropomyosin
C. Troponin
D. Melanin

273. The organ of Corti is found where?
A. Inner ear
B. Outer ear
C. Eyeball
D. Testes

274. Stimulation of the parasympathetic nerves excites the papillary sphincter, thereby decreasing the papillary aperture; this process is referred to as what?
A. Miosis
B. Mydriasis
C. Epistaxis
D. Astigmatism

275. A sensory nerve ending that responds to stimuli originating from within the body regarding movement and spatial position is called what?
A. Exteroceptor
B. Interoceptor
C. Proprioceptor
D. Neurocepturs

276. What is considered to be the most vital part of the entire brain and mediates the following reflexes?
- Blinking
- Swallowing
- Vomiting
- Coughing

A. Medulla oblongata
B. Cerebellum
C. Hypothalamus
D. Pons

277. Most of the nonessential amino acids derive their alpha-amino groups from which of the following?
A. Glutamate
B. Pyruvate
C. Oxaloacetate
D. Sucrose

278. Which two amino acids have sulfur containing side chains?
A. Lysine
B. Cysteine
C. Arginine
D. Glutamate
E. Methionine

279. Urea is synthesized where?
A. Kidney
B. Liver
C. Intestines
D. Gallbladder

280. A fluid into which normal body cells can be placed without causing either swelling or shrinkage of cells is said to be what?
A. Hypertonic
B. Isotonic
C. Hypotonic
D. Osmotic

281. Which of the following solutions has an osmotic pressure different from all the others?
A. 1 M glucose
B. 1 M sodium chloride
C. 1 M potassium nitrate
D. None of the above

282. Which of the following mechanisms explains how a single input signal to many neurons, lasting less than one millisecond, can be converted into a sustained output signal lasting many milliseconds?
A. Inhibition
B. Peripheral resistance
C. Synaptic delay
D. End-plate delay

283. Which muscle has a longer refractory period?

A. Ventricular muscle
B. Atrial muscle
C. Both are the same
D. None of the above

284. The average resting membrane potential of nerve and skeletal muscle fibers of mammals is what?

A. (+) 85 millivolts
B. (-) 85 millivolts
C. (-) 45 millivolts
D. (+) 45 millivolts

285. The following factors can cause what to happen to the enamel of developing teeth?

- Vitamin deficiency (A and D)
- Fluorosis
- Congenital syphilis
- Injury or trauma to the mouth
- Inadequate calcium intake

A. Hypoplasia
B. Hypermineralisation
C. Hypomaturatuon
D. All of the above

286. Iron, copper, iodine, manganese, cobalt, and zinc are all considered to be what type of minerals?

A. Major minerals
B. Trace minerals
C. O non-essential ions
D. None of the above

287. Avidin has a high affinity for which vitamin?

A. C
B. D
C. Riboflavin
D. Biotin

288. Which of the following vitamins act as a coenzyme in a fatty acid production and in the oxidation of fatty acids and carbohydrates?

A. C

B. Biotin
C. Cobalamin
D. D

289. What vitamin is important in the prevention of some visual disorders, especially cataracts?
A. D
B. Biotin
C. Ascorbic acid
D. Riboflavin

290. Which of the following is the active form of vitamin D?
A. Cholecalciferol
B. 25-hydroxycholecalciferol
C. 1,25-dihydroxycholecalciferol
D. Ergosterol

291. Which vitamin is essential for the synthesis of prothrombin in the liver?
A. Ascorbic acid
B. A
C. D
D. K

292. Which vitamin is essential for the metabolism of protein, fats and carbohydrates, normal blood formation, and neural function?
A. Vitamin B12
B. Ascorbic acid
C. Vitamin B6
D. Riboflavin

293. Pantothenic acid is what type of vitamin?
A. B
B. C
C. D
D. A

294. Which of the following enzymes is inactivated by phosphorylation of a specific serine residue?
A. Phosphorylase
B. Phosphorylase kinase

C. Glycogen synthetase
D. Enolase

295. What do all of the following have in common?
A. Phosphoenolpyruvte
B. Carbamoyl phosphate
C. Acetyl phosphate
D. Creatine phosphate
E. 1,3-diphosphoglyceric acid
Answer = they all are energy rich phosphate carriers.

296. What reaction do all of the following enzymes catalyze?
A. Pyridoxal phosphate (PLP)
B. Pyridoxamine phosphate (PMP)
C. Transaminase
Answer = they catalyse the reversible transfer of an amino group from an alpha amino acid to an alpha keto acid, especially alpha keto glutaric acid. Such processes are essential to metabolism.

297. Which enzyme is involved in bone mineralization, hydrolysis of phosphoric esters, and functions optimally at pH 9.3?
A. Creatine phosphatase
B. Alkaline phosphatase
C. Hyaluronidase
D. Acid phosphatase

298. The following signs are indicative of a deficiency in what?
- Lack of vigor and stamina
- Weakness
- Mental depression
- Poor resistance to infection
- Impaired healing of wounds
- Slow recovery from disease

A. Fats
B. Proteins
C. Hormones
D. Alcohol

299. The major site of amino acid degradation in mammals is where?
A. Kidney

B. Pancreas
C. Liver
D. Brain

300. Which of the following is a naturally occurring derivative of tryptophan found in platelets and in cells of the brain and the intestine?
A. Heparin
B. Serotonin
C. Histamine
D. Adrenaline

301. Which of the following is the best known stimuli for increasing the rate of thyroid-stimulating hormone secretion of the anterior pituitary?
A. Exposure to heat
B. Exposure to cold
C. Exposure to stress
D. All of the above

302. Which of the following pituitary hormones is under predominant inhibitory control by the hypothalamus?
A. Growth hormone
B. Antidiuretic hormone
C. Somatomedin
D. Prolactin
E. Thyroid-stimulating hormone

303. Which disease causes both extracellular and intracellular dehydration to develop?
A. Addison's disease
B. Diabetes
C. Hyperparathyroidism
D. None of the above

304. Ammonia is formed where?
A. Liver
B. Pancreas
C. Kidney
D. Brain

305. The kidneys regulate hydrogen ion concentration principally by increasing or decreasing the concentration of what in the body fluid?

A. Bicarbonate ion
B. Sodium ion
C. Ammonium ion
D. Calcium ion

306. The countercurrent theory is used to explain the functioning of what part of the kidneys?

A. Bowman's capsule
B. Distal tubule
C. Loops of Henle
D. None of the above

307. The following substances are all normal constituents of what fluid?

- Water
- Urea
- Sodium chloride
- Potassium chloride
- Phosphates
- Uric acid
- Organic salts
- Pigment urobilin

A. Blood
B. Urine
C. Serum
D. Bile

308. Which of the following are absorbed in the main segments of the loops of Henle?

A. Sodium and chloride
B. Potassium and water
C. Sodium and water
D. Potassium and chloride

309. The following signs and symptoms are indicative of what disorder?

A. Yellow discoloration of the skin and mucous membranes and sclerae of the eyes

B. Nausea
C. Vomiting
D. Abdominal pain
E. Dark urine
Answer = Jaundice

310. Where is the major site of production of acetoacetate and 3-hydroxy butyrate?
A. Stomach
B. Liver
C. Kidney
D. Lungs

311. Secretin is produced by cells that line which portion of the GI. tract?
A. Stomach
B. Duodenum and jejunum
C. Esophagus
D. Liver

312. Insulin is secreted by which cells?
A. Alpha cells of the Islets of Langerhans
B. Beta cells of the Islets of Langerhans
C. Gamma cells

313. All of the following can be categorized as what?
A. Pepsinogen
B. Chymotrypsinogen
C. Trypsinogen
D. Procarboxypeptidase
E. Proelastase
Answer = zymogens

314. Chylomicrons are synthesized where?
A. Small intestine
B. Liver
C. G.I. tract
D. Kidneys

315. What two gastrointestinal hormones are mainly responsible for acting on the following organs?
A. Stomach

B. Pancreas
C. Small intestine
D. Large intestine
E. Gall bladder
F. Liver
Answer = secretin and cholecystokinin

316. Which structure monitors the oxygen content of the blood and assists in regulating respiration?
A. Carotid body
B. Hypothalamus
C. Medulla oblongata
D. Pons

317. Which of the following is a proteolytic enzyme that dissolves fibrin?
A. Thrombin
B. Fibrinogen
C. Plasmin
D. None of the above

318. What is the name of the naturally occurring mucopolysaccharide that acts in the body as an antithrombin factor to prevent intravascular clotting?
A. Thrombin
B. Fibrin
C. Heparin
D. All of the above

319. Which enzyme causes fibrinogen to change to fibrin?
A. Enterokinase
B. Plasmin
C. Thrombin
D. Thromboplastin

320. Which of the following substances is found in all cells and is released in allergic, inflammatory reactions?
A. Heparin
B. Histamine
C. Glucose
D. Adrenaline

321. Which structure secretes the hormones progesterone and estrogen?
A. Adrenal cortex
B. Pituitary
C. Corpus luteum
D. Testes

322. Norepinephrine is synthesized naturally in what area?
A. Adrenal cortex
B. Adrenal medulla
C. Anterior pituitary
D. Pancreas

323. Which of the following is a life-threatening condition caused by partial or complete failure of adrenocortical function;
A. Addison's disease
B. Cretinism
C. Cushing's syndrome
D. None of the above

324. What steroid hormone produced by the adrenal cortex regulates sodium and potassium balance in the blood?
A. Aldosterone
B. Epinephrine
C. Vasopressin
D. Insulin

325. What causes the type of apnea which can occur after hyperventilation of an anesthetized patient?
A. Decreased oxygen tension
B. Increased carbon dioxide tension
C. Decreased carbon dioxide tension
D. Increased nitrogen tension

326. Which of the following is believed to be the basic stimulus for exciting the respiratory center?
A. Increased pH
B. Decreased pH
C. Decreased carbon dioxide concentration
D. None of the above

327. Which enzyme below catalyzes below catalyzes the transfer of carbon dioxide from the tissues into the blood and then to the alveolar air?

A. Enolase
B. Aldolase
C. Carbonic anhydrase
D. None of the above

328. The following clinical signs are indicative of what physiological state?

A. Reduced cardiac output
B. Circulating insufficiency
C. Tachycardia
D. Hypotension
E. Restlessness
F. Pallor
G. Diminished urinary output
H. Diminished glomerular filtration
I. Muscular weakness
Answer = shock

329. Antidiuretic hormone (vasopressin) is secreted by the cells of which organ?

A. Hypothalamus
B. Anterior pituitary
C. Adrenal cortex
D. Pancreas

330. Which of the following is a metabolic disorder owing to a deficiency of antidiuretic hormone?

A. Nephrogenic insipidus
B. Diabetes insipidus
C. Neither of the above
D. Diabetes mellitus

331. The rate of secretion of parathyroid hormone is controlled almost entirely by what?

A. Plasma phosphorus ion concentration
B. Plasma calcium ion concentration
C. Plasma potassium ion concentration
D. Urine calcium ion concentration

332. Calcitonin is secreted by which of the following cells?
A. Alpha cells
B. Beta cells
C. Parafollicular cells
D. Sertoli cells

333. Almost all secretions by the pituitary are controlled by signals transmitted from which of the following:
A. Cerebrum
B. Medulla
C. Hypothalamus
D. Pons

334. The following symptoms are characteristic of what disease?
A. Polyuria
B. Polydipsia
C. Weight loss
D. Polyphagia
E. Hyperglycemia
F. Weakness
G. Acidosis
H. Glycosuria
Answer = diabetes mellitus

335. The measurement of the amount of heat directly generated by any oxidative reaction (e.g., evaporation, radiation, conduction, convection) is defined as which one of the following:
A. Direct calorimetry
B. Indirect calorimetry
C. None of the above
D. Centrifugation

336. What is the name of the disorder that results from the incomplete metabolism of tyrosine, in which abnormal amounts of homogentisic acid are excreted?
A. Alkaptonuria
B. Phenylketonuria
C. Hyperammonemia
D. Cystinuria

337. In proteins, the alpha-carboxyl group of one amino acid is joined to the alpha-amino group of another amino acid by what type of bond?

A. Hydrogen bond
B. Hydrostatic bond
C. Peptide bond
D. Carbon-bond

338. The major site of cholesterol synthesis is where?

A. Liver
B. Pancreas
C. Appendix
D. Lung

339. The degradation and oxidation of fatty acids occurs where?

A. In the cytoplasm
B. In the mitochondria
C. In the nucleus
D. In endoplasmic reticulum

340. Prostaglandins are synthesized from what?

A. Saturated fatty acids
B. Unsaturated fatty acids
C. Carbohydrates
D. Hormone insulin

341. B-hydroxybutyric acid and aminoacetic acid are both called what?

A. Ketone bodies
B. Urate bodies
C. Transaminase intermediates
D. Calcium crystals

342. What are the following symptoms indicative of?

A. Ketonuria (ketones in urine)
B. Loss of potassium in urine
C. Fruity odor of acetone on the breath
Answer = ketosis

343. Which enzyme listed below is found in grains and vegetables and is involved in the hydrolysis of starch to maltose?

A. Alpha-amylase

B. Beta-amylase
C. Trans ketolase
D. Hydrolase

344. The arrangement of sugars into D- and L- configurations is based upon their resemblance to which monosaccharide?
A. Glyceraldehyde
B. Dihydroxyacetone
C. Glycine
D. Glucose

345. Another name for Coenzyme Q is what?
A. Adenyl cyclase
B. Ubiquinone
C. Biotin
D. Enolase

346. Aerobic glycolysis yields which of the following?
A. Pyruvic acid
B. Lactic acid
C. Acetic Acid
D. Homogentisic acid

347. In what anaerobic process do all of the following enzymes participate?
- Hexokinase
- Phosphoglucose isomerase
- Phosphofructokinase
- Aldolase
- Triose phosphate isomerase
- Glyceraldehyde 3-phosphate dehydrogenase
- Phosphoglycerate kinase
- Phosphoglyceromutase
- Enolase
- Pyruvate kinase

A. Glycolysis
B. Lipid metabolism
C. Fat catabolism
D. Kreb's cycle

348. Lactose is hydrolyzed to which of the following by the enzyme lactase?
A. Galactose and glucose

B. Glucose
C. Glucose and fructose
D. Fructose and galactose

349. Glucose 6-phosphatase is found most abundantly in which of the following organs?
A. Kidney
B. Liver
C. Intestine
D. Brain

350. Glucose released by the liver into the blood during muscular activity is taken up primarily by what two organs listed below?
A. Skeletal muscle
B. Heart
C. Brain
D. Kidney

351. The rate of glycolysis is primarily controlled by the level of activity of which enzyme?
A. Enolase
B. Aldolase
C. Phosphofructokinase
D. Hexokinase

352. Denaturing agents such as urea and guanidine hydrochloride disrupt which kind of bonds?
A. Covalent
B. Noncovalent
C. Hydrogen bond
D. Ionic bond

353. The major effect of acidosis on the body is what?
A. Increased respiration
B. Increased heart rate
C. Depression of the central nervous system
D. Decreased liver function

354. Which of the following is considered to be the normal hemoglobin?
A. Hemoglobin A
B. Hemoglobin C

C. Hemoglobin F
D. Hemoglobin S

Brain Diet and Self Assessment

1. **Name six highly distinctive and biologically crucial properties of enzymes?**
2. **A substance that alters the rate of an enzymatic reaction by interacting with the enzyme at a site other than the active site is called what?**
3. **Define km value of an enzyme.**
4. **What is the hallmark of competitive inhibition?**
5. **The first law of thermodynamics states what?**
6. **What is the pH of saliva?**
7. **Define isotope.**
8. **Tyrosine is a precursor of what two hormones?**
9. **What is the major bile salt?**
10. **What is the normal plasma concentration of glucose, calcium, and phosphorus?**
11. **What hormone acts to stimulate and to regulate the production of erythrocytes and is therefore able to increase the oxygen-carrying capacity of the blood?**
12. **Sixty-five percent of the total quantity of iron in the body is present in what form?**
13. **What two proteins are the oxygen carriers in vertebrates?**
14. **How will the following situations effect the release of oxygen from oxyhemoglobin?**
    A. Increase in arterial PCO_2
    B. Decrease in arterial PO_2
    C. Increased temperature
    D. Increase in arterial hydrogen ion concentration (pH)
15. **What process are all of the following involved in?**
    A. Calcium
    B. Fibrinogen
    C. Platelets
    D. Prothrombin.
    E. Tissue thromboplastin

Answer key to biochemistry

1	B	2	B	3	C	4	B
5	B	6	B	7	D	8	E
9	A	10	E	11	C	12	C, B
13	B	14	C	15	B	16	C
17	A, C	18	B	19	C	20	B
21	C	22	B	23	C	24	D
25	B	26	B	27	D	28	D
29	B	30	C	31	D	32	B
33	C	34	B	35	D	36	C
37	B	38	D	39	A	40	C
41	B	42	C	43	C	44	C
45	D	46	C	47	C	48	A, D
49	C	50	C	51	C	52	B
53	C	54	B, C	55	C	56	A, C
57	B	58	A	59	D	60	D
61	A	62	B, C	63	E	64	C
65	D	66	C	67	C	68	C
69	C	70	B	71	B	72	B
73	C	74	A	75	C	76	C
77	C	78	D	79	C	80	D
81	A	82	D	83	D	84	E
85	C	86	B	87	C	88	D
89	B	90	B	91	D	92	B
93	C	94	B	95	C	96	B
97	C	98	D	99	B	100	B
101	B	102	B	103	A	104	B
105	D	106	B	107	C	108	D
109	C	110	B	111	B	112	B
113	D	114	A	115	A	116	C
117	E	118	B	119	B	120	B
121	C	122	C	123	A	124	C
125	C	126	B	127	C	128	C
129	C	130	B, C	131	C	132	B
133	A	134	B	135	A	136	D
137	B	138	C	139	B	140	C
141	D	142	C	143	D	144	C
145	F	146	E	147	C	148	A

149	B	150	C	151	C	152	D
153	B	154	E	155	C	156	B
157	B	158	D	159	A	160	B
161	C	162	B	163	D	164	B
165	C	166	B	167	D	168	C
169	C	170	B	171	D	172	C
173	A	174	C	175	E	176	C
177	C	178	B	179	C	180	B
181	C	182	C	183	D	184	C
185	D	186	B	187	D	188	C
189	C	190	D	191	C	192	A
193	E	194	B	195	A	196	C
197	D	198	B	199	C	200	D
201	D	202	B	203	C	204	D
205	B	206	C	207	C	208	B
209	C	210	A	211	C	212	C
213	A	214	D	215	B	216	B
217	C	218	C	219	A	220	C
221	C	222	C, D	223	D	224	D
225	B	226	C	227	B	228	C
229	C	230	D	231	B	232	C
233	C	234	C	235	A	236	A
237	B	238	C	239	B	240	B
241	A, C	242	C	243	D	244	C
245	C	246	C	247	B	248	E
249	B	250	D	251	D	252	B
253	C	254	C	255	D	256	B
257	B	258	C	259	B	260	E
261	C	262	B	263	C	264	A
265	B	266	B	267	C	268	C
269	C	270	B	271	B	272	C
273	A	274	A	275	C	276	A
277	A	278	B, E	279	B	280	B
281	A	282	C	283	A	284	B
285	A	286	B	287	D	288	B
289	D	290	C	291	D	292	A
293	A	294	C	295	—	296	—
297	B	298	B	299	C	300	B
301	B	302	D	303	B	304	C

305	A	306	C	307	B	308	C
309	—	310	B	311	B	312	B
313	——	314	C	315	——	316	A
317	C	318	C	319	C	320	B
321	C	322	B	323	A	324	A
325	B	326	B	327	C	328	—
329	A	330	B	331	B	332	C
333	C	334	—	335	A	336	A
337	C	338	A	339	B	340	B
341	A	342	—	343	B	344	A
345	B	346	A	347	A	348	A
349	B	350	A	351	C	352	B
353	C	354	A				

Reader's Notes

3

Microbiology and Pathology

Part I

1. **Which of the following characteristics is the most reliable indicator of prognosis of malignant tumors?**
   A. Size of tumor
   B. The degree of differentiation
   C. The degree of localization
   D. Abnormal mitoses

2. **Humans may acquire *Toxoplasma gondii* by:**
   A. Airborne conidia
   B. Ingestion of cysts in poorly cooked meat
   C. Sustaining a dog bite
   D. Swimming in contaminated water.

3. **Which type of cancer listed below originates in the middle layer of the epidermis and is the most common type of oral cancer?**
   A. Basal cell carcinoma
   B. Malignant melanoma
   C. Squamous cell carcinoma
   D. Kaposi's sarcoma

4. Various species of the following bacteria produce the enzyme hyaluronidase, except:
A. Streptococcus
B. Clostridium
C. Staphylococcus
D. Neisseria

5. Quaternary ammonium compounds, which are widely used for skin antisepsis, are classified as:
A. Nonionic detergents
B. Anionic detergents
C. Cationic detergents
D. None of the above

6. All of the following are prokaryotic cells, except:
A. Bacteria
B. Chlamydia
C. Fungi
D. Mycoplasmas
E. Rickettsia

7. Capsules play important roles in all of the following diseases, except:
A. Haemophilus meningitis
B. Cryptococcoses
C. Gonorrhea
D. Pneumococcal pneumonia
E. Meningococcemia

8. Bacterial vaccines are composed of:
A. Capsular polysaccharides
B. Inactivated protein exotoxins (toxoids)
C. Killed bacteria
D. Live attenuated bacteria
E. All of the above

9. The enzymes superoxide dismutase and catalase are not present in:
A. Obligate aerobes
B. Facultative anaerobes
C. Obligate anaerobes
D. All of the above

10. The Hepatitis A virus, Poliovirus, and Rotavirus have which portal of entry listed below?
A. Respiratory tract
B. Gastrointestinal tract
C. Skin
D. Genital tract
E. Blood

11. Which of the following are respiratory enzymes capable of undergoing alternate reduction and oxidation?
A. Pyrimidine nucleotides
B. Cytochromes
C. Reductants
D. Surfactants

12. Phlebitis can occur in any vein in the body but most often effects the:
A. Veins of the upper extremities
B. Pulmonary veins
C. Hepatic veins
D. Veins of the lower extremities

13. Which syndrome listed below is also called Trisomy 21?
A. Down syndrome
B. Edward's syndrome
C. Patau's syndrome
D. All of the above

14. Anemia may be caused by:
A. Excessive bleeding
B. Decreased red blood cell production
C. Increased red blood cell destruction (hemolysis)
D. All of the above

15. Which cellular organelle listed below contains specialized enzymes whose functions involve hydrogen peroxide?
A. Mitochondria
B. Microbody
C. Nucleus
D. Golgi complex

16. Which genera of fungi listed below is not responsible for causing dermatophytosis?

A. Trichophyton
B. Microsporum
C. Histoplasma
D. Epidermophyton

17. The Ghon complex, a lesion in the lung and regional lymph nodes, is found in:

A. Actinomycosis
B. Primary tuberculosis
C. Blastomycosis
D. Histoplasmosis

18. Kidney stones (renal calculi) are a common complication in a patient with which disorder listed below?

A. Diabetes mellitus
B. Hyperthyroidism
C. Hyperparathyroidism
D. Hypopituitarism

19. Natural immunity (innate immunity) is resistance:

A. Acquired through contact with an antigen
B. Not acquired through contact with an antigen
C. Both of the above
D. None of the above

20. An injection of a drug into a patient who is allergic to this drug may lead to death due to:

A. Low levels of histamine
B. Hyperglobulinemia
C. Severe anaphylaxis (anaphylactic shock)
D. Localized anaphylaxis

21. The lipidoses are lipid storage disease caused by abnormalities in the enzymes that metabolize fat. They result in a toxic accumulation of fat by-products in tissue. Gaucher's diseases is a disorder of lipid metabolism caused by a deficiency of

A. Hexosaminidase A
B. Sphingomyelinase
C. Glucocerebrosidase
D. Alpha – L - iduronidase

22. All of the following statements concerning syphilis are true except :

A. It is a sexually transmitted disease caused by infection with treponema palidum (a spirochete)

B. Congenital infection in neonates and infants can occur.

C. It occurs in three stages: primary, secondary and tertiary

D. Gummas are lesions of primary syphilis

E. The prognosis is good if treated early, tertiary syphilis causes irreversible heart failure, dementia and disability

F. Parenteral penicillium G is the drug of choice for treating all stages.

23. Nephritic syndrome is a syndrome comprising the clinical symptoms of:

A. Nephritis

B. Hematuria

C. Hypertension

D. Renal failure

E. All of the above

24. Which of the following is a fungal infection that may develop in people who have poorly controlled diabetes?

A. Aspergillosis

B. Coccidioidomycosis

C. Mucormycosis

D. Crypttococcosis

25. Which type of leukemia listed below is the most common pediatric cancer?

A. Acute myeloid leukemia

B. Chronic myelocytic leukemia

C. Acute lymphocytic leukemia

D. Chronic lymphocytic leukemia

26. Which of the following are causes of ascites, the accumulation of fluid in the abdominal cavity?

A. Cirrhosis

B. Heart failure

C. Intra-abdominal cancer

D. Kidney failure

E. Tuberculosis

F. All of the above

27. Herpes Zoster (Shingles) is thought to be the adult counter - part of which of the following disease?
A. Rubella
B. Mumps
C. Smallpox
D. Chickenpox

28. Which type of Hepatitis is described below?
- It is spread by fecal-oral transmission; parenteral infection does not occur
- It has an incubation period of 21-45 days
- It does not cause a chronic carrier state
- It is also called infectious hepatitis

A. Hepatitis A
B. Hepatitis B
C. Non A non B hepatitis
D. Hepatitis E

29. Which of the following is also known as Vincent infection or trench mouth?
A. Juvenile gingivitis
B. Desquamate gingivitis
C. Acute necrotizing ulcerative gingivitis (ANUG)
D. Rapidly progressing periodontitis

30. A 19 year old man suffering from non-suppurative enlargement of the parotid glands and painful swelling of the testes. He also complains of pain while eating, headache and general malaise. This man is most likely suffering from?
A. German measles (Rubella)
B. Measles (Rubeola)
C. Mumps
D. Common cold
E. Influenza
F. Pharyngitis

31. Kaposi's sarcoma, a malignant tumor of vascular organ that appear painless and purple raised patches on the skin, frequently is associated with
A. Diabetes
B. Chronic renal failure

C. AIDS
D. Hypertension

32. The primary inflection with herpes simplex virus is characterized by all of the following except :
A. Average course of 2-3 weeks
B. A few lesions on the lips or the mouth that resolve over a week to 10 days
C. Fever chills and malaise (flu-like-symptoms)
D. Vesicle formation

33. Which of the following skin growths closely resembles squamous cell carcinoma
A. Dermatofibromas
B. Seborrhea Keratosis
C. Achrochordon
D. Keratoacanthoma
E. Actinic keratosis

34. Which two antifungal agents listed are also referred to as polyene antibiotics ?
A. Nystatin
B. Miconazole
C. Flucytosine
D. Amphotericin
E. Ketoconazole

35. All of the following statements concerning malignant melanoma are true except :
A. It originates in the pigment-producing cells of the skin (melanocytes)
B. It is considered of be the most severe type of skin cancer
C. It is most common in fair skinned persons
D. It is most often associated with excessive exposure to sunlight
E. It rarely spreads (metastasizes to distant parts of the body)

36. All of the following bacteria have been found to be the principal bacteria associated with juvenile periodontitis except:
A. Actino-bacillius actino-mycetamcomitans (AA)
B. Capnocytophaga ochraceus
C. Wolinella recta

D. Prevotella intermedius
E. Eikenella corodens

37. Which of the following is the drug of choice for treating Candidiasis?
A. Penicillin
B. Cephalosporins
C. Clindamycin
D. Nystatin

38. Which syndrome listed below is condition affecting girls, in which, one of the two X chromosomes is partially or completely missing?
A. Klinefelter's syndrome
B. Triple X syndrome
C. Turner syndrome
D. Down's syndrome

39. Which of the flowing immunodeficiency disorders is the most serious ?
A. Wiskott - Aldrich syndrome
B. Severe combined immunodeficiency disease (SCID)
C. Ataxia - Telangiectasia
D. Hyper – IgE syndrome

40. Which of the following is the proper time and temperature for autoclaving?
A. 350 F for 1 hour
B. 250 F for 15-20 minutes
C. 4500 F for 5 minutes
D. 890 F for 30 minutes

41. The area of the cytoplasm in prokaryotic cells in which DNA is located is called?
A. Granules
B. Nucleoid
C. Plastids
D. Transposons

42. All of the following statements concerning ethylene oxide sterilization are true except:
A. It is used extensively in hospitals for the sterilization of heat-sensitive materials such as surgical instrument and plastics

B. It kills by alkylating both proteins and nucleic acids
C. It is a fast process, 20 – 50 minutes depending on the material to sterilized
D. It is fairly toxic to humans and is also flammable

43 Gamma hemolytic streptococci can be differentiated from alpha & beta streptococci on blood agar plates by observing
A. A clear zone of hemloysis about the colony with no intact corpuscles
B. Small colonies surrounded by a greenish discoloration
C. No hemolysis
D. Small colonies surrounded by a zone of partial hemolyses and an outer clear zone

44. Which one of the following tests is abnormally prolonged in idiopathic thrombocytopenic purpura?
A. Partial thromb plastin time (PTT)
B. Thrombin time
C. Bleeding time
D. Prothrombin time (PT)

45. Acromegaly is
A. Excessive growth caused by the over-secretion of thyroid hormone
B. Excessive growth caused by the over-secretion of growth hormone
C. Excessive growth caused by the over-secretion of parathyroid hormone
D. Excessive growth caused by the over-secretion of epinephrine

46. Osgood - Schlatter disease is
A. Destruction of the growth plate in the neck of the thigh bone
B. Inflammation of the bone and cartilage at the top of the shinbone
C. A relatively common condition in which backache and humpback are caused by changes in the vertebrae
D. A rare form of inflammation of bone and cartilage affecting one of the small bones, the navicular bone, in the foot.

47. Which immunoglobulin antibody listed is some times referred to as the Secretory immunoglobulin?
A. Ig D

B. Ig E
C. Ig A
D. Ig M

48. All of the following abnormalities in parathyroid function are matched with the appropriate association except

A. Primary hyperparathyroidism; adenoma
B. Secondary hyperparathyroidism; liver disease
C. Tertiary hyperparathyroidism: hyperparathyroidism which persists after definitive therapy for secondary hyperparathyroidism.
D. Hypoparathyroidism; most commonly caused by accidental surgery excision during thyroidectomy
E. Pseudoparathyrodism: defective end organ responsiveness to PTH

49. Which of the following is the most important contributor to arterial thrombosis?

A. Pregnancy
B. Oral contraceptives
C. Atherosclerosis
D. Smoking

50. Generalized edema is known as:

A. Hydrothorax
B. Anasarca
C. Hydropericardium
D. Ascites
E. Exudate
F. Transudate

51. All of the following are amyloid-associated conditions, except:

A. Alzheimer's disease
B. Familial Mediterranean fever
C. Diabetes mellitus Type 2
D. Parkinson's disease
E. Senile amyloidosis

52. An infiltrate of which one of the following cells is most characteristic of the early stages of the acute inflammation?

A. Basophils
B. Eosinophils

C. Neutrophils
D. Monocytes

53. Which of the following is the most common type of peptic ulcer?
A. Esophageal ulcers
B. Gastric ulcers
C. Duodenal ulcers
D. Stress ulcers

54. Which type of necrosis listed below is the basic and most common type?
A. Liquefaction necrosis
B. Gangrenous necrosis
C. Caseous necrosis
D. Coagulative necrosis
E. Fat necrosis
F. Fibrinoid necrosis

55. The cause of most types of leukemia is:
A. Viral
B. Fungal
C. Bacterial
D. Unknown

56. The usual site of latency for the Herpes simplex virus type 2 is:
A. The cranial sensory ganglia
B. The lumbar or sacral sensory ganglia
C. The cranial or thoracic sensory ganglia
D. B - lymphocytes

57. Emphysema is associated with:
A. Pollutants
B. Genetic factors
C. Cigarette smoking
D. Infection
E. All of the above

58. Young plaque is dominated by which of bacteria listed below?
A. Gram-positive COCCI
B. Gram-positive rods

C. Gram-negative rods
D. Filaments

59. Which type of bronchogenic carcinoma listed below is the most aggressive?
A. Squamous cell carcinoma
B. Adenocarcinoma
C. Small cell (oat cell) carcinoma
D. Large cell carcinoma

60. Which of the following cancers is second in incidence only to carcinoma of the lung in men and third after breast and lung cancer in women?
A. Esophageal cancer
B. Stomach cancer
C. Colorectal cancer
D. Liver cancer

61. Which type of cancer listed below is the most common malignancy of women?
A. Bone cancer
B. Stomach cancer
C. Breast cancer
D. Ovarian cancer

62. Which of the following has been shown to be the most effective antimicrobial agent for reducing plaque and gingivitis long-term?
A. Stannous fluoride
B. Phenolic compounds
C. Chlorhexidine
D. Ouarternary ammonium compounds

63. Cephalosporins and penicillins both have which mode of action listed below?
A. Affect cell membrane
B. Interfere with protein synthesis
C. Affect cell wall
D. Interfere with normal biosynthetic pathways

64. Neoplastic epidermal cells, often with keratin pearls, characterize which type of skin cancer listed below?
A. Squamous cell carcinoma

B. Basal cell carcinoma
C. Malignant melanoma
D. None of the above

65. Which cells listed below are the most important phagocytic cells?
A. Eosinophils and basophils
B. Neutrophils and basophils
C. Neutrophils and macrophages
D. Macrophages and eosinophils

66. People with cystic fibrosis, burn victims, individuals with cancer, and patients requiring extensive stays in intensive care units are particularly at risk for infection with which species listed below?
A. Bacteroides
B. Fusobacterium
C. Pseudomonas
D. Streptococcus

67. A xenograft is:
A. A transfer of an individual's own tissue
B. A transfer of tissue between genetically identical individuals (identical twins)
C. A transfer of tissue between different species
D. A transfer of tissue between genetically different members of the same species (one human to another)

68. During phagocytosis, bacteria are ingested by the invagination of the neutrophil (PMN's) cell membrane around the bacteria to form a vacuole (phagosome). This engulfment is enhanced by the binding of IgG antibodies to the surface of the bacteria, a process called:
A. Transformation
B. Opsonization
C. Transduction
D. Recombination

69. An increase in the size of an organ or tissue due to an increase in the size of cells is known as
A. Hypertrophy
B. Atrophy

C. Hyperplasia
D. Hypoplasia
E. Metaplasia

70. Cytokines are soluble proteins secreted by which of the following cells?

A. Lymphocytes
B. Macrophages
C. Fibroblasts
D. Platelets
E. All of the above

71. Which myeloproliferative disorder listed below is characterized by an increased number of platelets?

A. Polycythemia vera
B. Myelofibrosis
C. Thrombocythemia
D. Chronic myelocytic leukemia

72. Histamine release within the body causes:

A. Increased capillary permeability
B. Increased gastric secretion
C. Bronchiolar constriction
D. Fall in blood pressure
E. All of the above

73. Carbon Monoxide

A. Attaches to the nucleus of red blood cells and blocks their capacity to replicate
B. Attaches to the cytoplasm membrane of red blood cells and causes lysis of the cell
C. Attaches to the hemoglobin of red blood cells and blocks their capacity to carry oxygen
D. Attaches t the cell membrane of red blood cells blocks their capacity to move within vessels

74. The most common bone lesion is a (an)

A. Osteochondroma
B. Fractures
C. Osteoma
D. Osteoblastoma

75. When gallstones are in the gallbladder the condition is know as:

A. Choledocholithiasis
B. Cholesterolosis, strawberry gall bladder
C. Cholelithiasis
D. Divertiuculosis of the gallbladder

76. All of the following statements concerning B cells are true except :

A. They mature in the bone marrow and migrate to lymphoid organs
B. They are found in the germinal centers of the spleen and lymph nodes
C. They are progenitors of plasma cells.
D. They involve in humoral antibody mediated and cell mediated immunity
E. They function to search out identity and bind with specific antigens

77. A serious condition in which the quantity of blood pumped by heart each minute (cardiac output) is insufficient to meet body normal requirements for oxygen and nutrients is called

A. Heart bock
B. Ventricular tachycardia
C. Congestive heart failure
D. Atrial fibrillation

78. Which of the following is the most frequently employed diagnostic laboratory technique for the microscopic detection of antigens in tissue secretion or in cell suspensions?

A. Immuofluorescence (Fluorescent antibody)
B. Agglutination
C. Radiommunoassay
D. Precipitation (Precepitin)
E. Enzyme Liked Immunosorbent Assay (ELISA)

79. Diabetes mellitus type –2 associated with all of the following characteristics except

A. Normal or increased insulin syntheses
B. Onset in adulthood
C. Autoimmune origin

D. Associated with obesity
E. Rare ketoacidosis

80. All of the following are characteristic of an exudates except:
A. Protein-rich
B. Low specific gravity
C. Glucose-poor
D. Cell-rich

81. Brief loss of consciousness and sometimes memory after an injury to the brain that doesn't cause obvious physical damage is called a
A. Hematoma
B. Infarction
C. Concussion
D. Meningioma

82. Malignant nephrosclerosis is a condition associated with
A. Server Hyperlipidemia
B. Severe high blood pressure
C. Severe hyper-albuminemia
D. Severe low blood pressure

83. Which of the following is the most common inherited disease leading to death among white people in the United States?
A. von Hippel Lindau disease
B. Cystic fibrosis
C. Marfan's syndrome
D. Familial hypercholesterolemia

84. All of the following statements concerning the rubella virus are true except:
A. It is a member of the toga virus family and is an enveloped virus; comprise of an icosahedral nucleocapsid and a positive – stranded single stranded RNA genome
B. It causes rubella (German Measles) and congenital rubella syndrome
C. It is transmitted by the bite of a rabid animal
D. Prevention involves immunization with the live, attenuated vaccine

85. Chronic bronchitis is primarily a disease of:
A. Alcoholics

B. Cigarette smokers
C. Miners
D. Patients with a family history of allergy

86. The cytopathic effect that is seen when a virus infects a specific cell culture
A. Is the same for most viruses
B. Is not useful in diagnostic virology
C. Is characteristic of each virus and can be used for detection of that virus
D. Does not affect the specific infected cells.

87. Acquired immunodeficiency syndrome (AIDS) is caused by an enveloped single stranded, linear, positive polarity RNA virus known as :
A. An arbovirus
B. A parvovirus
C. A retrovirus
D. An adenovirus

88. All of the following viruses are paramyxoviruses except:
A. Mumps virus
B. Measles virus
C. Influenza A, B, and C viruses
D. Respiratory syncytial virus (RSV)
E. Parainfluenza virus

89. Infections caused by certain nematodes cause
A. Marked neutrophilia
B. Marked eosinophilia
C. Marked basophilia
D. All of the above

90. Which of the following types of lymphoma is distinguished by a particular kind of cancer cell called a Reed – Sternberg cell which has a distinctive appearance under microscope?
A. Non –Hodgkin's lymphoma
B. Burkitt's lymphoma
C. Hodgkin's disease
D. Mycosis Fungicides

91. Which of the following is a powerful oxidizing agent that inactivates bacteria and most viruses by oxidizing free sulfhydryl groups?
A. Alcohol
B. Chlorine
C. Formaldehyde
D. Phenol

92. Two different pathways are involved in the metabolism of glucose one - anaerobic and one aerobic; the anaerobic process occurs in the
A. Mitochondria and is very efficient
B. Cytoplasm and is only moderately efficient
C. Mitochondria and is not efficient
D. Cytoplasm and is very efficient

93. A cell wall that contains teichoic acids and a thick peptido-glycans (murein) layer is characteristic of
A. Viruses
B. Gram positive bacteria
C. Fungi
D. Gram negative bacteria

94. Vaccines that contain a live virus whose pathogenicity has been attenuated are used against all of the following diseases except:
A. Measles
B. Mumps
C. Rabies
D. Rubella

95. Viruses that infect bacteria are known as :
A. Protoplasts
B. Saprophytes
C. Bacteriophages
D. Commensals

96. A laceration of the esophagus and the upper part of the stomach during forceful vomiting, retching, or hiccups is called:
A. Hiatal-Hernia
B. Mallory-Weiss syndrome

C. Achalasia
D. Acid reflux syndrome

97. All these organs get usually damaged from prolonged hypertension except?
A. Kidneys
B. Heart
C. Stomach
D. Brain

98. Which glands listed below fail to develop in children with the DiGeorge's anomaly (DiGeorge's syndrome)?
A. Thyroid gland
B. Thymus gland
C. Pituitary gland
D. Parathyroid glands
E. Adrenal glands

99. All of the following conditions are associated with a prolonged bleeding time except:
A. Idiopathic thrombocytopenic purpura
B. Von Willebrand's disease
C. Hemophilia
D. Patents taking anticoagulants (e.g. dicumarol, heparin etc.)
E. Long term treatment with aspirin

100. All of the following are examples of Type III hypersensitivity reactions (immune complex) except:
A. Arthus reaction
B. Farmer's lung
C. Myasthenia gravis
D. Cheesemaker's lung
E. Serum sickness
F. Rheumatoid arthritis

Answer key to Microbiology and Pathology part I

1	C	2	B	3	C	4	D
5	C	6	C	7	C	8	E
9	C	10	B	11	B	12	D
13	A	14	D	15	B	16	C
17	B	18	C	19	B	20	C
21	C	22	D	23	E	24	C
25	C	26	F	27	D	28	A
29	C	30	C	31	C	32	D
33	D	34	A, D	35	E	36	C
37	D	38	C	39	B	40	B
41	B	42	C	43	C	44	C
45	B	46	B	47	C	48	B
49	C	50	B	51	D	52	C
53	C	54	D	55	D	56	B
57	E	58	A	59	C	60	C
61	C	62	C	63	C	64	A
65	C	66	C	67	C	68	B
69	A	70	E	71	C	72	E
73	C	74	B	75	C	76	D
77	C	78	A	79	C	80	B
81	C	82	B	83	B	84	C
85	B	86	C	87	C	88	C
89	B	90	C	91	B	92	B
93	B	94	C	95	C	96	B
97	C	98	B, D	99	C	100	C

Part II

1. Which of the following is the most common cause of sudden, severe abdominal pain and abdominal surgery?
A. Ulcerative colitis
B. Acute appendicitis
C. Crohn's disease
D. Carcinoid tumor

2. Swollen bleeding gums accompanied by muscle joint and bone pain are characteristic of:
A. Pellagra
B. Scurvy
C. Beri-beri
D. Rickets

3. The main advantage of active immunity is that resistance is:
A. Available immediately
B. Short Term
C. Long term
D. None of the above

4. Which two enzymes listed below would be evaluated in the blood of a patient suffering from acute pancreatitis?
A. Alkaline phosphates
B. Acid phosphates
C. Lipase
D. Amylase
E. SGOT / SGPT

5. Three species of bacteria account for more than 80% of all cases of bacterial meningitis. Which species listed below is not one of them?
A. Neisseria meningitis
B. Hemophilus influenzae
C. Staphylococcus aureus
D. Sterptococcus pneumoniae

6. Urolithiasis is a condition resulting from the presence or formation of calculi in the urinary tract. Most of these calculi are:
A. Ammonium magnesium phosphate stones
B. Calcium stones
C. Uric acid stones
D. Cystine stones

7. Aflatoxins are produced by
A. Candida species
B. Coccidioides species
C. Aspergillus species
D. Histoplasma species

8. Jaundice refers to yellow discoloration of the skin, sclera and tissues caused by
A. Hyperlipidemia
B. Hyperglycemia
C. Hyperbilirubinemia
D. Hypocalcaemia

9. The most common cause of cirrhosis is :
A. Wilson's disease
B. Alcohol abuse
C. Bile duct obstruction
D. Hemochromatosis

10. Which species listed below has been implicated in the dental caries process?
A. Staphylococcus
B. Bacteroides
C. E. coli
D. Streptococcus

11. Which growth curve listed below describes the lytic reproduction cycle that releases a large number of phage simultaneously
A. One step growth curve
B. Two step growth curve
C. Horizontal growth curve
D. None of the above

12. Which system below is concerned chiefly with phagocytes and antibody formations?

A. Muscular system
B. Nervous system
C. Reticulo-endothelial system
D. Reticular activating system

13. All of the following statements concerning herpes simplex type 1 are true except:

A. Many children have a symptomatic primary infections
B. May be diagnosed by a Tzanck smear for rapid identification when skin lesions are involved
C. May involve a primary infection (e.g gingivo-stomatitis) or a recurrent infection (e.g. cold cores)
D. Can be treated prophylactically by vaccine

14. Which of the following is a neoplasm derived from all three germ cell layers?

A. Carcinoma
B. Sarcoma
C. Teratoma
D. APU Doma

15. The desired results in all surgical incisions is healing by :

A. Primary intention
B. Secondary intention
C. Tertiary intention
D. None of the above

16. Which cells listed below help to assist other T - cells and B - cells to express their immune function?

A. Cytotoxic (killer) cells
B. Plasma cells
C. T - helper cells
D. T - suppressor cells

17. All of the following are benign neoplasms except:

A. Papilloma
B. Adenoma
C. Sarcoma
D. Lipoma

18. Lactobacillus species are:
A. Gram negative rods that tend to form clusters
B. Gram negative cocci that tend to form clusters
C. Gram positive cocci that tend to form chains
D. Gram positive rods that tend to form chains

19. Which antibiotic listed below would be indicated for a patient requiring the administration of prophylactic antibiotic prior to dental treatment?
A. Tetracycline
B. Lincomycin
C. Amoxicilin
D. Chloramphenicol

20. All of the following are possible causes of tetany except:
A. Hypoparathyroidism
B. Rickets (Vitamin D deficiency)
C. Hypertension
D. Hyperventilation
E. Uremia

21. All of the following statements concerning X-linked agammaglobulinemia / Bruton's agammalobulinemia are true except :
A. It affects only boys
B. Result in decreased numbers or absence of B lymphocytes
C. Result in very low levels of antibodies
D. There is impaired resistance to viral infections
E. There is normal circulating T cells lymphocytes

22. The only *cold sterilizer solution* capable of destroying bacterial spores, viruses and vegetative bacteria is:
A. Quaternary ammonium compounds
B. Chlorhexidine
C. 90% isopropyl alcohol
D. 2% glutaraldehyde

23. All of the following bacteria produce a toxin that can be detected using the ELISA assay except.
A. E. coli
B. Vibrio cholera
C. Bacteroides
D. Staphylococcus aureus

24. Which type of pathogens provide the ultimate test for efficacy of sterilization?
A. Bacteria
B. Spore-forming
C. Virus
D. Fungi

25. All of the following species are found in saliva except
A. Actinomyces
B. Veillonella
C. Streptococcus
D. Staphylococcus

26. Anemia in a newborn can result form
A. Excessive blood loss during delivery
B. Excessive destruction of red blood cells
C. Impaired production of red blood cells
D. All of the above

27. Of the three types thyroiditis listed below, which one is the most common and the most common cause of hypothyroidism?
A. Hashimoto's thyroiditis
B. Sub acute granulomatous thyroiditis
C. Silent lympocyytic thyroiditis
D. All of the above

28. Which of the following is also known as marble bone disease or disease Albers - schonburg disease?
A. Fibrous dysplasia
B. Osteogenesis imperfecta
C. Osteopetrosis
D. Achondroplasia

29. Leukotriene C 4, D 4 and E 4 are collectively known as
A. Histamine
B. Slow reacting substances of anaphylaxis (SRS-A)
C. Heparin
D. Serotonin

30. Which of the following is an acute, self limited disease that occurs 6 - 8 days after the injection of a foreign protein (bovine albumin) and is characterized by fever, arthralgias, vasculitis and an acute glomerulonephritis?
A. Arthus reaction
B. Polyarteritis nodosa
C. Serum sickness
D. Systemic lupus Erythematosus

31. Which type of stock listed below most often associated with severe trauma to the CNS?
A. Hypovolemic shock
B. Cardiogenic shock
C. Septic Shock
D. Neurogenic Shock
E. Anaphylactic Shock

32. Which type of hypersensitive reaction listed below is characterized by a specific cytotropic antibody (IgE) that binds to receptors on basophils and mast cells and reacts with a specific antigen
A. Type I
B. Type II
C. Type III
D. Type IV

33. A nuclear change that involves the condensation and shrinkage of the cell nucleus with chromatin clumping is known as:
A. Pyknosis
B. Karyopyknosis
C. Karyolysis
D. Karyorrhexis

34. Impetigo (pyoderma) is a localized intraepidermal infection of the skin that is caused by
A. Streptococcus mutans and staphylococci epidermis
B. Streptococcus mitis & staphylococcus saprophyticus
C. Streptococcus pyogenes and staphylococcus aureus
D. Streptococcus pneumoniae and staphyloccous aureus

35. Gas gangrene is also called what?

A. Anthrax
B. Diphtheria
C. Myonecrosis
D. Pseudomebranous colitis

36. Which of the following statements is true concerning chronic leukemias?

A. They progress rapidly
B. They have a shorter, more devastating clinical course than the acute leukemias
C. They are characterized by proliferations of lymphoid or hematopoietic cells that are more mature than those of the acute leukemias
D. They constitute 75 % of all leukemias

37. Which group of viruses listed below possesses an RNA genome that does not function as positive or negative sense molecule but acts as a template for the viral DNA?

A. corona viruses
B. Picorna viruses
C. Retro viruses
D. Toga viruses

38. The average age of people who have chronic lymphocytic leukemia (CLL) is

A. 10 years old
B. 25 years old
C. 45 Years old
D. 60 Years Old

39. All of the following diseases are associated with adenoviruses except:

A. Acute respiratory infections
B. Acute contagious conjunctivitis (pink eye)
C. Generalized systemic disease with a maculo-papular rash
D. Pharyngo-conjunctival fever characterized by fever, pharyngitis, and conjunctivitis

40. All of the following are benign tumors of mesenchymal origin except

A. Leomyoma

B. Rhabdomyoma
C. Osteosarcoma
D. Fibroma
E. Chondroma

41. All of the following bacteria may be etiologically related to dental caries except:
A. Streptococcus mutans
B. Actinomyces viscous
C. Acitnobacillus actinomycetamcomitans
D. Streptococcus salivarius
E. Streptococcus sanguis

42. A single - celled parasite that causes amoebiasis in humans is:
A. Giardia lamblia
B. Entamoeba histolytica
C. Trachomonas vaginalis
D. Balantidium coli

43. The large majority (90%) of cancers of the lung are a consequence of:
A. Hereditary factors
B. Alcohol consumption
C. Cigarette smoking
D. Diet

44. Alcohol requires which concentration listed below to kill bacteria, given sufficient time?
A. 10% - 20%
B. 30% - 40%
C. 50% - 60%
D. 70% - 95%

45. Which of these bacteria are the principle bacteria associated with acute necrotizing ulcerative gingivitis / ANUG?
A. Streptoccccus sanguis
B. Prevotella intermedia
C. Spirochetes
D. Actinomyces israeli
E. Porphyromonas gingivalis

46. Mycobacterium cell walls contain a waxy substance composed of:
A. Resin acids
B. Chenic acids
C. Mycolic acids
D. Chenodeoxycholic acids

47. Which of the following are used in protective vaccines because of their antigenicity but have lost their toxicity?
A. Antitoxins
B. Toxoids
C. Mycotoxins
D. Endotoxins

48. All of the following bacteria have been found to be the principal bacteria associated with adult periodontitis except:
A. Porphyromonas gingivalis
B. Prevotella intermedia
C. Capnocytophaga ochraceus
D. Bacteroides forsythus
E. Campylobactor rectus

49. The rabies vaccine and clostridium tetani vaccine result in:
A. Naturally acquired passive immunity
B. Naturally acquired active immunity
C. Artificially acquired active immunity
D. Artificially acquired passive immunity

50. Renin is produced in the:
A. Liver
B. Intestines
C. Kidneys
D. Lungs

51. Pernicious anaemia is a megaloblastic anemia caused by the lack of
A. Vitamin C
B. Vitamin A
C. Vitamin B12
D. Vitamin K

52. All of the following statements concerning Peutz – Jeghers syndrome are true except :

A. It is a hereditary condition in which many small lumps called Juvenile polyps appear in a variety of sites in the GI tract, most commonly in the small intestine, esp in the jejunum
B. It only affect males
C. It is characterized by melanin pigmentation of the oral mucosa especially of the lips and gingiva
D. People with this syndrome are at increased risk for cancer of the pancreas, breast, lung, ovary and uterus.

53. The most common cause of secondary hypertension is

A. Hormonal disorder
B. Kidney disease
C. Drugs
D. Congenital anomalies

54. All of the following cells have the ability to retain a latent capacity for mitotic division except:

A. Bone marrow cells
B. Liver cells
C. Blood cells
D. Neurons in the brain or spiral cord

55. All of the following are clinical features of hyperthyroidism except:

A. Restlessness, irritability and fatigability
B. Heat intolerance (sweating) due to increased SMR
C. Tachycardia (a rapid heart rate)
D. Weight gain
E. Fine hair
F. Diarrhoea
G. Tremor (shakiness)

56. All of the following features are of rheumatoid arthritis except:

A. Serum anti – IgG antibodies ie rhematoid factors
B. Osteophyte formation
C. Subcutaneous rheumatoid nodules
D. Fatigue, malaise, anorexia, weight gain, fever and myalgias.
E. Symmetric polyarthritis

57. Reye's syndrome is a serious and potentially fatal complication that occurs most commonly in children during epidemics of

A. Mumps
B. Measles
C. Influenza – B
D. Common cold

58. All of the following are the motor symptoms / changes in the motor functions in multiple sclerosis condition except:

A. Tremors
B. Weakness, clumsiness
C. Difficulty in walking or maintaining balance
D. Double vision
E. Diarrhoea
F. Stiffness, unsteadiness and unusual tiredness

59. A small foreign molecule that is not immunogenic by itself but can react with specific antibody is called a / an :

A. Epitope
B. Hapten
C. Plasmid
D. Immunogen

60. The biologic consequences of compliment activation include

A. Chemotaxis of phagocytes
B. Immune adherence and opsonization
C. Anaphylatoxin activity
D. Membrane activity
E. All of the above

61. Pyelonephritis most commonly occurs as result of a (an)

A. Oral cavity infection
B. Urinary tract infection
C. Skin infection
D. Pulmonary infection

62. All of the following statements concerning fungal spores are true except:

A. Morphologic characteristics (e.g. the shape, color and arrangement) of conidia are useful and for the identification of fungi.

B. A fungal spore is as resistant to heat as bacterial spores
C. Fungal spores cause allergies in some people
D. A conidium is an asexually formed fungal spore.

63. Which of the following make up the triad of findings found in Sjogren's syndrome?
A. Associated connective tissue disorders e.g. rheumatoid arthritis
B. Xerostomia, dry mouth
C. Diabetes
D. Nephrosclerosis
E. Cirrhosis of the liver
F. Keratoconjunctivitis Sicca ie dry eyes

64. All of the following bacteria are negative, facultatively anaerobic rods except
A. Escherichia
B. Salmonella
C. Streptococcus
D. Proteus

65. Another name for acute glomerulo-nephritis is
A. Rapidly progressive glomerulonephritis
B. Goodpasture's syndrome
C. Post- streptococcal glomerulonephritis
D. Alport's syndrome

66. Which type of Hepatitis is described below?
- The three main modes of transmission are via blood, during sexual intercourse and parentally from mother to newborn
- It has an incubation period averaging 60-90 days
- It can result in a carrier state or chronic liver disease
- It also called Serum Hepatitis

A. Hepatitis A
B. Hepatitis B
C. Hepatitis C
D. Hepatitis D

67. A bacteriophage with the ability to form a stable, non – disruptive relationship within bacterium is called a :
A. Virulent phage
B. Plasmid

C. Temperate phage
D. Phage T4

68. Which virus listed below shows changes in the antigenicity of its hemagglutinin and neuramindase proteins?
A. Mumps virus
B. Measles Virus
C. Influenza Virus
D. Epstein Barr virus

69. All of the following statements concerning basal cell carcinoma are true, except
A. It is by far the most common malignant tumor of the skin
B. It originates in the lowest layer of the epidermis (Basel cell layer)
C. Usually develops on skin surface that are exposed to sunlight
D. Rather than spreading to distant parts of the body, it usually invades and destroys the surrounding tissues.
E. It is rarely cured by surgical resection

70. The infectious viral particle is called a
A. Viroid .
B. Virion
C. Prion
D. Neon

71. Differentiation is a measure of a tumor's resemblance to normal tissue. Anaplasia is
A. A high degree of differentiation
B. A moderate degree of differentiation
C. The absence of differentiation
D. Total differentiation

72. All of the following tissues regenerate except:
A. Bone
B. Intestinal mucosa
C. Liver
D. Striated muscle
E. Cartilage

73. The food and drug administration recommends the use of which antibiotic listed below to be reserved for serious anaerobic infections ?
A. Penicillin V
B. Tetracycline
C. Clindamycin
D. Cephalosporins

74. Most prominent symptoms of a pheochromocytoma is:
A. Diarrhea
B. Internal bleeding
C. High blood pressure
D. Hypoglycemia

75. The primary acidogenic microorganisms in the oral cavity are
A. Spirochetes
B. Streptococcus
C. Fusobacterium
D. Lactobacillus

76. Pseudomembranous colitis is a sign of toxicity for which antibiotic listed below ?
A. Cephalosporins
B. Tetracycline
C. Clindamycin
D. Carbenicillin

77. Which of the following is the proper time and temperature for dry heat sterilization?
A. 3200 F/ 160 C for 2 hours
B. 2500 for 20-30 minutes
C. 4500 F for 5 minutes
D. 890 F for 30 minutes

78. The enterotoxin produced by staphylococcus aureus causes
A. Bacterial dysentery
B. Gas gangrene
C. Food poisoning
D. Scarlet fever

79. The killing or removal of all microorganisms including bacterial spores is called?

A. Disinfection
B. Cleaning
C. Sterilization
D. Wiping

80. During which growth phase of the typical growth curve of a bacterial culture is the cell increasing in mass or cell number?

A. Lag phase
B. Log phase
C. Secondary phase
D. Death phase

81. Osteomyelitis is a bone infection usually caused by:

A. Parasites
B. Viruses
C. Bacteria
D. Fungi

82. All of the following statements concerning erythema multiforme are true except

A. It is a disorder characterized by patches of red raised skin that often look like targets and are usually distributed symmetrically over the body
B. It is usually a reaction to a drug, most often penicillins or infectious agent and is commonly associated with herpes simplex infection
C. It is an uncommon disorder with a peak incidence in the first decade of life
D. It usually heals on its own but Stevens Johnson syndrome (Which is a very severe form) can be fatal

83. Paget's disease of bone / osteitis deformans is characterized by :

A. High serum calcium, low serum phosphate, high serum alkaline phosphatase
B. Normal serum calcium, phosphorous and alkaline phosphatase
C. Normal serum calcium and phosphorus with a markedly increased serum alkaline phosphatase
D. Normal serum phosphorus, low serum calcium, high serum alkaline phosphatase

84. Which blood group listed below has neither antigen A or B?

A. A
B. B
C. O
D. AB

85. Characteristics of systemic lupus erythematosus include all of the following except:

A. "Butterfly rash" on the face
B. Skin rash
C. Sensitivity to light
D. Fluid around the lungs, heart or other organs
E. Blindness
F. Arthritis
G. Kidney, nerve, or brain dysfunction

86. Metabolic acidosis occurs in which stage of shock?

A. Non-progressive (early) stage
B. Progressive stage
C. Irreversible stage
D. May occur in any stage

87. An embolus is usually:

A. Fat
B. Amniotic fluid
C. A blood clot
D. An air bubble

88. Which of the following is the classic lesion of rheumatic fever

A. The Barr body
B. The brush field body
C. The Aschoff body
D. The charcot - Leyden body

89. Anaphylatoxins

A. Produce inflammation
B. Cause enhanced capillary permeability
C. Induce smooth muscle contraction
D. Cause hypertension
E. All of the above

90. An abscess is

A. Tumor composed of granulation tissue

B. An abnormal sac containing air or fluid
C. An accumulation of pus
D. Considered to be pre-malignant

91. Decreased melanin pigmentation is seen in
A. Addison's disease
B. Jaundice
C. Albinism and vitiligo
D. Hemosiderosis

92. Granulomatous inflammation is typical of the tissue response elicited by all of the following except:
A. Fungal infections
B. Tuberculosis
C. Acute meningitis
D. The presence of foreign material e.g. suture or talc
E. Leprosy
F. Sarcoidosis

93. A specific chromosome marker characterizes which type of leukemia listed bellow:
A. Acute lymphocytic leukemia
B. Chronic myelocytic leukemia
C. Acute myeloid leukemia
D. Chronic lymphocytic leukemia

94. All of the following are RNA enveloped viruses except
A. Picorna-viruses
B. Human immunodeficiency virus (HIV)
C. Measles, mumps, rubella and hepatitis - C viruses
D. Respiratory viruses

95. Chronic obstructive pulmonary disease COPD is a group of disorders characterized by airflow obstruction during respiration. Which one those listed below is marked by dyspnea and wheezing expiration caused by episodic narrowing of the airways?
A. Bronchial asthma
B. Chronic bronchitis
C. Emphysema
D. Bronchiectasis

96. Which of the following DNA enveloped viruses are the largest and most complex?
A. Herpes viruses
B. Hepatitis B virus
C. Pox viruses
D. Rabies virus

97. A malignant tumor of skeletal muscle is know as ?
A. A fibroma
B. A rhabdomyosarcoma
C. A rhabdomyoma
D. A leiomyoma

98. The principal oral site for the growth of spirochetes, fusobacteria and other gram negative anaerobes is
A. Saliva
B. Calculus
C. The gingival margin
D. The gingival sulcus

99. Which of the following can cause mutation?
A. Ultraviolet light
B. Chemicals
C. Radiations
D. Viruses
E. All of the above

100. Which antibiotic listed below is considered to be a broad spectrum antibiotics?
A. Ampicillin
B. Penicillin G
C. Cephalosporins
D. Penicillin V

Answer key to microbiology and pathology part II

1	B	2	B	3	C	4	C,D
5	C	6	B	7	C	8	C
9	B	10	D	11	A	12	C
13	D	14	C	15	A	16	C
17	C	18	D	19	C	20	C
21	D	22	D	23	C	24	B
25	D	26	D	27	A	28	C
29	B	30	C	31	D	32	A
33	A	34	C	35	C	36	C
37	C	38	D	39	C	40	C
41	C	42	B	43	C	44	D
45	B, C	46	C	47	B	48	C
49	C	50	C	51	C	52	B
53	B	54	D	55	D	56	B
57	C	58	E	59	B	60	E
61	B	62	B	63	A,B,F	64	C
65	C	66	B	67	C	68	C
69	E	70	B	71	C	72	D
73	C	74	C	75	B	76	C
77	A	78	C	79	C	80	B
81	C	82	C	83	C	84	C
85	E	86	B	87	C	88	C
89	E	90	C	91	C	92	C
93	B	94	A	95	A	96	C
97	B	98	D	99	E	100	C

Part III

1. Which subtypes of non-Hodgkin's lymphoma listed below closely linked to the Epstein Barr virus ?
A. Mycosis fungicides
B. Burkitt's lymphoma
C. None of the above
D. Both of the above

2. Various strains of which species listed below produce the enzyme penicillinase:
A. Streptococcus
B. Pseudomonas
C. Staphylococcus
D. Mycobacterium

3. Which malabsorption syndrome listed below is an inherited disorder in which an allergic intolerance to gluten, a protein, cause changes in the intestine that result in malabsorption
A. Tropical sprue
B. Celiac disease
C. Intestine lymphangiectasia
D. Whipple disease

4. Transcription
A. Is the synthesis of mRNA from RNA by RNA dependent DNA polymerase
B. Is the synthesis of mRNA from DNA by RNA dependent DNA polymerase
C. IS the synthesis of mRNA from DNA by DNA dependent RNA polymerase
D. IS the synthesis of mRNA from RNA by RNA dependent RNA polymerize

5. Mis-sense mutations
A. Stop protein synthesis prematurely
B. Result in the substitution of one amino acid for another
C. Generates a termination codon
D. Almost always destroy protein function

6. Endotoxins are the lipopolysaccharide component of the cell wall of
A. Gram-positive bacteria
B. Gram negative bacteria
C. Mycoplasma
D. Viruses

7. All of the following statements concerning serotonin are true except
A. It is widely considered to be a neurotransmitter
B. It is present in the brain
C. It is believed to play a role in temperature regulation sensory perception and in the onset of sleep
D. It is synthesized from the amino acid argenine

8. All of the following concerning sickle cell anemia are true except:
A. It is an inherited condition characterized by sickle shaped red blood cells and chronic hemolytic anemia
B. The red blood cells contain an abnormal form of hemoglobin that reduces the amount of oxygen in the cells causing them to become crescent or sickle shaped
C. It affects whites almost exclusively
D. The sickle shaped cells block and damage the capillaries in the spleen, kidneys, brain, bones and other organs reducing their oxygen supply

9. Osteomalacia is caused by a :
A. Vitamin B deficiency in adults
B. Vitamin C deficiency in children
C. Vitamin D deficiency in adults
D. Vitamin A deficiency in children

10. All of the following are characteristics of gout except
A. Most often affects the joint at the base of the big toe, condition called podagra
B. Higher incidence in women
C. Hard lumps of urate crystals (tophi) are deposited under the skin around joints
D. An abnormally high uric acid level in the blood (hyperuricemia)

11. Hay fever and allergies to certain foods are examples of :

A. Antibody dependent cytotoxic hypersensitivity reactions
B. Immune complex mediated hypersensitivity reactions
C. Atopic allergies
D. Cell mediated or delayed hypersensitivity reactions

12. All of the following statements concerning infectious mononucleosis are true except:

A. It is caused by the Epstein bar versus (EBV)
B. It is a disease of old age
C. It is sometime called kissing disease
D. It is associated with the production of typical lymphocytes and IgM heterophile antibodies identified by the heterophile test

13. Which of the following is the most common cause of death in the early hours following the onset of a myocardial infarction/ heart attack ?

A. Cardiogenic shock
B. Arrhythmias
C. Ventricular rupture
D. Mural thrombosis

14. The most serious complication of pericarditis is

A. Infection
B. Fever
C. Cardiac tamponade
D. Leukocytosis

15. Which of the following is the most common joint disorder?

A. Rheumatoid arthritis
B. Psoriatic arthritis
C. Osteoarthritis
D. Systemic lupus erythematosus
E. Discoid lupus erythematosus

16. An infection is epidemic if:

A. It has a worldwide distribution
B. It is constantly present at a low level in a specific population
C. It occurs much more frequently than usual
D. It is highly communicable

17. The characteristic cell components of chronic inflammation include all of the following except:
A. Lymphocytes
B. Plasma cells
C. Polymorphonuclear leukocytes
D. Macrophages

18. Which of the following may cause blood in the urine / hematuria?
A. Bladder or kidney disease
B. Glomerulonephritis
C. Kidney stones
D. Kidney cysts
E. Sickle cell anemia
F. Hydronephrosis
G. All of the above

19. Which cystic disease of the kidney listed below is the most common inherited disorder of the kidney?
A. Adult polycystic kidney disease
B. Infantile pilocystic kidney disease
C. Medullary cystic disease
D. Medullary sponge kidney

20. Which of the following is most commonly caused by left ventricular failure (congestive heart failure)?
A. Bronchiectasis
B. Chronic bronchitis
C. Ateclectasis
D. Pulmonary edema

21. Which of the following predispose people to pneumonia?
A. Alcoholism
B. Cigarette smoking
C. Diabetes
D. Heart failure
E. Chronic objectives pulmonary disease (COPD)
F. All of the above

22. Usually the main symptoms of lung cancers
A. A persistent cough
B. Diarrhea

C. A low grade fever
D. A skin rash

23. Lymphomas principally involve which of the following
A. Lymph nodes
B. Spleen
C. Liver
D. Bone narrow
E. All of the above

24. Which type of cancer listed below is the second most common cause of cancer death?
A. Liver cancer
B. Bone cancer
C. Prostate cancer
D. Testicular cancer

25. Which two antibiotics listed below are usually prescribed in the treatment of Rickettsial disease?
A. Tetracycline
B. Polymixin B
C. Erythromycin
D. Chloramphenicol

26. Which term listed below is an interactive associations between two populations of different species living together, in which one population benefits from the association while the other is not affected—
A. Latency
B. Mutualism
C. Symbiosis
D. Commensalisms

27. Which toxin or enzyme listed below produced by Group A Streptococcus (S pyogenes) activates plasminogen to form plasmin which dissolves fibrin in clots, thrombi and emboli?
A. Streptokinase
B. Streptodornase
C. Hyaluronidase
D. Erythrogenic toxin
E. Streptolysin O

28. Freund's adjuvant is a mixture composed of
A. Mineral oil
B. Lanolin
C. Killed mycobacteria
D. All of the above

29. All of the following are formed via the cyclo-oxygenase pathway except
A. Prostaglandins
B. Prostacyclin
C. Leukotrienes
D. Thromboxanes

30. All of the following are considered to be the risk factors for developing atherosclerosis except
A. Increased age
B. High blood cholesterol levels
C. Diabetes
D. Smoking
E. Drug use

31. Lysozyme degrades
A. Peptidoglycans
B. RNA – polymerase
C. Lipopolysaccharide
D. Chitin

32. Very severe hypothyroidism in adults is called?
A. Cretinism
B. Plummer's Syndrome
C. Myxoedema
D. Graves disease

33. Which cellular organelle listed below contains digestive enzymes?
A. Ribosome
B. Inclusions
C. Lysosome
D. Mitochondria

34. All of the following statements concerning Ludwig's angina are true, except:
A. Most cases appear to be a mixed infection

B. It is often caused by normal oral flora gaining access through an infected tooth
C. It can cause severe swelling in the floor of the mouth, even forcing the tongue upward blocking the airway
D. Fever and malaise are usually not present

35. The classic symptom of coronary artery disease is:
A. Coughing
B. Venous congestion
C. Angina pectoris
D. Dizziness

36. Rheumatic fever is:
A. Inflammation of joints (arthritis) and the spleen (splenomegaly) resulting from a staphylococcal infection, usually of the throat
B. Inflammation of joints (arthritis) and the parotid glands (parotitis) resulting from a streptococcal infection, usually of the middle ear
C. Inflammation of the joints (arthritis) and the heart (carditis) resulting from a streptococcal infection, usually of the throat
D. Inflammation of the joints (arthritis) and the thyroid gland (goiter) resulting from a staphylococcal infection, usually of the blood

37. Which type of infection listed below often causes leukocytosis?
A. Parasitic
B. Viral
C. Bacterial
D. Fungal

38. The vascular phase of the acute inflammation involves all of the following cells except:
A. Platelets
B. Tissue mast cells
C. Eosinophils
D. Basophils

39. The increased excretion of calcium in the kidneys results in:
A. Jaundice
B. Nephrolithiasis

C. Polycystic kidney disease
D. Diabetes

40. Who would be at risk for black lung disease?
A. Aerospace workers
B. Farmers
C. Coal workers
D. Sandstone or granite cutters

41. Infection with the Epstein-Barr virus can cause infectious mononucleosis, which may be characterized by the appearance of :
A. Koplik's spots
B. Owl's eye inclusions
C. Heterophile antibodies
D. Cowdry type A inclusions

42. Almost all patients with a lung abscess present with
A. Diarrhea
B. Malaise
C. Cough and fever
D. Weight loss

43. Which of the following statements describes the herpes viruses?
A. Large-sized enveloped viruses with an icosahedral nucleocapsid containing circular, single-stranded DNA.
B. Medium sized enveloped viruses with an icosahedral nucleocapsid containing linear double-stranded RNA.
C. Small-sized enveloped viruses with an icosahedral nucleocapsid containing circular, double stranded DNA.
D. Medium-sized enveloped viruses with an icosahedral nucleocapsid containing linear double-stranded DNA.

44. Which herpes simplex virus listed below causes acute herpetic gingivostomatitis, recurrent herpes labialis, cancre sores, keratoconjunctivitis and encephalitis?
A. Herpes simplex virus type 1 (HSV – 1)
B. Herpes simplex virus type 2 (HSV – 2)
C. Epstein Barr virus
D. None of the above

45. Which of the following is a constituent of gram-negative microorganisms and has been suggested as an important agent in the pathogenesis of inflammatory periodontal disease?

A. Carbohydrates
B. Lipids
C. Exotoxin
D. Endotoxin

46. All of the following statements concerning Respiratory Synctial Virus (RSV) are true, except:

A. It belongs to the orthomyxovirus family
B. Its surface spikes are fusion proteins, not hemagglutinins or neuraminidases.
C. It is the most important cause of severe pneumonia and bronchiolitis in infants.
D. Transmission occurs via respiratory droplets and by direct contact of contaminated hands with the nose or mouth

47. Reoviruses:

A. Have a unique single-shelled capsid that contains a non-segmented double stranded DNA genome.
B. Have a unique double-shelled capsid that contains a segmented single stranded RNA genome
C. Have a unique double-shelled capsid that contains a segmented double stranded RNA genome.
D. Have a unique single-shelled capsid that contains a segmented Single stranded DNA genome.

48. Which bacteria listed below has a THICK murein layer that makes up the cell wall?

A. Gram-positive bacteria
B. Gram-negative bacteria
C. Both of the above
D. None of the above

49. Esophageal varices are the result of which of the following?

A. Kidney stones
B. Portal hypertension
C. Ulcers
D. Diverticulosis

50. Which of the following organs undergoes regeneration?
A. Heart
B. Brain
C. Kidney
D. Liver

51. Which of the following describes the lytic reproduction cycle that releases a large number of phage simultaneously?
A. Two-step growth curve
B. One-step growth curve
C. Horizontal growth curve
D. None of the above

52. Which of the following is the term used to describe the synthesis of mRNA, rRNA, and tRNA from a DNA template?
A. Translation
B. Transcription
C. Transduction
D. Transversion

53. All of the following are benign neoplasms except?
A. Adenoma
B. Fibroma
C. Fibrocarcinoma
D. Hemangioma
E. Lipoma

54. A tumor of striated muscle that may occur in the uterus, vagina, pharynx, and tongue is called what?
A. Fibroma
B. Leiomyoma
C. Rhabdomyoma
D. Lipoma

55. Which of the following types of skin cancer is the most common?
A. Squamous cell carcinoma
B. Basal cell carcinoma
C. Malignant melanoma
D. Oat cell carcinoma

56. Endotoxins are the lipopolysaccharide of the cell wall of which bacteria?
A. Gram-positive bacteria
B. Gram-negative bacteria
C. Fungi
D. Viruses

57. Which of the following induces or forms toxic free—radicals, which cause chemical reactions disruptive to the biochemical organization of microorganisms?
A. Ultraviolet light
B. Ionizing radiation
C. Disinfectants
D. Autoclaving

58. Which of the following bacteria are gram-negative, facultatively anaerobic-rods, motile by means of peritrichous or polar flagella, and divided into five tribes?
A. Enterobacteria
B. Mycobacterium
C. Neisseria
D. Bacteroides

59. Which of the following bacteria form unusual acids, called mycolic acids, that are associated with their cell walls?
A. Escherichia coli
B. Lactobacillus casei
C. Mycobacterium tuberculosis
D. Streptococci

60. Which of the following viruses have spikes that are involved in the absorption of the virus to the host cell?
A. Papovaviruses
B. Adenoviruses
C. Iridoviruses
D. Poxvirus

61. The coxsackie virus is classified under which family name?
A. Togaviridae
B. Orthomyxoviridae
C. Picornaviridae
D. Retroviridae

62. Which virus below is known for its antigenic shift?
A. Rubeola
B. Rubella
C. Influenza
D. Mumps

63. Which of the following is a highly contagious infection of the respiratory tract caused by a myxovirus and transmitted by airborne droplet infection?
A. Anthrax
B. Influenza
C. Gas gangrene
D. Hepatitis B

64. A fetus with the following triad of complications i.e. Cataracts, Cardiac malformations, Deafness probably was infected with what virus?
A. Rubella
B. Herpes simplex
C. Herpes zoster
D. EB virus

65. Which form of hepatitis is characterized by rapid onset of acute signs and symptoms?
A. Hepatitis B
B. Hepatitis A
C. Non A non B
D. Hepatitis D

66. Which group of viruses listed below is frequently found as the causative agent of gastroenteritis?
A. Coxsackie virus
B. Epstein-Barr virus
C. ECHO virus
D. Herpes simplex

67. Which of the following disorders displays the characteristic "Butterfly" rash?
A. Rheumatoid arthritis
B. Systemic lupus erythematosus
C. Myasthenia gravis
D. None of the above

68. Which syndrome below is characterized by multiple intestinal polyps and abnormal mucocutaneous pigmentation, usually over the lips and buccal mucosa?

A. Sjogren's syndrome
B. Peutz-Jeghers syndrome
C. Stevens-Johnson syndrome
D. All of the above

69. Which drug listed below is the drug of choice for treatment of trichomoniasis?

A. Penicillin
B. Metronidazole
C. Nystatin
D. Amphotericin B

70. The drug of choice in treating Candidiasis is which of the following?

A. Penicillin
B, Erythromycin
C. Nystatin
D. Chloramphenicol

71. A group of diverse, widespread unicellular and multicellular eukaryotic organisms, lacking chlorophyll and usually bearing spores and often filaments are what?

A. Bacteria
B. Viruses
C. Fungi
D. All of the above

72. Which genus of fungi listed below infects skin, hair, and nails?

A. Blastomyces
B. Trichophyton
C. Histoplasma
D. Coccidioides

73. Which two protozoans listed below are found in the oral cavity?

A. Giardia
B. Entamoeba
C. Plasmodium
D. Trichomonas

74. Which of the following fungal diseases is seen primarily in patients with chronic debilitating, especially uncontrolled diabetes mellitus?

A. Actinomycosis
B. Histoplasmosis
C. Zygomycosis / mucormycosis
D. Coccidioidomycosis

75. Which of the following is a genus of fungi that is a common contaminant in the laboratory and a cause of nosocomial infections?

A. Blastomyces
B. Coccidiodies
C. Aspergillus
D. None of the above

76. Which of the following is an infectious disease caused by a yeast-like fungus that usually affects only the skin but may invade the lungs, kidneys, central nervous system, and bones?

A. Histoplasmosis
B. Blastomycosis
C. Candidiasis
D. None of the above

77. Which of the following is referred to as valley fever or San Joaquin fever?

A. Coccidioidomycosis
B. Actinomycosis
C. Blastomycosis
D. Mucormycosis

78. All of the following antibiotics are classified as cell-wall inhibitors except?

A. Penicillins
B. Tetracylines
C. Cephalosporins
D. Vancomycin
E. Bacitracin
F. Chloramphenicol
G. Cycloserine

79. Which of the following antibiotics is considered a broad-spectrum antibiotic?
A. Penicillin
B. Cephalosporins
C. Ampicillin
D. Amoxicillin

80. The antibiotic of choice for prophylactic therapy covering dental procedures in a patient with a heart valve abnormality is which of the following?
A. Tetracycline
B. Amoxicillin
C. Erythromycin
D. Lincomycin

81. Aplastic anemia is a sign of toxicity for which antibiotic listed below
A. Pencillin
B. Clindamycin
C. Chloramphenicol
D. Carbencillin

82. Which antibiotic listed below is most efficient in treating infection due to Bacteroides and fusobacterium species?
A. Penicillin
B. Erythromycin
C. Clindamycin
D. Tetracycline

83. The use of vaccines for preventing clinical symptoms after introduction of the virus is most likely to be effective against which two viruses listed below?
A. Influenza
B. Herpes Zoster
C. Rabies
D. Clostridium tetani
E. Rhinoviruses

84. Which class of anti bodies provides the defense against environmental antigens?
A. IgA
B. IgD

C. IgE
D. IgG
E. IgM

85. An injection of a drug into a patient who is allergic to this drug may lead to death due to which of the following
A. Low levels of histamines
B. Anaphylactic shock
C. Hyperglobulinemia
D. Cardiogenic shock

86. Which two antibiotics are usually prescribed in the treatment of rickettsial diseases?
A. Lincomycin
B. Polymyxin B
C. Tetracycline
D. Chloramphenicol

87. An increase in the size of a cell or a group of cells is called what
A. Atrophy
B. Hypertrophy
C. Hyperplasia
D. Dysplasia

88. Cells of which of the following do not have the ability to retain a latent capacity for mitotic division
A. Blood
B. Bone marrow
C. Liver
D. Neurons in the brain

89. A person with the following clinical signs is probably in what physiological state?
A. Reduced cardiac output
B. Circulatory insufficiency
C. Tachycardia
D. Hypotension
E. Pallor and restlessness
F. Diminished urinary output

90. Which type of chronic inflammation is highly cellular and destructive?
A. Granulomatous
B. Banal
C. Agranulomatous
D. All of the above

91. A slowly developing localized thickening of the outer layers of the skin as a result of chronic excessive exposure to the sun is called what?
A. Actinic keratosis
B. Verruca vulgaris
C. Seborrheic keratosis
D. Squamous cell carcinoma
E. None of the above

92. Which of the following is most commonly found in the ovaries or testes
A. An adenoma
B. A teratoma
C. A sarcoma
D. A lipoma

93. Which of the following types of skin cancer most often arises from keratinocytes in the epidermis of elderly individuals who have been excessively exposed to the sun?
A. Malignant melanoma
B. Squamous cell carcinoma
C. Basal cell carcinoma
D. Ameloblastoma

94. The most common place for malignancy of the GI tract to occur is where
A. Stomach
B. Colon
C. Esophagus
D. Anus

95. Neolithic cells characteristically resemble prickle cells and form keratin pearls on the surface of lesions in which of the following
A. Adenocarcinoma

B. Squamous cell carcinoma
C. Basal cell carcinoma
D. Malignant melanoma

96. Which of the following types of skin cancer is considered to be the most severe?
A. Basal cell carcinoma
B. Squamous cell carcinoma
C. Malignant melanoma
D. All of the above

97. Which of the following is the most common malignancy in women?
A. Breast cancer
B. Lung cancer
C. Brain cancer
D. Colon cancer

98. A patient with a painless enlarged lymph node or nodes in the neck who complains of weakness, fever and weight loss is probably suffering from what?
A. Legionnaire's Disease
B. Tay Sach Disease
C. Malignant Lymphoma
D. Leukoplakia

99. Any of several bleeding disorders characterized by hemorrhage into the tissues particularly beneath the skin or mucous membrane, which then produces ecchymoses or petechiae is called what?
A. Purpura
B. Hemophilia
C. Aplastic anemia
D. Agranulocytosis

100. Productive cough, often with wheezing, is universal factor of which disease?
A. Emphysema
B. Lung cancer
C. Chronic bronchitis
D. Asthma

Answer key to microbiology and pathology part III

1	B	2	C	3	B	4	C
5	B	6	B	7	D	8	C
9	C	10	B	11	C	12	B
13	B	14	C	15	C	16	C
17	C	18	G	19	A	20	D
21	F	22	A	23	E	24	C
25	A, D	26	D	27	A	28	D
29	C	30	E	31	A	32	C
33	C	34	D	35	C	36	C
37	C	38	C	39	B	40	C
41	C	42	C	43	D	44	A
45	D	46	A	47	C	48	A
49	B	50	D	51	B	52	B
53	C	54	C	55	B	56	B
57	B	58	A	59	C	60	B
61	C	62	C	63	B	64	A
65	B	66	C	67	B	68	B
69	B	70	C	71	C	72	B
73	B, D	74	C	75	C	76	B
77	A	78	B, F	79	B	80	B
81	C	82	C	83	C, D	84	C
85	B	86	C, D	87	B	88	D
89	Shock	90	A	91	A	92	B
93	B	94	B	95	B	96	C
97	A	98	C	99	A	100	C

Part IV

1. **Which of the following is defined as the accumulation of extravascular fluid in lung tissues and alveoli caused most commonly by congestive heart failure**
   A. Bronchiectasis
   B. Pulmonary emboli
   C. Pulmonary edema
   D. Atelectasis
2. **Which of the following is a closed sac in or under the skin lined with epithelium and containing fluid semisolid material?**
   A. A granuloma
   B. A cyst
   C. An abscess
   D. All of the above
3. **Which of the following bacteria are often responsible for lung abscess?**
   A. Clostridium
   B. Staphylococcus
   C. Bacillus .
   D. Streptococcus
4. **Which bacteria listed below produces the enzyme collagenase?**
   A. Streptococcus pyogenes
   B. Clostridium perfringens
   C. Staphylococcus aureus
   D. Streptococcal sanguis
5. **Which bacteria listed below has been found predominately in cases of advanced periodontitis?**
   A. Bacillus anthracis
   B. Bacteroids melaninogenicus
   C. Streptococcus
   D. Veillonella alcalescens
6. **Which of the following bacteria are notable for their fluorescent pigments and their resistance to disinfectants and antibiotics**
   A. Bacteroides

B. Pseudomonas
C. Staphylococci
D. Treponema

7. Which of the following bacteria produces a toxin that can be detected using the ELISA assays?
A. Bacteroides
B. E. coli
C. Neisseria
D. Eikenella

8. Which of the following bacteria is the most common cause of urinary tract infection?
A. Staphylococcus
B. Bacteroides
C. Escherichia
D. Streptococcus

9. Organisms belonging to which of the following genera can tolerate the lowest pH?
A. Proteus
B. Clostridium
C. Lactobacillus
D. Pseudomonas

10. Which of the following is a group of gram-positive, asporogenic, regularly shaped rods that produce lactic acid as a major fermentation product?
A. Bacteroides
B. Neisseria
C. Lactobacillus
D. Salmonella

11. Which of the following is a genus of nonmotile, spherical, gram-positive bacteria which may cause severe, purulent infections or produce an enterotoxin, which may cause nausea, vomiting and diarrhea?
A. Streptococcus
B. Staphylococcus
C. Neisseria
D. Salmonella

12. Which virus listed below can cause herpes zoster lesions along sensory nerve roots in later life?
A. Poxvirus
B. Epstein-Barr virus
C. Varicella virus
D. HSV I virus

13. An infection or inflammation of the membranes covering the brain and spinal cord is called what?
A. Meningitis
B. Encephalitis
C. Meningism
D. None of the above

14. Cytopathic effects (CPE) are due to infection by which of the following?
A. Fungi
B. Viruses
C. Spirochetes
D. All of the above

15. Which of the following species is known to produce the enzyme penicillinase?
A. Streptococcus
B. Bacillus
C. Neisseria
D. Staphylococcus

16. The erythrogenic toxin produced by streptococcus pyogenes causes which disease?
A. Gas gangrene
B. Bacterial dysentery
C. Scarlet fever
D. Tetanus

17. Dental caries is initiated at the tooth surface as a result of the growth of which species listed below?
A. Staphylococcus
B. Pseudomonas
C. Streptococcus
D. Bacteroides

18. Which two bacteria listed below are referred to as lactic acid bacteria?
A. Streptococcus
B. Lactobacillus
C. Staphylococcus
D. Bacteroids

19. What two bacteria listed below cause impetigo?
A. Streptococcus
B. Neisseria
C. Staphylococcus
D. Bacteroides

20. Which bacteria listed below is penicillin-resistant?
A. Streptococcus pyogenes
B. Streptococcus fecalis
C. Streptococcus pneumoniae
D. None of the above

21. The majority of bacterial pneumonias are caused by which etiologic agent listed below?
A. Streptococcus
B. Klebsiella
C. Haemophilus influenza
D. Clostridium

22. Chemical agents that kill microorganisms are called what?
A. Germicides
B. Microbiostatic agents
C. Disinfectants
D. Antiseptics

23. IgE is involved in which of the four types of hypersensitivity reactions?
A. Type 1
B. Type 2
C. Type 3
D. Type 4

24. All of the following diseases are classified as what?
A. Serum sickness
B. Systemic lupus-erythematosus
C. Glomerulonephritis

D. Autoimmune hemolysis
E. Rheumatoid arthritis
Answer = immune complex diseases

25. Which of the following is a mixture of leukotrienes that acts as a potent bronchial constrictor?
A. Heparin
B. Histamine
C. Slow-reacting substance of anaphylaxis
D. Dopamine

26. Which of the following cell types is found in great abundance at the inflamed site?
A. Macrophages
B. Basophils
C. Eosinophils
D. Neutrophils

27. Which of the following is the principal chemical mediator located in the granules of mast cells and basophils?
A. Bradykinin
B. Plasmin
C. Histamine
D. Complement

28. Which of the following refers to a disease or microorganism that is indigenous to a geographic area or population?
A. Endemic
B. Pandemic
C. Epidemic
D. Epizootic

29. Which of the following is defined as a modified protein exotoxin that has lost its toxicity but has retained its specific antigenicity?
A. Antitoxin
B. Toxoid
C. Hapten
D. None

30. The enzyme catalase is contained in which organelle within a cell?
A. Nucleus

B. Microbodies
C. Golgi apparatus
D. Lysosomes

31. Which of the following is a nonproteinaceous substance that acts as antigen by combining with particular bonding sites on an antibody?
A. Lipids
B. Plasmids
C. Haptens
D. Flagella

32. Which of the following is an interactive association between two populations of different species living together in which one population benefits from the association, while the other is not affected?
A. Symbiosis
B. Mutualism
C. Commensalisms
D. Latency

33. A chronic infectious disease of the eye characterized by inflammation, pain, photophobia, and lacrimation is called what?
A. Pink eye
B. Trachoma
C. Inclusion conjunctivitis

34. Urethritis, dysuria, purulent, greenish-yellow urethral or vaginal discharge, red or oedematous meatus, and itching, burning, or pain around the vagina or urethral orifice are characteristic of which disease?
A. Syphilis
B. Gonorrhea
C. Herpes
D. HIV

35. Primary syphilis produces which of the following on the genitalia?
A. Rash
B. Chancre
C. Bruise
D. Gummas

36. Anthrax, botulism, gas gangrene, and tetanus are caused by which type of bacteria?

A. Spore-forming
B. Nonspore-forming
C. Fungi
D. Viruses

37. Which of the following statements describes the herpes viruses?

A. Large-sized viruses containing circular, single-stranded DNA
B. Medium-sized viruses containing linear, double-stranded DNA
C. Small-sized viruses containing circular, double-stranded DNA
D. Small-sized viruses containing circular, single-stranded RNA

38. The common cold, influenza, measles, mumps, chicken pox and infections mononucleosis are all caused by which type of pathogen ?

A. Viral
B. Bacteria
C. Fungal
D. Rickettsial

39. Short term immunity brought about by the transfer of preformed antibody from an immune subject to a non - immune subject is called what

A. Autoimmunity
B. Passive immunity
C. Hypersensitivity
D. Natural Immunity

40. Leukocytes often accompany which type of infection?

A. Viral
B. Bacterial
C. Fungal
D. Parasitic

41. The following biochemical mediators are called what?

A. Macrophage chemotactic factor
B. Migration inhibitory factor
C. Interlukin-1
D. Interlacing - 2

E. Platelet activating factor
Answer = lymphokines

42. The following elements make up what system?
A. Macrophages
B. Kupffer cells of the liver
C. Reticulum cells of lungs
D. Bone marrow
E. Lymph nodes and spleen
Answer = reticuloendothelial system

43. Which of the following is an abnormal condition in which the kidneys are enlarged and contain many sacs
A. Glomerulonephritis
B. Polycystic kidney
C. Secondary amyloidosis
D. All of the above

44. Which of the following is a progressive megaloblastic, macrocytic anemia affecting mainly older people ?
A. Thalassemia major
B. Thalassemia minor
C. Pernicious anemia
D. Aplastic anemia

45. Which of the following types of hemophilia is also called the Christmas diseases?
A. Hemophilia - A
B. Hemophilia B
C. Hemophilia C
D. None of the above

46. A patient taking dicumarol can be expected to have which of the following ?
A. Normal blood clotting
B. Delayed blood clotting
C. Enhanced blood clotting

47. Which of the following is an aggregation of blood platelets, fibrin, clotting factor and cellular elements that forms in the heart in the process of dying?
A. Mural thrombus
B. Agonal thrombus

C. White thrombus
D. Red thrombus

48. Which of the following is a naturally occurring derivative of tryptophan found in platelets and in cells of the brain and the intestine
A. Histamine
B. Bradykinin
C. Serotonin
D. Plasma

49. Which blood group listed below has agglutinins neither A or B?
A. A
B. B
C. O
D. AB

50. Which 2 enzymes of the following are elevated in a patient suffering from acute pancreatitis?
A. Alkaline phosphatase
B. Acid phosphatase
C. Lipase
D. Amylase

51. Which of the following complications of peptic ulcers is the most infrequent and accounts for nearly two thirds of all deaths in peptic ulcer patients?
A. Hemorrhage
B. Obstruction of the GI tract from edema scars
C. Perforation
D. Atresia

52. Vomiting of bright red blood indicating rapid upper gastrointestinal bleeding is called what ?
A. Hematomyelia
B. Hematuria
C. Hematemesis
D. Hemosiderosis

53. The most likely diagnosis for a patient with hemoptyses, pain in the chest, weight loss, anorexia, nausea, vomiting and a history of heavy smoking is what ?
A. Carcinoma of the larynx

B. Laryngeal polyps
C. Carcinoma of the lungs
D. Basal cell carcinoma

54. Which of the following is the fragmentation of chromatin filaments and distribution of it through the cytoplasm as result of nuclear disintegration?
A. Karyopyknosis
B. Pyknosis
C. Karyolysis
D. Karyorrhexis

55. A patient with the following symptom is probably suffering from what disorder?
A. Polyuria
B. Polydipsia
C. Hyperglycemia
D. Glycosuria
E. Weight loss
F. Polyphagia
Answer = diabetes mellitus

56. Which of the following is described as the deposition of calcium salt in previously undamaged tissues?
A. Dystrophic calcification
B. Metastatic calcification
C. Calcinosis
D. Tophi

57. Which of the following is the most common form of cancer in men over the age of 50 aside from skin cancer ?
A. Lung
B. Prostate
C. Liver
D. Bone

58. Which of the following is a severe infection of one or more of the five major lobes of the lungs which if untreated eventually result in consolidation of lung tissue?
A. Bronchopneumonia
B. Emphysema

C. Lobar Pneumonia
D. Asthma

59. A chronic lung disease that results in the development of alveolar, interstitial and pleural fibrosis is called as:
A. Anthracosis
B. Asbestosis
C. Berylliosis
D. Silicosis

60. Burton's congenital agammaglobulinemia results in the failure of which cell to differentiate and produce antibodies?
A. T - cells
B. Macrophage
C. Monocytes
D. B - Cells

61. A sex linked inherited condition characterized by the absence of gamma globulin in the blood is called as?
A. Hodgkin's disease
B. Bruton's agammaglobulinemia
C. Thalassemia major
D. None of the above

62. Which of the following is a rare & severe illness of unknown cause mostly affecting young males and characterized by severe uveitis and retinal vasculitis?
A. Multiple myeloma
B. Bahcet's disease
C. Rubeola
D. Pernicious anemia

63. Reversible oxidation - reduction carriers in respiration are called as?
A. Pyramidine nucleotides
B. Cytochromes
C. Reductant
D. Surfactants

64. When nitrate or sulfate serves as the terminal electron acceptor, the metabolic pathway is called what
A. Aerobic respiration
B. Anaerobic respiration

C. Fermentation
D. None of the above

65. An increased serum alkaline phosphatase level is clinically significant and aids in the diagnosis of which of the following condition
A. Hyperparathyroidism
B. Paget's disease of bone
C. Prostate carcinoma
D. Hepatitis B

66. Haberden's nodes are diagnostic of which type of arthritis ?
A. Rheumatoid arthritis
B. Osteoarthritis
C. Hyperuricemia
D. None of the above

67. Anemia, hemorrhage, splenomegaly, lymphadenopathy, and localized tumefactions over bones are usually present in which disease
A. Multiple myeloma
B. Lettere Siwe disease
C. Hand Schuller Christian disease
D. Osteoradionecrosis

68. A patient with increased bone density / marble bone, hydrocephalus, blindness, deafness, dental caries and facial palsies is most likely suffering from what
A. Osteopetrosis
B. Osteogenesis imperfecta
C. Achondroplasia
D. Fibrous dysplasia

69. A malignant tumor developing from bone marrow, usually in long bones or the pelvis of adolescent boys is called what?
A. Myeloma
B. Ewing's sarcoma
C. Osteogenic sarcoma
D. Squamous cell carcinoma

70. Which of the following is the physiological function of Vitamin A?
A. Hemopoiesis

B. Collagen formation
C. Production of rhodopsin
D. Absorption of calcium

71. Which of the following vitamins functions in collagen formation?
A. B
B. C
C. D
D. A

72. The Philadelphia chromosome is present in myeloblasts in most patients with which disease listed below?
A. Multiple myeloma
B. Chronic myelocytic leukemia
C. Aplastic anemia
D. Gaucher's disease

73. There is no conclusive evidence of a causative infectious agent to which disease listed below?
A. Herpes
B. Infectious Mononucleosis
C. Hodgkin's disease
D. Mumps

74. Which of the following is a characteristic of malignancy?
A. Dysplasia
B. Anaplasia
C. Metaplasia
D. Aplasia

75. Which of the following is a malignant, usually bronchogenic epithelial neoplasm consisting of small, tightly packed, round, oval, or spindle-shaped epithelial cells that stain darkly & contain neurosecretory granules and little or no cytoplasm?
A. Adenocarcinoma
B. Squamous cell carcinoma
C. Oat cell carcinoma
D. Basal cell carcinoma

76. Which syndrome listed below is a condition found in males with one or more extra X chromosomes?
A. Klinefelter's syndrome
B. Turner 's syndrome

C. Down's syndrome
D. None of the above

77. Secondary hyperparathyroidism results from which of the following?
A. Adenoma
B. Hypertension
C. Chronic renal disease
D. Diabetes

78. Name the condition that is associated with hypertension in which there is necrosis of the renal arterioles.
A. Acute nephritis
B. Nephrosclerosis
C. Chronic pyelonephritis
D. Nephrosis

79. Which of the following lesions is most common in the adrenal medulla of young children?
A. Malignant melanoma
B. Basal cell carcinoma
C. Neuroblastoma
D. Squamous cell carcinoma

80. Renal calculi occur in approximately 75 percent of all patients with which disorder?
A. Polycystic kidney
B. Glomerulonephritis
C. Hyperparathyroidism
D. Hypoparathyroidism

81. Which two glands listed below fail to develop in children with the DiGeorge syndrome?
A. Thyroid
B. Adrenal
C. Thymus
D. Pituitary
E. Parathyroid

82. Compression of the heart produced by the accumulation in the pericardial sac of fluid or of blood resulting from the rupture of a blood vessel of the myocardium is called what?
A. Constrictive pericarditis

B. Mitral stenosis
C. Cardiac tamponade
D. Hypertension

83. Which three organs below get damaged by prolonged hypertension?
A. Heart
B. Intestine
C. Brain
D. Stomach
E. Kidneys

84. Tissue from another species used as a temporary graft in certain cases, as in treating a severely burned patient, is called what?
A. Xenograft
B. Autograft
C. Allograft
D. Isograft

85. Which healing process of a wound listed below would contain granulation tissue?
A. First intention
B. Second intention

86. A chronic metabolic condition characterized by a gradual, marked enlargement and elongation of the bones of the face, jaw, and extremities afflicting middle-aged adults is called what?
A. Acromegaly
B. Gigantism
C. Cretinism
D. None of the above

87. Which of the following is a proteolytic enzyme, produced by & stored in the juxtaglomerular apparatus that surrounds each arteriole as it enters a glomerulus?
A. Plasmin
B. Lysozyme
C. Renin
D. Pepsin

88. The acid fast stain may be performed on many clinical specimens but is most commonly used in examining sputum for which bacteria listed below

A. Escherichia coli
B. Streptococcus pneumonia
C. Clostridium botulinum
D. Mycobacterium tuberculosis

Answer key to microbiology and pathology part IV

1	C	2	B	3	B	4	B
5	B	6	B	7	B	8	C
9	C	10	C	11	B	12	C
13	A	14	B	15	D	16	C
17	C	18	A, B	19	A, C	20	B
21	A	22	A	23	A	24	=
25	C	26	D	27	C	28	A
29	B	30	B	31	C	32	C
33	b	34	B	35	B	36	A
37	B	38	A	39	B	40	B
41	=	42	=	43	B	44	C
45	B	46	B	47	B	48	C
49	D	50	C, D	51	C	52	C
53	C	54	D	55	=	56	B
57	B	58	C	59	B	60	D
61	B	62	B	63	B	64	B
65	B	66	B	67	B	68	A
69	B	70	C	71	B	72	B
73	C	74	B	75	C	76	A
77	C	78	B	79	C	80	C
81	C, E	82	C	83	A,C,E	84	A
85	B	86	A	87	C	88	D

Reader's Notes

4

Pharmacology

1. All of the following are currently accepted as neurotransmitters in the CNS *except*

A. Acetylcholine
B. Dopamine
C. Nor epinephrine
D. Reserpine
E. Serotonin
F. GABA (gamma-aminobutyric acid)
G. Opioid peptides (beta endorphin enkephalins and dynorphin)
H. Glycine
I. Glutamate and aspartate

2. What are the four criteria to consider when selecting an analgesic agent for a patient?

A. Type of pain
B. Location of pain
C. Age of patient
D. Sex of patient
E. Patient's mental state
F. Concurrent medication
G. Pregnancy

3. An IV injection of histamine results in all of the following except.

A. A fall in systemic blood pressure
B. An increase in gastric acid secretion

C. Constriction of CNS blood vessels
D. Bronchoconstriction
E. Dilation of terminal arterioles

4. All of the following statements concerning rennin are true *except*.
A. Renin is an enzyme that is produced by and stored in the granular cells of the juxtaglomerular apparatus of the kidneys.
B. It is released by granular cells of the kidney into the blood in response to sodium depletion and/or low blood volume
C. Renin converts angiotensin I to angiotensin II
D. High levels of renin in the blood may indicate Addison's disease, cirrhosis, essential hypertension, hypokalemia, malignant hypertension of Barter's syndrome

5. The prototype tricyclic antidepressant drug is
A. Imipramine
B. Amitriptyline
C. Desipramine
D. Nortriptyline
E. Clomipramine
F. Doxepin
G. Protriptyline

6. Chloramphenicol is active against all of the following except
A. Gram-positive bacteria
B. Gram-negative bacteria
C. Anaerobic bacteria
D. Fungi
E. Rickettsia

7. Which of the following is a contraindication or precaution to the use of prilocaine ?
A. Biliary tract disease
B. Imipenem hypersensitivity
C. Benzyl alcohol hypersensitivity
D. Hepatic disease

8. All of the following anti epileptic drugs are effective in treating absence seizures (formerly called petitmal) except.
A. Ethosuximide
B. Valproic acid

C. Phenytoin
D. Clonazepam

9. All of the following are important effects of aspirin (acetylsalicylic acid) except
A. The reduction of fever
B. The reduction of prostaglandin synthesis in inflamed tissue
C. The reduction of the tendency to bleed
D. Respiratory stimulation when taken in toxic dosage
E. Tinnitus and vertigo

10. All of the following are anti-muscarinic agents except
A. Atropine
B. Scopolamine
C. Glycopyrrolate
D. Mecamylamine
E. Methantheline
F Propantheline

11. Poisoning with an organophosphate cholinesterase inhibitor can be treated with
A. Edrophonium
B. Carbachol
C. Pralidoxime
D. Nicotine

12. Which of the following can develop during therapy with phenobarbital
A. Drowsiness
B. Dizziness
C. Lethargy
D. Headache
E. Vertigo
F. Severe depression
G. Anxiety
H. Irritability
I. All of the above

13. The drug of choice in anaphylaxis is
A. Nor epinephrine
B. Terbutaline
C. Epinephrine
D. Phenycephrine

14. Of the following, which is a clinically significant adverse reaction due to Metoprolol?
A. Alopecia
B. Dry mouth
C. Dysarthria
D. Folliculits

15. The most common adverse effect associated with the benzodiazepines include all of the following except
A. Ataxia
B. CNS depression (drowsiness and sedation)
C. Confusion
D. Disorientation
E. Dry mouth
F. GI disturbances (nausea, vomiting and diarrhoea)

16. Which of the drugs are considered to be anti arrhythmic agents?
A. Sodium channel blockers
B. Beta-adrenergic blockers
C. Potassium channel blockers
D. Calcium channel blockers
E. All of the above

17. All of the following statements concerning propoxyphene are true except
A. Proxyphene is a synthetic opiate agonist
B. Structurally, propoxyphene is more similar to morphine than to methadone
C. Compared with codeine propoxyphene is one half to two thirds as potent an analgesic
D. Propoxyphene exerts little or no antitussive activity

18. Which schedule of drugs listed below would include a drug that is considered to have a strong potential for abuse or addiction but which has legitimate medical use?
A. Schedule I
B. Schedule II
C. Schedule III
D. Schedule IV
E. Schedule V

19. Inhaled ammonia is the drug of choice for acting against
A. Anaphylaxis
B. Heart attack
C. Syncope
D. Urticaria

20. All of the following are useful in the treatment of gout *except*:
A. Allopurinol
B. Aspirin
C. Colchicine
D. Indomethacin
E. Probenecid

21. The major natural mineralocorticoid in humans is:
A. Aldosterone
B. Cortisol
C. Dexamethasone
D. Prednisone

22. Amyl nitrite is used in the emergency treatment of cyanide poisoning because it:
A. Oxidizes hemoglobin
B. Irreversibly binds cyanide
C. Competes with cyanide for binding of cytochromes
D. Inhibits tubular reabsorption of cyanide

23. A pharmacologic antagonist drug:
A. Has no affinity for a receptor and no intrinsic activity
B. Has affinity for a receptor but no intrinsic activity
C. Has affinity for a receptor and intrinsic activity
D. Has no affinity for a receptor but has intrinsic activity

24. When a drug is administered repeatedly, a higher concentration of the drug than is desired may be achieved. The effect of this excessive accumulation is known as:
A. Additive effect
B. Synergistic response
C. Cumulative action
D. Idiosyncrasy

25. The currently available ganglionic blockers for clinical use include:
A. Mecamylamine

B. Hexamethonium
C. Tetraethylammonium
D. Trimethaphan

26. All of the following are phenothiazines except.
A. Chlorpromazine
B. Haloperidol
C. Prochlorperzine
D. Triflupromazine
E. Promazine
F. Trifluoperazine

27. All of the following drugs are used to the treatment of Parkinson's disease *except*.
A. Levodopa
B. Bromocriptine
C. Pergolide
D. Haloperidol
E. Amantadine

28. Methylphenidate is a central nervous system stimulant that is chemically similar to the:
A. Benzodiazepines
B. Amphetamines
C. Phenothiazines
D. Tranquilizers

29. The Controlled Substance act of 1970 uses which criteria listed below for inclusion of a drug into one of the five schedules?
A. Potential for abuse
B. Medical usefulness
C. Degree to which it produces one of physiological dependence
D. Degree to which it produces physical dependence
E. All of the above

30. Which of the following statements are true concerning the occupation theory of drug receptor interaction?
A. It is one of the few theoretical and unifying concepts in pharmacology
B. It follows the law of mass action

C. The theory states that the maximum effects of a drug occurs when all receptors are occupied
D. The theory also states that the magnified of the effect of a drug is proportional to the number of receptors occupied
E. All of the above statements

31. Which of the following drugs can be used in cases of hypotension associated with shock?
A. Prednisone
B. Norepinephrine
C. Pseudoephedrine
D. Lithium

32. Of the following, which is a clinically significant adverse reaction to Cocaine?
A. Epiphyseal closure
B. Hyperkalemia
C. Headache
D. Epistaxis

33. Which of the following are true statements about protein binding?
A. Albumin is the main plasma protein that binds drugs
B. Only bound drugs can interact with receptors to produce therapeutic or toxic effects
C. Drugs can be considered highly protein bound when over 90% of the total drug in plasma is protein-bound.
D. None of the above

34. All of the following statements concerning edrophonium are true except:
A. It is a direct-acting cholinergic agonist (cholinomimetic)
B. It is a rapid-acting, short-duration, parental cholinesterase inhibitor
C. It is the drug of choice for diagnosing myasthenia gravis because of its rapid onset of action and reversibility
D. It is also useful in differentiating a myasthenic crisis from a cholinergic crisis

35. All of the following are macrolide antibiotics except:
A. Erythromycin
B. Azithromycin

C. Clarithromycin
D. Clindamycin

36. Opioid drugs are used therapeutically as all of the following except:
A. Analgesics
B. Antitussives
C. Antiemetics
D. Antidiarrhoeals

37. All of the following drugs are adrenergic agonist except
A. Dopamine
B. Epinephrine
C. Clonidine
D. Phenoxybenzamine
E. Terbutaline
F. Albuterol

38. A contraindication or precaution to the use of propranolol is:
A. Achalasia
B. Renal failure
C. Collagen-vascular disease
D. Near sightedness

39. The most preferable antibiotic for the treatment of a non-penicillinase producing gram positive staphylococcal infection is :
A. Tetracycline
B. Clindamycin
C. Penicillin G or V
D. Ampicillin

40 All of the following drugs are amphetamines except:
A. Benzedrine
B. Dexedrine
C. Morphine
D. Methedrine

41. The penicillinase -resistant drugs are active against aerobes but they are reserved for treating:
A. Candida infections
B. Streptococcal infections

C. Staphylococcal infections
D. Meningococcal infections

42. The brief duration of action of an ultra short acting barbiturate is due to:
A. The slow rate of metabolism in the liver
B. A low lipid solubility, resulting in a minimal concentration in the brain
C. A high degree of binding to plasma proteins
D. A rapid rate of redistribution from the brain due to its high liposolubility
E. A slow rate of excretion by the kidneys

43. All of the following drugs are known to produce orthostatic hypotension as an adverse reaction except:
A. Levodopa
B. Meperidine
C. Chlorpromazine
D. Indomethacin

44. All of the following are optimum alkaloids except
A. Meperidin
B. Morphine
C. Codeine
D. Heroin

45. Which of the following is a contraindication or precaution to the use of Tobramycin
A. Sunlight (UV) exposure
B. Scleroderma
C. Myasthenia gravis
D. Syphilis

46. A therapeutic dose of morphine produces all of the following except.
A. Miosis
B. Decreased GI motility
C. CNS depression
D. Hyperventilation

47. Which antiarrhythmic drug listed below is effective only on the ventricles and is useful in acute ventricular arrhythmias?
A. Quinine

B. Lidocaine
C. Flecainide
D. Propranolol

48. Tetracycline's are the drugs of first choice in the treatment of :
A. Mycoplasma Pneumonia
B. Chlamydia infection
C. Rickettsial infections
D. Vibrio infections
E. All of the above

49. All of the following are components of the typical local anesthetic molecule *except*.
A. An aromatic group
B. A heme group
C. An intermediate chain
D. A secondary or tertiary amino group

50. Buspirone is classified as a (an)
A. Benzodiazepine
B. Azaspirodecanedione
C. Barbiturate
D. Phenothiazine

51. Which of the following is often Co-administered with antibiotics to delay the renal clearance of the antibiotic
A. Aztreonam
B. Imipenem
C. Probenecid
D. Reserpine

52. Alkylating agents are most effective in treating:
A. Chronic leukemias
B. Lymphomas
C. Myelomas
D. Carcinomas of the breast and ovary
E. All of the above

53. All of the following are catecholamines except:
A. Epinephrine
B. Norepinephrine
C. Methyldopa

D. Isoproterenol
E. Dopamine
F. Dobutamine

54. The autonomic nervous system has cholinergic fibers that secrete:
A. Acetylcholine
B. Dopamine
C. Epinephrine
D. Norepinephrine

55. The positive inotropic effect of Digoxin:
A. Is dependent upon a normal cardiac rhythm
B. Directly increases the force of myocardial contractions
C. Is antagonized by beta-blockers
D. All of the above

56. Ethyl alcohol causes a well-marked diuresis by inhibiting the production of:
A. Growth hormone
B. Insulin
C. Antidiuretic hormone (ADH)
D. Epinephrine

57. All of the following are antifungal agents except:
A. Amphotericin B
B. Flucytosine
C. Ketoconazole
D. Polymyxin B
E. Fluconazole
F. Itraconazole

58. All of the following penicillins are acid stable except:
A. Cloxacillin
B. Dicloxacillin
C. Methicillin
D. Nafcillin
E. Oxacillin
F. Pencillin V

59. All of the following are antihistamine H_1 blockers except:
A. Astemizole (Hismanal)
B. Chlorpheniramine (Chlor-Trimeton)

C. Cimetidine
D. Diphenhydramine (Benadryl)
E. Terfenadine (Seldane)

60. Which of the following is most likely to cause cholestasis as an adverse reaction?
A. Ampicillin
B. Diphenhydramine
C. Promethazine
D. Ranitidine

61. Local anesthetics theoretically should be less effective in acutely inflamed tissue than in normal tissue because in inflamed tissue:
A. The pH decreases, thus significantly reducing the concentration of the free-base form of the local anesthetic
B. The pH remains the same, however, the extracellular fluids inactivate the local anesthetic.
C. The pH rises, thus inactivating the anesthetic
D. The pH rises, thus significantly reducing the concentration of the free-base form of the local anesthetic

62. The maximum recommended dose of a local anesthetic that can be administered to a child is determined by:
A. Age
B. Weight
C. Height
D. Gender

63. The dilation of vessels in muscle, the constriction of vessels and a positive inotropic and chronotropic effect on the heart are all action of :
A. Acetylcholine
B. Epinephrine
C. Isoproterenol
D. Metaproterenol

64. Epinephrine reversal is a predictable result of the use of epinephrine in a patient who has received a (an)
A. Beta-blocker
B. Alpha blocker

C. Adrenergic agonist
D. All of the above

65. All of the following statements concerning codeine are true except

A. Codeine is an opiate agonist with chemical structure and effects similar to morphine
B. Codeine is available as phosphate or scuffle salt both of which can be administered by the oral, subcutaneous or intramuscular route
C. Codeine is much more potent than morphine
D. Codeine is the standard of centrally acting narcotic antitussives
E. Codeine has less analgesic respiratory depressive and other side effect than morphine but is a more effective antitussive agent.

66. A teaspoon contains

A. 5 milliliters
B. 10 milliliters
C. 15 milliliters
D. 20 milliliters

67. Tetracycline's should not be used in patient who have

A. Cataracts
B. Leucopenia
C. Severe renal impairment
D. Cardiac disorders

68. Erythromycin is well known to cause adverse :

A. CNS effects
B. GI effects
C. Hematological effects
D. Renal effects

69. All of the following drugs are beta - blockers except

A. Acebutotol
B. Metoprolol
C. Nadolol
D. Prazosin
E. Timolol

70. Adrenaline (epinephrine) stimulates :
A. Alpha 1 receptors
B. Beta 1 receptors
C. Both alpha 1, 2 and beta 1, 2 receptors
D. Alpha 1 and beta 1 receptors only

71. All of the following statements concerning barbiturates are true except.
A. Barbiturates may increase the half lives of drugs metabolized by the liver
B. Barbiturates depress neuronal activity by increasing membrane ion conductance (primarily chloride), reducing glutamate induced depolarization and potentiating the inhibitory effects of GABA
C. Compared with benzondiazepines the barbiturates exhibit a steeper dose response relationship
D. Barbiturates may precipitate acute porphyrias in susceptible patient

72. Of the following penicillin which one has the widest or broadest spectrum of activity?
A. Penicillin G
B. Carbenicillin
C. Oxacillin
D. Cloxacilin

73. Antibiotics administered for angioplasty therapy include
A. Dactinomycin
B. Doxorubicin
C. Bleomycin sulfate
D. Mitomycin
E. All of the above

74. Which of the following species is a catalase positive gram positive bacterium that produces the enzyme beta-lactamase and has been implicated in hospital acquired infections since the 1950's
A. Streptococcus
B. Staphylococcus
C. Mycobacterium
D. Lactobacillus

75. The major clinical use of an opioid antagonist is :

A. In the management of acute alcohol poisoning
B. In the management of status asthmatics
C. In the management of acute opioid overdose
D. In the management of anaphylaxis

76. The term bio-availability of a drug refers to:

A. The movement of a drug into the body tissues over time
B. The dissolution of a drug in the GI tract
C. The measurement of the rate and amount of therapeutic active drug that reaches the systemic circulation
D. The relationship between the physical and chemical properties of a drug and the systemic absorption of the drug
E. The amount of drug destroyed by the liver prior to systemic absorption from GI tract

77. Clindamycin is an antibiotic structurally similar to:

A. Azithromycin
B. Clarithromycin
C. Erythromycin
D. Lincomycin

78. Which of the following are considered to be first-line agents in the treatment of tuberculosis?

A. Isoniazid (INH)
B. Ethambutol
C. Pyrazinamide (PZA)
D. Rifampicin

79. Verapamil is useful for the treatment of :

A. Angina
B. Hypertension
C. Supraventricular tachyarrhythmia
D. All of the above

80. All of the following drugs are monoamine oxidase inhibitors (MAOIs) except

A. Phenelzine
B. Isocarboxazid
C. Imipramine
D. Tranylcypromine

81. Local anesthetics act directly on the membrane by :
A. Increasing K^+ flux
B. Increasing nerve membrane permeability to sodium
C. Decreasing nerve membrane permeability to sodium
D. Increasing membrane excitability

82. The Ester local anesthetics are hydrolyzed primarily in the:
A. Liver
B. Lungs
C. Kidney
D. Plasma

83. An antidiarrheal drug related to meperidine is :
A. Omeprazole
B. Sucralfate
C. Loperamide
D. Metoclopramide

84. The prototype depolarizing neuromuscular blocking agent is :
A. Tubocurarine
B. Mivacurium
C. Vecuronium
D. Succinylcholine
E. Atracurium
F. Rocuronium

85. Biotransformation is also called :
A. Drug elimination
B. Drug Metabolism
C. Drug bioavailability
D. Drug half life

86. The specificity of a drug is most commonly accomplished by altering
A. The solubility
B. The molecular structure
C. The dose
D. The concentration

87. The drug of choice for treating candidiasis is :
A. Chloramphenicol
B. Clindamycin

C. Nystatin
D. Penicillin

88. The antibiotic of choice for prophylactic coverage for the prevention of bacterial endocarditis is:
A. Tetracycline
B. Lincomycin
C. Erythromycin
D. Amoxicillin

89. A vial contains 3.6 ml of a 2% solution of lidocaine with 1:100, 000 epinephrine. How much Lidocaine and epinephrine does this vial contain?
A. 7.2 mg of lidocaine & 0.36 mg of epinephrine
B. 7.2 mg of lidocaine & 0.036 g of epinephrine
C. 72 mg of lidocaine & 0.36 mg of epinephrine
D. 72 mg of lidocaine & 0.036 mg of epinephrine

90. Local anesthetics depress which of the following fibers first?
A. Large myelinated fibers
B. Small unmyelinated fibers
C. Small myelinated fibers
D. Large unmyelinated fibers

91. All of the following statements concerning pilocarpine are true except
A. It is a choline ester
B. It is a direct acting cholinergic agonist (Cholinomimetic)
C. It is lipid soluble
D. The duration of action range from 30 minutes to two hours

92. Which of the following agents has little value in treating acute inflammation
A. Ibuprofen
B. Aspirin
C. Acetaminophen
D. Naproxen

93. The major natural glucocorticoid is:
A. Triamcinolone
B. Cortisol (Hydrocortisone)
C. Dexamethasone (Decadron)
D. Prednisolone (Prelone)

94. All of the following statements concerning Methohexital (Brevital) are true except:

A. It is an ultrashort-acting barbiturate similar to Thiopental
B. It has a faster onset of action and recovery time than does Thiopental
C. It is not as potent as Thiopental
D. It can be used along as an anesthetic for short procedures that are relatively painless, as an inducing agent, or as an adjunct to regional anesthesia
E. Post - anesthesia excitatory phenomena occur more frequently with Methohexital than with Thiopental.

95. Oral contraceptives exert their primary effect by inhibiting:

A. Follicle formation
B. Ovulation
C. Follicle Growth
D. All of the above

96. For a patient who is taking anticoagulants, what is the most valuable test used in evaluating this patient as a surgical risk?

A. PTT (Partial thromboplastin Time)
B. PT (Prothrombin Time)
C. Platelet count
D. Hemoglobin

97. All of the following statements concerning heparin are true except:

A. Heparin inhibits several steps in the intrinsic pathway of blood clotting
B. Heparin is used when anticoagulation is needed immediately
C. It is often used 1 to 2 weeks immediate following a heart attack
D. It passes the placental barrier
E. Increased bleeding is the most common adverse effect of heparin

98. Disulfiram (Antabuse) is used in the management of :

A. Nicotine abuse
B. Ethanol abuse
C. Opioid abuse
D. NSAID abuse

99. Which of the following is a pharmacological antagonist of aldosterone in the collecting tubule?

A. Mannitol
B. Glycerin
C. Isosorbide
D. Urea
E. Spironolactone

100. All of the following are skeletal muscle spasmolytic drugs except

A. Methocarbamol
B. Cyclobenzaprine
C. Baclofen
D. Succinycholine
E. Dantrolene

101. Which of the following has a clinically significant drug interaction with Amoxicillin?

A. Dorzolamide & Timolol
B. Methotrexate
C. Calcitrol
D. Candesartan

102. A drug that acts in a way opposite to the sympathetic nervous system is called a:

A. Sympathomimetic
B. Sympatholytic
C. Sympathetic
D. Adrenergic agent

103. Antipsychotic drugs include:

A. Phenothiazines
B. Thioxanthenes
C. Butyrophenones
D. All of the above

104. All of the following are cholinergic actions except:

A. Slowing of the heart
B. Dilation of the pupils
C. The stimulation of the smooth muscles of the bronchi, GI tract, gallbladder, bile duct, bladder and ureters
D. The stimulation of sweat, salivary, tear and bronchial glands

105. Which agent listed below is used as an antiseptic in mouthwashes and skin wound cleansers?
A. Dexamethasone
B. Hexylresorcinol
C. Epinephrine
D. Penicillin

106. All of the following drugs are alpha blockers except:
A. Doxazosin
B. Phenoxybenzamine hydrochloride
C. Phentolamine hydrochloride
D. Propranolol
E. Terazosin

107. Nitroglycerin either directly or through reflexes result in all of the following except:
A. Increased heart rate
B. Increased venous capacity
C. Decreased cardiac force
D. Decreased after-load

108. Aluminum salt used as antacids include:
A. Hydroxide
B. Carbonate
C. Phosphate
D. Amino acetate
E. All of the above

109. Pain that has no organic basis and is fixed upon some portion of the anatomy is referred to as:
A. Intractable pain
B. Referred pain
C. Psychogenic pain
D. Phantom pain

110. All of the following are effects of insulin except:
A. Decreased gluconeogenesis
B. Increased triglyceride storage
C. Decreased protein synthesis
D. Increased glycogen synthesis

111. Tissue thromboplastin is considered to be coagulation factor
A. I

B. II
C. III
D. IV

112. Prominent toxic effects of mercury include all of the following except
A. Acute renal failure
B. Tremors
C. Salivation
D. Mydriasis
E. Slurred speech
F. Loosened teeth

113. All of the following are angiotensin - converting enzyme (ACE) inhibitors except
A. Captopril
B. Hydralazine
C. Enalapril
D. Lisnopril

114. If norepinephrine or epinephrine were to stimulate or combine with the alpha - receptors in the eye, which response listed below would you except?
A. Miosis (Contraction of the pupil)
B. Mydriasis (dilation of the pupil)
C. Neither of the above; nor - epinephrine and epinephrine do not stimulate or combine with alpha receptors in the eye

115. Which antibiotic listed below is used cautiously due to its side effects pseudomembranous colitis (severe GI upset)?
A. Clindamycin
B. Cloxacillin
C. Erythromycin
D. Vancomycin

116. Which of the following side effects are most common with the use of Diazepam (Valium)?
A. Rash, itch
B. Mouth, throat ulcers
C. Drowsiness, fatigue
D. Difficulty with urination

117. Which of the following is a contraindication or precaution to the use of Cefotaxime?
A. Scoliosis
B. Bronchitis
C. Aortic Stenosis
D. Breast-feeding

118. The amide local anesthetics are metabolized primarily in the:
A. Lungs
B. Plasma
C. Liver
D. Kidney

119. All of the following are benzodiazepines except
A. Lorazapam
B. Oxazepam
C. Alprazolam
D. Carbamazepine
E. Midazolam

120. Ethosuximide is effective in treating absence seizures by causing
A. Sodium channel blockade
B. Neuronal membrane hyperpolarization
C. Calcium channel blockade
D. GABA-chloride channel blockade

121. Sulfonamides are structurally similar to :
A. Penicillin
B. PABA (para aminobenzoic acid)
C. Salicylic acid
D. Ergotamine

122. Which alpha - adrenergic blocker listed below is used for persistent pulmonary hypertension of the newborn and for treating peripheral vasoplastic disorders in adults
A. Prazosin
B. Terazosin
C. Tolazolin
D. Doxazosin
E. Phentolamine
F. Phenoxybenzamine (dibenzylene)

123. Local anaesthetics

A. Greatly decreases the resting potential of peripheral nerves
B. Act on the extracellular surface of the nerve membrane in the uncharged state
C. Prevent the development of the action potential of a nerve
D. Block nerve conduction by interfering with calcium conductance

124. A drug with a high LD_{50} and a Ed_{50} has a

A. High therapeutic index and is therefore very dangerous
B. High therapeutic index and is therefore relativity safe
C. Low therapeutic index and is therefore very dangerous
D. Low therapeutic index and is therefore relativity safe

125. All of the following drugs are cardiac glycosides (cardio - tonics) except:

A. Amrinone
B. Deslanoside
C. Digoxin
D. Propranolol
E. Digitoxin
F. Ouabain

126. Which term listed bellows is a compulsive, uncontrollable dependence on a substance, habit or practice to such a degree that cessation causes severe emotional mental or physiological reactions?

A. Habituation
B. Tolerance
C. Addiction
D. None of the above

127. An international Unit of a substance is:

A. The amount that is eliminated by the kidneys
B. The amount that produces a specific biological result
C. The amount that produces toxicity
D. The amount that is bound to protein

128. Acyclovir can be used to treat

A. Tuberculosis
B. Varicella - zoster virus infections
C. Atrial fibrillation
D. Anticholinergic syndrome

129. The body contains three types of endogenous opioids which one of the following is not one of them?
A. Beta-endorphins
B. Morphine
C. Enkephalins
D. Dynorphins

130. All of the following fibers are cholinergic except
A. Preganglionic sympathetic fibers
B. Preganglionic parasympathetic fibers
C. Postganglionic sympathetic fibers
D. Postganglionic parasympathetic fibers

131. Which from of a local anesthetic can readily penetrate tissue membrane?
A. Ionized form
B. Non-ionized free base form
C. Ionized and non-ionized form
D. None of the above

132. Which of the following presents the greatest danger of penicillin therapy?
A. GI upset
B. CNS irritation
C. An allergic reaction
D. Renal damage

133. Alpha receptors are located on:
A. Vascular smooth muscle
B. Presynaptic nerve terminals
C. Blood platelets
D. Fat cells
E. Neurons in the CNS
F. All of the above

134. All of the following statements concerning toxicity are true except
A. Toxicity is often an extension of the desired drug effect
B. Toxicity is dose dependent but not time dependent
C. Toxicity can be anything ranging from nausea to death
D. Toxicity can be caused by even minimal concentrations of a drug

135. Acetazolamide is a:
A. Loop diuretic
B. Carbonic anhydrase inhibitor
C. Thiazide diuretic
D. Potassium sparing diuretic

136. All of the following are choline esters except:
A. Pilocarpine
B. Methacholine
C. Bethanechol
D. Carbachol

137. For which of the following conditions can ranitidine be used?
A. Prostatitis
B. Pyrosis (heart burn)
C. Toxic-shock syndrome
D. Renal failure

138. Cephalosporins have which of the following mode of action?
A. Affect cell membrane
B. Interfere with protein synthesis
C. Affect cell wall
D. Interfere with normal biosynthetic pathways

139. Which insulin zinc suspension listed below has the longest duration of action
A. Ultra-lente insulin
B. Semilente insulin
C. Lente insulin
D. None of the above

140. The treatment of the pseudomembranous colitis caused by clindamycin is
A. Penicillin
B. Streptomycin
C. Tetracycline
D. Vancomycin

141. All of the following are CNS stimulants except:
A. Pentylenetetrazol
B. Doxapram
C. Phenobarbital
D. Nikethamide

E. Picrotoxin
F. Strychnine

142. The heart is generally considered to have predominantly which type of adrenergic receptors
A. Alpha 1
B. Alpha 2
C. Beta 1
D. Beta 2

143. All of the following drugs are neuronal blockers except:
A. Guanethidine
B. Guanadrel
C. Clonidine
D. Reserpine

144. The prototype penicillin is :
A. Penicillin V
B. Penicillin G
C. Ampicillin
D. Nafcillin

145. Clinically, Scopolamine is used to:
A. Prevent motion sickness
B. Reduces salivation and excess bronchial secretion prior to surgery
C. Reduces spastic states in Parkinsonism
D. Treat iritis and uveitis
E. All of the above

146. Of the following which is a clinically significant adverse reaction due to Diphenhydramine (Benadryl)?
A. Hypovitaminosis
B. Paresthesia
C. Contact dermatitis
D. Delirium

147. All of the following are anti - HIV agents except:
A. Didanosine
B. Ganciclovir
C. Ritonavir
D. Lamivudine
E. Indinavir

148. The maximal recommended adult dose of Lidocaine is 300 mg. How many milliliters of 2% Lidocaine need to be given to reach this level?
A. 7.5 milliliters
B. 10 milliliters
C. 15 milliliters
D. 20 milliliters

149. Lithium is the drug of choice in treating:
A. Unipolar disorders
B. Bipolar affective disorder
C. Migraines
D. Pain

150. All of the following contain aspirin except:
A. Darvon Compound-65
B. Fiorinal
C. Tylenol
D. Empirin with Codeine # 3 or # 4
E. Diflunisal

151. Which of the following are broncho-dilators:
A. Theophylline
B. Aminophylline
C. Epinephrine
D. Terbutaline
E. Albuterol
F. All of the above.

152. All of the following statements concerning ibuprofen are true except:
A. It has a half-life of about 2 hours
B. It is relatively safe
C. It produces more GI disturbances than does aspirin
D. It is well absorbed after oral administration and is excreted via the kidney
E. It is the least expensive of the newer NSAID's (Naproxen, Indomethacin, etc.)
F. It is available in low-dose over the counter formulations

153. All of the following are cholinesterase inhibitors except:
A. Physostigmine

B. Neostigmine
C. Edrophonium
D. Methacholine
E. Pyridostigmine

154. The physiochemical properties of drugs that influence their passage across biologic membranes are:
A. Lipid solubility
B. Degree of ionization
C. Molecular size and shape
D. All of the above

155. The major disadvantages with the use of opioid analgesics is:
A. Allergic response
B. Nausea
C. Vomiting
D. Respiratory depression

156. Growth hormone is also called:
A. Vasopressin
B. Aldosterone
C. Somatotropin
D. Dopamine

157. Antimetabolites are cell cycle-specific drugs, acting primarily in the:
A. G 0 phase or resting phase of the cell cycle
B. S phase of the cell cycle
C. G 1 phase of the cell cycle
D. G 2 phase of the cell cycle

158. Which route of drug administration listed below will give the most rapid onset of pharmacological effect?
A. Oral administration
B. Subcutaneous injection
C. Intravenous injection
D. Intramuscular injection

159. All of the following are pharmacologic effects of glucocorticoids except:
A. A decrease in gluconeogenesis
B. A decrease in the utilization of glucose

C. The inhibition of protein synthesis
D. An increase in protein catabolism
E. A decreased resistance to infection

160. Which route of administration of a drug listed below is most known for its significant hepatic "first pass" metabolism?
A. Intramuscular
B. Inhalation
C. Sublingual
D. Oral

161. All of the following sites are generally accepted for IM injections except:
A. The buttocks
B. The biceps muscle
C. The deltoid muscle
D. The anterior thigh

162. Quinacrine is an oral anti-protozoal agent used most commonly in the treatment of:
A. Chronic bronchitis
B. AIDS
C. Giardiasis
D. Leprosy

163. The only nonbarbiturate sedative-hypnotic agent that is indicated in the practice of dentistry is:
A. Pentobarbital
B. Secobarbital
C. Chloral hydrate
D. Meperidine

164. Which of the following is a contraindication or precaution to the use of Procainamide?
A. Polycystic ovary syndrome
B. Ester local anesthetic hypersensitivity
C. Thrombocytopenia
D. Acute myocardial infarction

165. Which of the following is a pharmacologic antagonist of aldosterone in the collecting tubule?
A. Mannitol
B. Glycerin

C. Spironolactone
D. Isosorbide
E. Urea

166. All of the following are skeletal muscle spasmolytic drugs except:
A. Methocarbamol
B. Cyclobenzaprine
C. Baclofen
D. Succinylcholine
E. Dantrolene

167. All of the following drugs are indirect-acting adrenergic agonists except:
A. Tyramine
B. Amphetamine
C. Epinephrine
D. Methamphetamine
E. Hydroxyamphetamine

168. The safest and easiest route for drug administration is:
A. Oral
B. IV
C. Rectal
D. Inhalation

169. Which of the following routes of drug administration is generally used for local drug effects?
A. Topical administration
B. Oral ingestion
C. Subcutaneous injection
D. Intravenous injection

170. Which of the following refers to the efficacy of a drug?
A. The relative concentrations of two or more drugs that produce the same drug effect
B. The ability of a drug to produce a desired therapeutic effect regardless of dosage
C. The dose of a drug that will kill a patient
D. None of the above

Answer key to pharmacology

1	D	2	ACFG	3	C	4	C
5	A	6	D	7	D	8	C
9	C	10	D	11	C	12	I
13	C	14	A	15	E	16	E
17	B	18	B	19	C	20	B
21	A	22	A	23	B	24	C
25	A,D	26	B	27	D	28	B
29	E	30	E	31	B	32	C
33	A, C	34	A	35	D	36	C
37	D	38	B	39	C	40	C
41	C	42	D	43	D	44	A
45	C	46	D	47	B	48	E
49	B	50	B	51	C	52	E
53	C	54	A	55	B	56	C
57	D	58	C	59	C	60	C
61	A	62	B	63	B	64	B
65	C	66	A	67	C	68	B
69	D	70	C	71	A	72	B
73	E	74	B	75	C	76	C
77	D	78	A, D	79	D	80	C
81	C	82	D	83	C	84	D
85	B	86	B	87	C	88	D
89	D	90	B	91	A	92	C
93	B	94	C	95	B	96	B
97	D	98	B	99	E	100	D
101	B	102	B	103	D	104	B
105	B	106	D	107	C	108	E
109	D	110	C	111	C	112	D
113	B	114	B	115	A	116	C
117	D	118	C	119	D	120	C
121	B	122	C	123	C	124	B
125	D	126	C	127	B	128	B
129	B	130	C	131	B	132	C
133	F	134	B	135	B	136	A
137	B	138	C	139	A	140	D
141	C	142	C	143	C	144	B
145	E	146	C	147	B	148	C

149	B	150	C	151	F	152	C
153	D	154	D	155	D	156	C
157	B	158	C	159	A	160	D
161	B	162	C	163	C	164	B
165	C	166	D	167	C	168	A
169	A	170	B				

Reader's Notes

5

Dental Anatomy

1. **Bilateral contraction of the posterior fibers of the temporalis muscles results in which mandibular movement listed below?**
   A. Retrusion
   B. Protrusion
   C. Opening
   D. Closing

2. **How does the distoincisal angle of most anterior teeth compare to the mesioincisal angle?**
   A. It is straighter
   B. It is more rounded
   C. There is no difference
   D. None of the above

3. **All of the following teeth are non-succedaneous, except:**
   A. The permanent maxillary and mandibular premolars
   B. The permanent maxillary and mandibular first molars
   C. The permanent maxillary and mandibular second molars
   D. The permanent maxillary and mandibular third molars

4. **What percentage of dentin is organic?**
   A. 5-10%
   B. 20%

C. 30%
D. 60%

5. **Which primary mandibular tooth listed below does not resemble any other primary or permanent tooth?**
A. Primary mandibular canine
B. Primary mandibular lateral incisor
C. Primary mandibular first molar
D. Primary mandibular second molar

6. **The triangular space between adjacent teeth cervical to the contact area is called as:**
A. Dead space
B. Freeway space
C. Interproximal space
D. Inter-radicular space

7. **The chewing surface of posterior teeth is referred to as the:**
A. Anatomic crown
B. Clinical crown
C. Incisal edge
D. Occlusal surface

8. **Gingival fibers are found within the:**
A. Attached and free gingiva
B. Attached gingiva
C. Free gingiva
D. Mucogingival junction

9. **Which tooth listed below is very often a developmental anomaly with only a slight resemblance to other permanent teeth?**
A. Maxillary first molar
B. Mandibular second molar
C. Maxillary third molar
D. Mandibular first premolar

10. **When viewed from the mesial or distal, mandibular molar crowns appear to be**
A. Tilted buccally
B. Tilted lingually
C. Straight
D. None of the above

11. During typical empty mouth swallowing, the mandible is braced in which jaw position below to allow for proper stabilization?

A. Centric relation (CR)
B. Intercuspal position (ICP)
C. Retruded contact position (RCP)
D. Protruded contact position (PCP)

12. Which of the following teeth may have a pulp chamber that will be triangular?

A. Permanent mandibular second premolars
B. Permanent maxillary molars
C. Permanent maxillary lateral incisors
D. Permanent mandibular canines

13. In an ideal intercuspal position, the mesiobuccal cusp of the permanent maxillary second molar opposes what?

A. The buccal groove of the mandibular second molar
B. The developmental-groove between the distobuccal and distal cusps of the mandibular first molar
C. The distobuccal groove of the mandibular first molar
D. The mesiobuccal groove of the mandibular second molar
E. The mesiobuccal groove of the mandibular first molar

14. The lateral pterygoid muscles help perform which two mandibular movements listed below?

A. Closing
B. Opening
C. Retrusion
D. Protrusion

15. The mandible functions as which type of lever?

A. Class I
B. Class II
C. Class III
D. Class IV

16. In the early stage of lateral movement, the condyle appears to rotate with a slight lateral shift in the direction of the movement. This movement is called the Bennett movement and it refers to the:

A. Non- working side condyle only

B. Working side condyle only
C. Both the nonworking and working side condyles
D. None of the above

17. Which tooth listed below may have a pulp chamber that is somewhat triangular as opposed to oval
A. Maxillary central incisor
B. Mandibular central incisor
C. Maxillary lateral incisor
D. Mandibular lateral incisor

18. The primary maxillary canine typically erupts around what age?
A. 7 months old
B. 10 month old
C. 18 month old
D. 24 month old

19. The character of occlusal contacts in the unworn dental arch are all of the following except:
A. Point-to-Point
B. Edge-to-edge
C. Edge-to-area
D. Area-to-area

20. The pulp is composed of:
A. Loose connective tissue (collagen and reticulin fibers)
B. Cells (fibroblasts, odontoblasts, histocytes, and lymphocytes)
C. Blood vessels (arteries and veins)
D. Nerves
E. Lymphatic
F. Ground substance
G. All of the above

21. Which of the following is the main function of cementum?
A. Compensation for tooth wear
B. Reparative
C. To attach the principal fibers of the periodontal ligament to the tooth
D. Protection

22. Which primary mandibular molar listed below has a prominent transverse ridge that unites the mesiobuccal and mesiolingual cusps?

A. Primary mandibular first molar
B. Primary mandibular second molar
C. Primary maxillary first molar
D. Primary maxillary second molar

23. What is the minimum number of lobes from which any tooth may develop?

A. Two
B. Three
C. Four
D. Five

24. All posterior teeth have how many line angles?

A. Two
B. Four
C. Six
D. Eight

25. All of the following statements concerning the mandibular lateral incisor are true, except:

A. The mandibular lateral incisor is a little larger in all dimensions than the mandibular central incisor
B. The crown of the mandibular lateral incisor is not as bilaterally symmetrical as the mandibular central incisor
C. The cingulum is directly in the center of the lingual surface
D. The root is very narrow mesiodistally

26. Oversized anomalies are more common with which tooth listed below?

A. Maxillary third molar
B. Mandibular third molar
C. Mandibular second premolars
D. Maxillary first molars

27. The excessive formation of cementum around the root of a tooth after it has erupted is known as:

A. Gomphosis
B. Ankylosis

C. Hypercementosis
D. Osteodontosis

28. Occlusocervically, the height of the distal marginal ridge of a permanent maxillary first molar is the same height as:
A. The distal marginal ridge of a permanent maxillary second premolar
B. The mesial marginal ridge of a permanent mandibular first molar
C. The mesial marginal ridge of a permanent maxillary second molar
D. The mesial marginal ridge of a permanent maxillary second premolar

29. Drug with teratogenic effects can produce:
A. An abnormal fetus
B. Hyperglycemia
C. Renal toxicity
D. Tumors

30. In an ideal intercuspal position, the facial cusp tips of permanent maxillary premolars oppose what?
A. The facial embrasure between their class counterpart and the tooth mesial to it
B. The facial embrasure between their class counterpart and the tooth distal to it
C. The opposing central fossae
D. The opposing mesial marginal ridge

31. All of the following types of oral mucosa are non-keratinized except:
A. Buccal mucosa
B. Inferior surface of the tongue
C. The soft palate
D. Floor of the mouth
E. Hard palate

32. Of the choices listed below, which one describes the boundaries that define the attached gingiva?
A. From the gingival margin to the interdental groove
B. From the free gingival groove to the gingival margin
C. From the mucogingival junction to the free gingival groove
D. From the epithelial attachment to the cementoenamel junction

33. The mesial and distal aspect (or surfaces) of all anterior teeth have a

A. Trapezoidal outline
B. Triangular outline
C. Square outline
D. Oval shape

34. Which of the following are the three cardinal rules regarding the eruption of teeth

A. Boys before girls
B. Girls before boys
C. Maxillary before mandibular
D. Mandibular before maxillary
E. Slender before stocky
F. Stocky before slender

35. On the lingual surface of all maxillary and mandibular posterior teeth, the height of contour (crest of curvature) is located in the:

A. Occlusal third
B. Middle third
C. Cervical third
D. Gingival third

36. Ordinarily, a 6-year-old child would have what teeth clinically visible in the mouth?

A. All (20) primary teeth and 4 permanent first molars
B. 18 Primary teeth and 2 permanent mandibular central incisors
C. 18 primary teeth, 2 permanent mandibular central incisors and 4 permanent first molars.
D. None of the above

37. Which of the following is the main function of the dental pulp?

A. Nutritive
B. Sensory
C. Protective
D. Formative

38. Which of the following is formed very rapidly in response to irritants?

A. Primary dentin

B. Secondary dentin
C. Reparative dentin
D. Sclerotic dentin

39. Which statement below is *true?*
A. The sum of the mesiodistal widths of the *primary molars* in any one quadrant is equal to the permanent teeth that succeed them (*premolars*)
B. The sum of the mesiodistal widths of the *Primary Molars* in any one quadrant is less than the permanent teeth succeed them *(premolars)*
C. The sum of the mesiodistal widths of the *Primary Molars* in any one quadrant is *greater than* the permanent teeth that succeed them (premolars)
D. None of the above

40. The difference b/w the sum of MD widths of primary c, d, e teeth and that of permanent 3, 4, 5 teeth is known as?
A. Free way space
B. Lee way space of Nance
C. Inter-occlusal distance
D. E – space

41. The distance b/w the occlusal surfaces of upper arch and lower arch at rest position is called as:
A. Free way space
B. Lee way space
C. E – space
D. None of the above

42. A *mesiolingual* developmental groove is a positive ID for which tooth listed below?
A. Maxillary first premolar
B. Mandibular first premolar
C. Maxillary second premolar
D. Mandibular second premolar

43. Which tooth listed below is the *most stable* and self-cleansing?
A. Mandibular central incisor
B. Mandibular first premolar
C. Maxillary canine
D. Maxillary lateral incisor

44. A *small elevation of enamel* found on the crown portion of a tooth would be classified as what?
A. Tubercle
B. Mamelon
C. Ridge
D. Developmental depression

45. The lobes of anterior teeth are always separated by which of the following?
A. Sulci
B. Developmental depressions
C. Inclined planes
D. Developmental artefact

46. Which cusp on permanent maxillary molars generally is the one that gets progressively smaller as you go posterior in the arch?
A. Mesiobuccal
B. Distobuccal
C. Mesiolingual
D. Distolingual

47. The wearing away of tooth structure by mechanical means is known as:
A. Attrition
B. Erosion
C. Abrasion
D. Ablation

48. The mandibular molars have a decided inclination in which direction?
A. Facially
B. Lingually
C. Neither facially or lingually
D. Distally

49. Caries is usually found on all of the following areas, except:
A. Proximal surfaces
B. Pits and grooves
C. Cusp tips
D. Cervical thirds

50. In the intercuspal position, *the distobuccal cusp of a permanent* mandibular first molar occludes where?

A. The interproximal marginal ridge between maxillary second bicuspid and first molar
B. Central fossa of the maxillary first molar
C. Central fossa of the maxillary second molar
D. The interproximal marginal ridge area between maxillary first molar and second molar

51. Which permanent teeth listed below occlude with only one tooth in the opposite jaw assuming that an ideal relation ship exists?

A. Maxillary canines
B. Maxillary central incisors
C. Mandibular central incisors
D. Mandibular third molars

52. Which component of the free gingiva listed below fills the embrasure space between the area of tooth contact?

A. Free gingival groove
B. Gingival sulcus
C. Interdental gingiva
D. Gingival margin

53. Which group of gingival fibers listed below resists rotational forces that are applied to a tooth?

A. Trans-septal fibers
B. Dento-gingival fibers
C. Alveolo-gingival fibers
D. Circumferential fibers
E. Dentoperiosteal fibers

54. Which teeth listed below typically have trifurcations?

A. Mandibular molars
B. Maxillary molars
C. Mandibular premolars
D. Maxillary first premolars

55. On a maxillary molar the largest, longest and strongest of the three roots is the

A. Mesiobuccal
B. Distobuccal

C. Palatal
D. Mesiolingual

56. When a mandibular movement to the left is performed, which condyle moves anteriorly, downward and medially, and also rotates at the same time?
A. Working condyle (left)
B. Nonworking condyle (right)
C. Both of the above
D. Nothing happens

57. When do the deciduous (primary) teeth begin to form in utero?
A. One week
B. Three week
C. Six weeks
D. Ten weeks

58. Which stage in the life cycle of a tooth listed below includes final shaping of the tooth?
A. Initiation (Bud stage)
B. Proliferation (Cap stage)
C. Differentiation (Bell stage)
D. Apposition

59. Which of the following cells form cementum?
A. Ameloblasts
B. Cementoblasts
C. Cementoclasts
D. Odontoblasts

60. Which teeth listed below when viewed from the facial resemble a pentagon (five-sided)?
A. Canines
B. Centrals
C. Laterals
D. Molars

61. Which of the following are primary centers of calcification?
A. Ridges
B. Lobes
C. Grooves
D. Pearls

62. Any linear elevation on the surface of a tooth is called what?
A. An incline
B. A prominence
C. A ridge
D. A tuberosity

63. Which tooth listed below is most often restored, extracted, or replaced
A. Maxillary first molar
B. Mandibular first molar
C. Mandibular first premolar
D. Maxillary first premolar

64. Which maxillary premolar listed below is distinguished by having many accessory grooves on the occlusal surface?
A. First premolar
B. Second premolar
C. Both of the above
D. None of the above

65. As a general rule, root tips tend to curve which way
A. Towards the mesial
B. Towards the distal
C. Towards the mesial on maxillary teeth and toward the distal on mandibular teeth
D. Toward the distal on maxillary teeth and toward the mesial on mandibular teeth

66. The term "homodont" means what?
A. Teeth are continually being replaced
B. Teeth differ from one another
C. Teeth are all alike
D. Long teeth

67. How does mandibular arch generally compare in length with the maxillary arch?
A. It is exactly the same
B. It is slightly longer
C. It is slightly shorter
D. None of the above

68. In the intercuspal position, the mesiolingual cusp of a permanent maxillary second molar occludes where?

A. Central fossa of the mandibular first molar
B. Central fossa of the mandibular second molar
C. The interproximal marginal ridge areas between the mandibular first and second molars
D. The interproximal marginal ridge areas between the mandibular second and third molars

69. All of the following statements concerning supporting cusps are true, except

A. They contact the opposing tooth in the intercuspal position
B. They support the vertical dimension of the face
C. They are nearer the facio-lingual center of the tooth than the non-supporting cusps
D. Their outer incline has a potential for contact
E. They have narrower and sharper cusp ridges than non-supporting cusps

70. In the absence of periodontal disease, the configurations of the crest of the interdental alveolar septa are determined by which of the following?

A. The relative positions of the contact points between teeth
B. The relative positions of the adjacent cementoenamel junctions
C. The relative positions of the heights of contour between adjacent teeth
D. None of the above

71. Which group listed below of the principle fibers of the periodontal ligament runs perpendicular from the alveolar bone to the cementum and resists lateral forces?

A. Alveolar crest
B. Horizontal
C. Oblique
D. Apical

72. The cemento- enamel junction (cervical line) of teeth curves in which two directions?

A. Towards the apex on the facial and lingual surfaces
B. Away from the apex on the facial and lingual surfaces

C. Towards the apex on the mesial and distal surface
D. Away from the apex on the mesial and distal surfaces

73. How many planes of movement can the mandible move in ?
A. One
B. Two
C. Three
D. Four

74. The connective tissue between the cementum of a tooth and the alveolar bone is called the
A. Gingival sulcus
B. Periodontal ligament
C. Periosteum
D. Pulp

75. All of the following are characteristics common to all mandibular anterior teeth, except:
A. Indistinct cingula with smooth lingual anatomy without grooves and pits
B. Incisal edges are lingual to the root axis line
C. The facial surfaces are marked by pronounced labial ridges
D. Continuous convexity inciso-apically on the facial surface

76. A maxillary right canine may be distinguished from a maxillary left canine because
A. The root always curves to the distal in the apical one-third.
B. The distal half of the canine shows more convexity than the mesial half.
C. **Labially**, the cusp tip is placed distal to a line which bisects the crown and root.
D. **Lingually,** the cervical line slopes mesially.

77. Of the two mandibular incisors, which has a root that is larger in all dimensions?
A. Mandibular central incisor
B. Mandibular lateral incisor
C. Both have equal roots
D. None of the above

78. Which cusp ridge listed below is longest on the permanent canines?
A. Labial

B. Lingual
C. Mesial
D. Distal

79. Which of the following is the fundamental morphologic unit of enamel?
A. Enamel tuft
B. Enamel spindle
C. Enamel rod
D. Enamel lamellae

80. All of the following statements are true, except:
A. The primary teeth are darker in color than the permanent teeth
B. The pulp cavities are proportionately large in the primary teeth
C. In general, the crowns of primary teeth are more bulbous and constricted than the permanent counterpart
D. The crown surface of all primary teeth are much smoother than the permanent teeth (in other words, there is less evidence of pits and grooves)

81. A sharply defined, shallow, linear depression formed during tooth development which usually separates the primary parts of the crown is called a:
A. Supplemental groove
B. Developmental groove
C. Transverse ridge
D. Triangular ridge

82. Any union of two triangular ridges produces a single ridge, which is called as:
A. A cusp ridge
B. A marginal ridge
C. A transverse ridge
D. A proximal ridge

83. Part of the free gingiva include all of the following except:
A. Gingival margin
B. Free gingival groove
C. Mucogingival junction
D. Gingival sulcus
E. Interdental (interproximal) gingiva

84. **Which tooth listed below is the smallest and the narrowest (mesial to distal) of all permanent teeth?**
   A. Mandibular central incisor
   B. Mandibular lateral incisor
   C. Maxillary central incisor
   D. Maxillary lateral incisor

85. **Which ligament below is the only one that gives direct support to the capsule of the TMJ?**
   A. Sphenomandibular ligament
   B. Stylohyoid ligament
   C. Stylomandibular ligament
   D. Temporomandibular ligament

86. **All of the following muscles are involved in elevating the mandible (closing the mouth), except:**
   A. Masseter muscles
   B. Medial pterygoid muscles
   C. Lateral pterygoid muscles
   D. Temporalis muscles

87. **Rotational movements take place in which compartment of the TMJ?**
   A. Upper (mandibular fossa-disc) compartment
   B. Lower (condyle-disc) compartment
   C. Both of the above
   D. None of the above

88. **Cervical line contours are closely related to the attachment of gingival at the neck of the tooth. The greatest contours of the cervical lines and gingival attachments occur on which of the following surfaces?**
   A. Distal surfaces of anterior teeth
   B. Distal surfaces of posterior teeth
   C. Mesial surfaces of anterior teeth
   D. Mesial surfaces of posterior teeth

89. **The permanent mandibular lateral incisor typically erupts around what age?**
   A. 5 Years old
   B. 7 Years old
   C. 10 Years old
   D. 12 Years old

90. The distal contact area of a permanent mandibular canine is usually located where?

A. Incisal third
B. Middle third
C. Junction of the incisal and middle third
D. None of the above

91. The tooth germ is composed of all the three structures listed below except?

A. Enamel organ
B. Dental sac
C. Dental papilla
D. Hertwig's epithelial root sheath

92. Which structure listed below is the first formed by the tooth germ and remains in evidence in the formed tooth?

A. Cemento-enamel junction (CEJ)
B. Dentino-enamel junction (DEJ)
C. Cemento-dentinal junction (CDJ)
D. Mucogingival junction (MGJ)

93. For every contact area there are how many embrasures?

A. One
B. Two
C. Three
D. Four

94. "Primate spaces" in the primary dentition are found in which two locations?

A. In the, maxillary arch, the primate space is located between the central incisors and lateral incisors
B. In the maxillary arch, the primate space is located between the lateral incisors and canines
C. In the mandibular arch, the primate space is located between the canines and first molars
D. In the mandibular arch, the primate space is located between the lateral incisors and canines

95. The temporomandibular joint is which type of joint?

A. Hinge joint
B. Gliding (sliding) joint
C. Combined hinge and gliding (sliding) joint
D. None of the above

96. Which of the following molars is the most symmetrical?
A. Maxillary second molar
B. Maxillary first molar
C. Mandibular first molar
D. Mandibular second molar

97. Which anterior tooth listed below is most likely to have a bifurcated root?
A. Maxillary central incisor
B. Mandibular canine
C. Mandibular incisor
D. Maxillary canine

98. How many root are visible from the buccal aspect of a maxillary first molar?
A. One roots
B. Two roots
C. Three roots
D. Four

99. A child with an anterior open bite of the moderate severity should be presumed to have what habit until proven otherwise?
A. Mouth breathing
B. Thumb sucking
C. Pencil biting
D. Night time milk drinking

100. Which tooth listed below has a mesial marginal ridge that is distinctly shorter in length and less prominent in height than the distal marginal ridge?
A. Maxillary first molar
B. Mandibular first premolar
C. Mandibular second premolar
D. Maxillary canine

101. Which premolar listed below is the only one that has a mesial buccal cusp ridge that is longer than its distal buccal cusp ridge?
A. Maxillary first premolar
B. Maxillary second premolar

C. Mandibular first premolar
D. Mandibular second premolar

102. All of the muscles are considered to be extrinsic muscles of the tongue except:
A. Genioglossus muscle
B. Longitudinal muscle
C. Hyoglossus muscle
D. Palatoglossus muscle

103. The surfaces of which teeth listed below have a trapezoid outline?
A. Lingual and labial of posterior teeth
B. Lingual and facial of all teeth
C. Proximal surfaces of anterior teeth
D. Proximal surfaces of all posterior teeth

104. All of the following are the theoretical determinants needed for restoring a complete and functional occlusal surface of a tooth except:
A. The amount of vertical overlap of the anterior teeth
B. The contour of the articular eminence
C. The amount and direction of lateral shift in the working side condyle
D. The position of the tooth in the arch
E. The height of the pulp horn of that particular tooth.

105. When posterior teeth are in a normal ideal relationship, which of the following cusps are considered to be supporting cusps?
A. Maxillary lingual cusps
B. Maxillary buccal cusps
C. Mandibular lingual cusps
D. Mandibular buccal cusps
E. All of the above

106. Which succedaneous teeth are usually the last to erupt?
A. Maxillary canines
B. Mandibular canines
C. Mandibular second premolars
D. None of the above

107. When the mandible is in its physiologic rest or postural position, contact of teeth is :
A. Maximum
B. Not present
C. Premature
D. Slight

108. Which of the following decreases with age in the dental pulp?
A. Number of collagen fibers
B. Number of reticulin fibers
C. The size of the pulp
D. Calcifications within the pulp

109. The permanent mandibular first molar has a morphology closely resembles which primary tooth listed below?
A. Primary mandibular first molar
B. Primary mandibular second molar
C. Primary maxillary first molar
D. None of the above

110. Which of the following encloses the TMJ like a tube?
A. Bowman's capsule
B. Crosby capsule
C. Fibrous capsule
D. Glisson's capsule

111. A diarthrodial joint is:
A. A joint that permits no movement at all
B. A joint that permits relatively free movement
C. Joint that permits slight movement
D. None of the above

112. Which permanent tooth listed below (other than the third molars) varies in form more than any other tooth?
A. Maxillary centrals
B. Mandibular centrals
C. Maxillary laterals
D. Mandibular lateral

113. Which tooth below may show three types of occlusal surfaces?
A. Maxillary first premolar
B. Mandibular second premolar

C. Mandibular first premolar
D. Maxillary second premolar

114. Which premolar listed below is usually the largest?
A. Maxillary first
B. Maxillary second
C. Mandibular first
D. Mandibular second

115. All of the following muscles are infrahyoid muscles, except the:
A. Thyrohyoid muscle
B. Sternohyoid muscle
C. Omohyoid muscle
D. Mylohyoid muscle
E. Sternothyroid muscle

116. Which of the following is a hereditary dental defect in which the enamel of the teeth is soft and undercalcified in context, yet of normal quantity?
A. Enamel hypoplasia
B. Enamel hypocalcification
C. Fluorosis
D. Enamel hypomaturation

117. Which muscle listed below plays a subsidiary role in mastication?
A. Masseter
B. Lateral pterygoid
C. Buccinator
D. Medial pterygoid
E. Temporalis

118. If a maxillary first molar has a fourth canal, it will be located where?
A. In the palatal root
B. In the distobuccal root
C. In the mesiobuccal root
D. In the distal furcation

119. The determinants of occlusion include
A. The right temporomandibular joint and its suspensory ligaments

B. The left temporomandibular joint and its suspensory ligaments
C. The occlusal surfaces of the teeth
D. The neuromuscular system
E. All of the above

120. In an ideal intercuspal position, the mesiolingual cusps of permanent mandibular molars oppose what?
A. The opposing central fossae
B. The lingual embrasure between their class counterpart and the tooth distal to it
C. The opposing distal marginal ridge
D. The lingual embrasure between their class counterpart and the tooth mesial to it

121. The periodontium includes
A. The gingiva
B. The periodontal ligament
C. The cementum
D. The alveolar and supporting bone
E. All of the above

122. All of the following anterior teeth have a cingulum which is located in the center of the lingual surface, except:
A. Maxillary lateral incisor
B. Mandibular canine
C. Maxillary canine
D. Mandibular central incisor

123. The permanent maxillary canine is most likely to occlude with which of the following mandibular teeth?
A. Lateral incisor and canine
B. Canine only
C. Canine and first premolar
D. First premolar only

124. When viewed from a buccal or lingual aspect the crowns of all mandibular and maxillary incisors appear to have a :
A. Triangular outline
B. Trapezoidal outline
C. Rhomboidal outline
D. Rectangular outline

125. Which of the following is the first deciduous (primary) tooth to erupt?
A. Mandibular central incisor
B. Mandibular first molar
C. Maxillary central incisor
D. Maxillary first molar

126. Which of the following is the hardest substance in the body?
A. Enamel
B. Dentin
C. Cementum
D. Bone

127. All of the following are the four distinct layers of the enamel organ except?
A. Outer enamel epithelium
B. Inner enamel epithelium
C. Stratum granulosum
D. Stratum intermedium
E. Stellate reticulum

128. Mamelons are found on newly erupting
A. Molars
B. Canines
C. Premolars
D. Incisors

129. Which ridge listed below is found only on maxillary molars?
A. Labial ridge
B. Marginal ridge
C. Oblique ridge
D. Transverse ridge

130. The periodontal ligament is made up of all of the following except:
A. Collagenous fibers
B. Nerves
C. Lymphatics
D. Blood vessels
E. Cartilages

131. The roots of all but one anterior are likely to have longitudinal grooves on the mesial and distal surfaces. Which tooth listed below doesn't have these grooves?
A. Maxillary canine
B. Maxillary lateral incisor
C. Maxillary central incisor
D. Mandibular lateral incisor

132. Which tooth listed below has a small DL cusp that can be absent, creating a three-cups tooth?
A. Mandibular second molar
B. Maxillary first molar
C. Mandibular first premolar
D. Maxillary second molar

133. A fissured groove is most frequently found on which surface listed below
A. Facial of maxillary molars
B. Lingual of maxillary molars
C. Facial of mandibular molars
D. Lingual of mandibular molars

134. During working side movement of the mandible, the oblique ridge of a maxillary first molar passes through which sulcus listed below of a permanent mandibular first molar?
A. Mesiobuccal sulcus
B. Distobuccal sulcus
C. Mesiolingual sulcus
D. Distolingual sulcus

135. The prime mover in effecting a left working-side movements is :
A. The right medial pterygoid muscle
B. The left medial pterygoid muscle
C. The right lateral pterygoid muscle
D. The left lateral pterygoid muscle

136. A patient with a paralyzed right lateral pterygoid muscle is instructed to open his mouth wide. Which direction will the mandible deviates to upon opening?
A. To the right
B. To the left

C. It will not deviate to right or left
D. None of the above

137. Which of the following terms refers to tooth contacts while the mandibular is in action, such as during mastication and swallowing?
A. Centric relation
B. Centric occlusion
C. Functional occlusion
D. Malocclusion

138. Which three mandibular teeth listed below are so aligned that when viewed from the occlusal, a straight line may be drawn that will bisect all contact areas?
A. Central incisor, lateral incisor and canine
B. Canine, first premolar and second premolar
C. Second premolar, first molar, and second molar
D. None of the above

139. A child 19 months old will have how many teeth?
A. Four
B. Eight
C. Twelve
D. Sixteen
E. Twenty

140. When viewed from the facial, all premolars have their contacts where?
A. Middle third
B. Junction of the occlusal and middle third
C. Occlusal third
D. Cervical third

141. Morphologically, the primary maxillary second molar strikingly resembles which permanent tooth listed below?
A. Permanent maxillary third molar
B. Permanent maxillary second molar
C. Permanent maxillary first molar
D. Permanent mandibular second molar

142. Which of the following is the first layer of dentin formed?
A. Mantle dentin
B. Peritubular dentin

C. Intertubular dentin
D. Interglobular dentin

143. A long depression or a V-shaped valley on the occlusal surface of a posterior tooth located between ridge and cusps is called a:
A. Pit
B. Sulcus
C. Fossa
D. Fissure

144. Which primary molar listed below is the most atypical of all the molars, primary and permanent and appears to be intermediate in form and development between a premolar and molar?
A. Primary mandibular first molar
B. Primary maxillary first molar
C. Primary mandibular second molar
D. Primary maxillary second molar

145. What is the term used to describe the triangularly shaped spaces located between the proximal surfaces of adjacent teeth?
A. A contact area
B. An occlusal curvature
C. A gingival space
D. An embrasure

146. The articular disc (meniscus) is a fibrous saddle-shaped structure that separates:
A. The condyle and the sphenoid bone
B. The condyle and the ethmoid bone
C. The condyle and the temporal bone
D. The condyle and the occipital bone

147. The cusp of Carabelli is often on which permanent tooth listed below?
A. Maxillary second molar
B. Maxillary first molar
C. Mandibular first molar
D. Mandibular second molar

148. Which tooth listed below has a mesial development depression?
A. Mandibular first premolar
B. Maxillary second premolar
C. Maxillary first premolar
D. Mandibular second premolar

149. The mental foramen is located most closely to the apex of which tooth listed below?
A. Mandibular canine
B. Mandibular second premolar
C. Mandibular first molar
D. Maxillary first premolar

150. The parotid duct opens on the oral surface of the cheek through a small opening opposite which tooth listed below?
A. Maxillary first premolar
B. Maxillary second molar
C. Mandibular first molar
D. Mandibular second molar

151. Which of the following is a developmental abnormality characterized by the total absence of teeth?
A. Hypodontia
B. Anodontia
C. Diphyodontia
D. Hypsodontia

152. All of the following are suprahyoid muscle, except the :
A. Geniohyoid muscle
B. Mylohyoid muscle
C. Stylohyoid muscle
D. Digastric muscle
E. Omohyoid muscle

153. Which of the following is a hereditary dental defect in which the enamel of the teeth is soft and undercalcified in context yet normal in quantity?
A. Enamel hypoplasia
B. Enamel hypocalcification
C. Fluorosis
D. None of the above

154. Which cusp listed below of the permanent maxillary first molar serves as a reference point in identifying Angle's Class I, II, and III occlusion?

A. Distobuccal
B. Distolingual
C. Mesiobuccal
D. Mesiolingual

155. The periodontal ligament fibers are anchored into cementum and bone by :

A. Gray fibers
B. Purkinje's fibers
C. Sharpey's fibers
D. Spindle fibers

156. Which structure listed below is the inner layer of cells of the junctional epithelium and attaches the gingiva to the tooth?

A. Mucogingival junction
B. Free gingival groove
C. Epithelial attachment
D. Gingival pocket

157. Which of the following provides the most common criterion for differentiating permanent mandibular central incisors from permanent mandibular lateral incisors?

A. Difference in root length
B. Difference in ratio of crown length to root length
C. Degree of slope of the incisal edge when viewed facially
D. Difference in rotation of the crown on the root

158. Which teeth listed below are the only ones have labial ridges?

A. Centrals
B. Laterals
C. Canines
D. Molars

159. The RCP is what type of the position?

A. Tooth guided
B. Ligament guided
C. Muscle guided
D. None of the above

160. The character of occlusal contacts in the unworn dental arch are all of the following except

A. Point-to –Point
B. Point-to-Area
C. Edge-to-edge
D. Edge-to-area
E. Area-to-area

161. A small elevation resulting from overproduction of enamel (enamel pearls) would be classified as what?

A. Cusp
B. Tubercle
C. Mamelon
D. Ridge

162. A pinpoint depression at the junction or terminus of grooves is called what?

A. Fossae
B. Fissure
C. Pit
D. Sulcus

163. In the intercuspal position, the distobuccal cusp of a permanent mandibular first molar occludes where?

A. The interproximal marginal ridge area between maxillary second bicusid and first molar
B. Central fossa of the maxillary first molar
C. Central fossa of the maxillary second molar
D. The interproximal marginal ridge area between maxillary first molar and second molar

164. In the intercuspal position, the mesiolingual cusp of permanent maxillary second molar occludes where?

A. Central fossa of the mandibular first molar
B. Central fossa of the mandibular second molar
C. The interproximal marginal ridge areas between mandibular second and third molars
D. The distal fossa of first molar

165. The axial surfaces of which teeth listed below have a rhomboid outline?

A. Buccal of mandibular posterior teeth

B. Buccal of maxillary posterior teeth
C. Lingual of maxillary posterior teeth
D. Mesial and distal of mandibular posterior teeth
E. Mesial and distal of maxillary posterior teeth

166. All teeth have how many line angles?
A. Two
B. Four
C. Six
D. Eight

167. The divergence of two proximal surfaces from the area of contact, facially, lingually, occlusally, and gingivally, creates a space, which is called as?
A. A contact area
B. A gingival space
C. An embrasure
D. An occlusal curvature

168. The primary first molar is usually exfoliated between what ages?
A. 6-8 years
B. 7-9 years
C. 10-12 years
D. 12-14 years

169. A primary centre of growth or calcification on a tooth is called what?
A. Lobe
B. Ridge
C. Cingulum
D. Groove

170. The interproximal space is a triangular area. The base and the sides of this triangle are represented by which of the following?
A. Buccal embrasure
B. Lingual
C. Alveolar bone
D. Proximal surfaces of the teeth
E. Occlusal embrasure

171. The height of contour are located where on the lingual surface of all maxillary molars?
A. Occlusal third
B. Middle third
C. Cervical third
D. None of the above

172. When viewed from the facial, all molars have their contacts where?
A. Middle third
B. Junction of the occlusal and middle third
C. Occlusal third
D. All of the above

173. Which of the following cusps are referred to as "stamp cusps"?
A. Maxillary lingual cusps
B. Maxillary buccal cusps
C. Mandibular lingual cusps
D. Mandibular buccal cusps

174. When posterior teeth are in normal ideal relationship, which of the following cusps are considered supporting cusps?
A. Maxillary lingual
B. Maxillary facial
C. Mandibular lingual
D. Mandibular facial

175. Which mandibular deciduous tooth does not resemble any permanent tooth?
A. Deciduous canine
B. Deciduous lateral
C. Deciduous first molar
D. Deciduous second molar

176. Which primary molar listed below is the most atypical of all the molars, primary and permanent, and appears to be intermediate in form and development between a premolar and a molar
A. Mandibular first primary molar
B. Maxillary first primary molar
C. Mandibular second primary molar
D. Maxillary second primary molar

177. Name two ridges which are present on all teeth.
A. Triangular ridges
B. Mesial and distal cusp ridges
C. Oblique ridge
D. Mesial and distal marginal ridges
E. Buccal ridge

178. The surfaces of which teeth listed below have a triangular outline?
A. Mesial and distal of anterior teeth
B. Mesial and distal of posterior maxillary teeth
C. Mesial and distal of posterior mandibular teeth
D. Labial of anterior teeth
E. Lingual of anterior teeth

179. Which of the following provides the most reliable criterion for differentiating permanent mandibular central incisors from permanent mandibular lateral incisors?
A. Difference in root length
B. Difference in ratio of crown length to root length
C. Degree of slope of the incisal edge when viewed facially
D. Difference in rotation of the crown on the root

180. The cingulum of most anterior teeth is located where?
A. In the centre of the lingual surface.
B. In the mesial portion of the lingual surface.
C. In the distal portion of the lingual surface.
D. Near the incisal edges of the teeth

181. Oversized anomalies are more common with which tooth listed below?
A. Maxillary third molar
B. Mandibular third molar
C. Maxillary premolars
D. Mandibular lateral incisors

182. The only anterior tooth which occasionally shows three developmental depressions on its labial surface is which of the following?
A. Maxillary central
B. Maxillary lateral
C. Maxillary cuspid

D. Mandibular cuspid
E. Mandibular lateral

183. Which of the premolars is usually the largest?
A. Maxillary first
B. Maxillary second
C. Mesial surface of anterior teeth
D. Mandibular second

184. A mesiolingual developmental groove is a positive ID for what tooth?
A. Maxillary first premolar
B. Mandibular first premolar
C. Maxillary second premolar
D. Mandibular second premolar

185. The region of the pulp that is relatively cell poor is called what?
A. Coronal pulp
B. Zone of Weil
C. Radicular pulp
D. Central zone

186. Lobes of teeth are usually separated by which of the following?
A. Depressions
B. Developmental grooves
C. Sulci
D. Depressions or developmental groove
E. Developmental groove or sulci

187. A linear elevation on the surface of a tooth is called what?
A. Incline
B. Prominence
C. Ridge
D. Tuberosity

188. The wearing away of the incisal or occlusal surfaces is referred to as?
A. Erosion
B. Attrition
C. Abrasion
D. Ablation

189. The largest embrasure associated with the adjacent teeth in contact is which of the following?
A. Occlusal
B. Labial
C. Lingual
D. Buccal

190. What is the minimum number of lobes from which any tooth may develop?
A. Two
B. Three
C. Four
D. Five

191. What is the percentages of dentin that is inorganic?
A. 2-5%
B. 10-15%
C. 20-30%
D. 50-60%
E. 70-80%

192. Give the name for the curve, which runs in a mesial-distal direction along the cusps of lower teeth?
A. Curve of Wilson
B. Curve of Spee
C. Curve of Monson
D. None of the above

193. The gingiva is normally attached to the tooth by what structure?
A. Frenum
B. Epithelial attachment
C. Free gingiva
D. Attached gingiva

194. Which of the following listed below gives rise to the cementum and the periodontal ligament?
A. Dental sac
B. Enamel reticulum
C. Dental papilla
D. Enamel organ

195. Which of these terms describes the tissue formed in response to irritational stimuli produced by carious or mechanical penetration of a tooth?
A. Primary dentin
B. Secondary dentin
C. Dead tracts
D. Sclerotic dentin

196. The primary function of the dental pulp is to:
A. Respond to irritation by its inflammatory reaction
B. Furnish nutrition to the tooth
C. Form dentin
D. Provide sensation

197. What is the fundamental morphological unit of enamel?
A. Enamel prism
B. Enamel tufts
C. Enamel spindles
D. Enamel lamellae

198. What is the percentage of water in fully development enamel?
A. 4%
B. 10%
C. 50%
D. 70%

199. A freely movable joint in which contiguous bony surfaces are covered by articular cartilage and connected by ligaments lined with synovial membrane is referred to as what type joint?
A. Amphi-arthroidal
B. Synarthroidal
C. Diarthroidal
D. None of the above

200. Of the choices listed below, one describes the boundaries that define the attached gingiva?
A. Form the gingival crest to the interdental groove
B. From the free gingival groove to the gingival crest
C. From the mucogingival junction to the free gingival groove
D. From the epithelial attachment to the cementoenamel junction

201. **Which tooth listed below has a mesial development depression?**
A. Mandibular first premolar
B. Maxillary second premolar
C. Maxillary first premolar
D. Mandibular second premolar

202. **When a mandibular movement to the left is performed, which condyle moves anteriorly, downward and medially, and also rotates at the same time?**
A. Working condyle (left)
B. Nonworking condyle (right)
C. Both the condyles
D. No movement at all as said above

203. **A patient with a paralyzed left genioglossus muscle is instructed to bring his tongue out. Which direction will be tongue take on opening?**
A. To the right
B. To the left
C. Straight
D. Downwards

204. **Constriction of the posterior fibers of the temporalis muscle results in what mandibular movement?**
A. Retrusion
B. Protrusion
C. Opening with translation
D. Closing

205. **The combined pull of the two lateral pterygoid muscles along with the anterior bellies of the two digastric and other suprahyoid muscles will result in what mandibular movement?**
A. Protrusion
B. Retrusion
C. Closing
D. Opening

206. **When the mandible is in its physiologic rest or postural position, contact of teeth is:**
A. Maximum

B. Not present
C. Premature
D. Slight

207. Which of the following will have a pulp chamber that will be triangular?
A. Permanent mandibular second premolar
B. Permanent mandibular molars
C. Permanent maxillary molars
D. Permanent maxillary lateral incisors

208. Occlusocervically, the height of the distal marginal ridge of a permanent maxillary first molar is at the same height as which of the following listed below?
A. Mesial marginal ridge of a maxillary second premolar
B. Mesial marginal ridge of a mandibular first molar
C. Mesial marginal ridge of a maxillary second molar
D. Distal marginal ridge of a maxillary second premolar

209. The permanent maxillary canine is most likely to occlude with which of the following mandibular teeth?
A. Lateral incisor and canine
B. Canine only
C. Canine and first premolar
D. First premolar and second premolar.

210. Which of the following muscles is the prime mover in effecting a right working movement?
A. Right lateral pterygoid
B. Right medial pterygoid
C. Left lateral pterygoid
D. Left medial pterygoid

211. Which position listed is one in which there is a relative muscular equilibrium?
A. Retruded contact position
B. Postural position
C. Protruded contact position
D. Intercuspal position

212. Which tooth below may show three types of occlusal surfaces?
A. Maxillary first premolar

B. Mandibular second premolar
C. Mandibular first premolar
D. Maxillary second premolar

213. Which of the following teeth has a mesial marginal ridge that is distinctly shorter in length and less prominent in height than the distal marginal ridge?
A. Maxillary first molar
B. Mandibular first premolar
C. Mandibular first molar
D. Maxillary first premolar

214. The smallest permanent tooth and the narrowest mesial to distal width, is which tooth?
A. Mandibular central incisor
B. Mandibular lateral incisor
C. Maxillary lateral incisor
D. Mandibular canine

215. The roots of all but one anterior tooth are likely to have longitudinal grooves on the mesial and distal surfaces, which tooth doesn't have these grooves?
A. Maxillary canine
B. Maxillary lateral incisor
C. Maxillary central incisor
D. Mandibular lateral incisor

216. A maxillary right canine may be distinguished from a maxillary left canine because:
A. The root always curves to the distal in the apical one-third
B. The distal half of the canine shows more convexity than the mesial half
C. Labially, the cusp tip is placed distal to a line which bisects the crown and root.
D. Lingually, the cervical line slopes mesially.

217. Pits in the occlusal surfaces of molars and premolars are at the junction of which of the following?
A. Marginal ridges and inclined planes
B. Inclined planes and cusp tips
C. Developmental grooves
D. Facial and mesial surfaces

218. The surface of a premolar or molar located within the marginal ridges which contact the corresponding surfaces of antagonists during closure of the posterior teeth is called what?

A. Occlusal table
B. Clinical crown
C. Occlusal surface
D. Height of contour

219. Which primary molar has a prominent transverse ridge that unites the mesiofacial and mesiolingual cusps?

A. First primary mandibular molar
B. Second primary mandibular molar
C. First primary maxillary molar
D. Second primary maxillary molar

220. Which teeth listed below should ideally provide the predominant guidance through the full range of movement in lateral mandibular excursions?

A. Premolars
B. First molars
C. Incisors
D. Canines

QUESTIONS FOR BRAIN DIET AND SELF ANSWERING

1. Listed below are the usual events in the histogenesis of a tooth. Place them in their correct sequence (from what happens first to what happens last).

A. Deposition of the first layer of dentin
B. Differentiation of odontoblasts
C. Deposition of the first layer of enamel
D. Elongation of the inner enamel epithelial cells

2. The axial surfaces of which teeth listed below have a rhomboid outline?

A. Mesial and distal of maxillary posterior teeth
B. Mesial and distal of mandibular posterior teeth
C. Lingual of maxillary posterior teeth
D. Buccal of maxillary posterior teeth
E. Buccal of mandibular posterior teeth

3. During typical empty mouth swallowing, the mandible is braced in what position to allow for proper stabilization?
4. What is the Bennett movement?
5. The vertical overlap of the maxillary incisors to the mandibular incisors is called what?
6. What is anterior guidance?
7. List four theoretical determinants needed for restoring a complete and functional occlusal surface of a tooth.
8. List the four features of the human dentition, which directly affect the health of the periodontal ligament and its hard tissue anchorage in term of resisting occlusal force?
9. Which are the basic principles for occlusal adjustment?
10. How does the maxillary alveolar bone differs from the mandibular bone?

Answer key to the dental anatomy

1	A	2	B	3	A	4	B
5	C	6	C	7	D	8	C
9	C	10	B	11	B	12	B
13	A	14	B, D	15	C	16	B
17	A	18	C	19	D	20	G
21	C	22	A	23	C	24	D
25	C	26	B	27	C	28	C
29	A	30	B	31	E	32	C
33	B	34	B, D, E	35	B	36	A
37	D	38	C	39	C	40	B
41	A	42	B	43	C	44	A
45	B	46	D	47	C	48	B
49	C	50	B	51	C	52	C
53	D	54	B	55	C	56	B
57	C	58	C	59	B	60	A
61	B	62	C	63	B	64	B
65	B	66	C	67	C	68	B
69	E	70	B	71	B	72	A
73	C	74	B	75	C	76	B
77	B	78	D	79	C	80	A
81	B	82	C	83	C	84	A
85	D	86	C	87	B	88	C

89	B	90	C	91	D	92	B
93	D	94	C	95	C	96	D
97	B	98	C	99	B	100	B
101	A	102	B	103	B	104	E
105	A, D	106	A	107	B	108	B, C
109	B	110	C	111	B	112	C
113	B	114	A	115	D	116	B
117	C	118	C	119	E	120	D
121	E	122	B	123	C	124	B
125	A	126	A	127	C	128	D
129	C	130	E	131	C	132	D
133	B	134	B	135	C	136	A
137	C	138	C	139	D	140	B
141	C	142	A	143	B	144	B
145	D	146	C	147	B	148	C
149	B	150	B	151	B	152	E
153	B	154	C	155	C	156	C
157	D	158	C	159	B	160	E
161	B	162	C	163	B	164	B
165	D	166	D	167	C	168	C
169	A	170	C	171	B	172	A
173	A, D	174	A	175	C	176	B
177	D	178	A	179	D	180	C
181	B	182	C	183	B	184	B
185	B	186	D	187	C	188	B
189	A	190	C	191	E	192	B
193	B	194	A	195	B	196	C
197	A	198	A	199	C	200	C
201	C	202	B	203	B	204	A
205	D	206	B	207	C	208	C
209	C	210	C	211	B	212	B
213	B	214	A	215	C	216	B
217	C	218	C	219	A	220	D

Reader's Notes

6

General Medicine

1. **Bilateral lower motor neurone facial palsy can be caused by:**
   A. Leprosy
   B. Mumps
   C. Sarcoidosis
   D. Tabes dorsalis

2. **During CPR, the effectiveness of cardiac massage is indicated by:**
   A. Increase in pulse rate more than 60 per minute
   B. Increase in pulsation in great veins
   C. Disappearance of cyanosis
   D. Pulsations appear and the constriction of pupil starts

3. **Parkinsonism can be indicated which of the following:**
   A. Lead pipe rigidity
   B. Positive Romberg's sign
   C. Loss of position sense
   D. Loss of fine touch

4. **A viral infection which responds to antibiotics is:**
   A. Chickenpox
   B. Lymphogranuloma venerum
   C. Measles
   D. Mumps

5. Which of the following is not seen in hyperaldosteronism:
A. ↑ Calcium
B. Hypertension
C. Hypokalemia
D. Polyuria

6. Which of the following is not a sex-linked disease:
A. Duchenne type myopathy
B. G-6-P D deficiency
C. Galactosemia
D. Hemophilia

7. All of the following can be seen in zinc deficiency except:
A. Acrodermatitis
B. Decreased wound healing
C. Goitre
D. Hypogonadism

8. Hyperkalemia is treated with:
A. Glucagon
B. Insulin
C. Corticosteroids
D. Ringer lactate

9. In resistant congestive heart failure, diuretic of choice is:
A. Triamterene
B. Spironolactone
C. Furosemide
D. Acetazolamide

10. Which of the following is true about HLA:
A. It can be changed with immunosuppresives
B. It is determined on neutrophils
C. It is not useful for determining paternity
D. It is useful to determine paternity

11. Treatment of ventricular fibrillation is:
A. Immediate electrical cardio-version
B. Intravenous digoxin
C. Intravenous propranolol
D. Intravenous soda bicarbonate

12. Left ventricular failure is indicated, if pulmonary artery wedge pressure exceeds:
A. 5 mm Hg
B. 10 mm Hg
C. 15 mm Hg
D. 20 mm Hg

13. Following is the most important factor in the management of shock:
A. Blood pressure
B. Cardiac output
C. CVP to 8 cm of water
D. Deficiency of effective circulating blood volume

14. SABE does not occur in:
A. ASD
B. Small VSD
C. Fallot's Tetralogy
D. Mitral valve prolapse.

15. Gram negative septic shock is most commonly due to infection of:
A. Biliary tract
B. Genitourinary tract
C. GIT
D. Respiratory tract

16. Which statement is true for staphylococcal pneumonia:
A. Common after viral infection
B. Interstitial long tissue involved
C. Multiple lung abscesses common
D. Resolution occurs without scar
E. Upper posterior lobe most often involved

17. Congenitally passed immunity is not observed with:
A. Chickenpox
B. Mumps
C. Poliomyelitis
D. Rubella
E. Whooping cough

18. Ideal treatment for thalassemia is:
A. Packed cells
B. Platelets
C. Washed cells
D. Whole blood

19. Chvostek' and Trousseau's signs positive and hyperreflexia denote the deficiency of:
A. Calcium
B. Magnesium
C. Potassium
D. Sodium

20. The following disease is most likely to cause syncope and angina in the same patient:
A. Ischemic Heart Disease
B. Aortic stenosis
C. Mitral valve prolapse
D. Vertebro-basilar artery insufficiency

21. K^+ depletion occurs is:
A. Addison's disease
B. Diarrhoea
C. Pheochromocytoma
D. Renal failure

22. Of the HLA, most significant is:
A. HLA—A
B. HLA—B
C. HLA—C
D. HLA—D

23. Hemiplegia is most often caused by thrombosis of:
A. Anterior cerebral artery
B. Basilar artery
C. Middle cerebral artery
D. Posterior cerebral artery

24. Marfan's Syndrome involves all of the following except:
A. Abnormalities of eyes
B. Long tapering fingers
C. Marked obesity
D. Dissecting aneurysm

25. Sturge-Weber syndrome is:
A. An outcome of bilateral temporal lobes ablation
B. A tumor of pituitary with gigantism
C. A sequela of head injury
D. Multiple angiomas over face, eyes and brain

26. Drug of choice in chronic myeloid leukaemia is:
A. Busulphan
B. Chlorambucil
C. Leukeran
D. Melphalan

27. The treatment of hypoxic hypoxia is:
A. Bronchodilators
B. Hyperbaric oxygen
C. Pure oxygen
D. Vasodilators

28. Most specific urinary finding in acute glomerulonephritis is:
A. Cellular (RBC's) casts
B. WBC's casts
C. Albuminuria
D. Serum creatinine

29. In thalassemia following are seen except:
A. Target cells
B. Mongoloid facies
C. ↑ Osmotic fragility
D. Microcytic hypochromic anemia

30. Which is not a feature of diabetic ketoacidosis:
A. Kussmauli's breathing
B. Ataxia
C. Tremors
D. Severe dehydration

31. HLA—DR 4 is marker of:
A. Rheumatoid arthritis
B. Sarcoidosis
C. Seronegative gouty arthritis
D. Psoriasis

32. Earliest symptom of myasthenia is:
A. Diplopia + ptosis
B. Fatigue
C. Respiratory weakness
D. Palatal palsy

33. Petecheal haemorrhages seen in the gums is due to the deficiency of:
A. Vitamin K
B. Ascorbic acid
C. Cholecalciferol
D. Nicotinic acid

34. Diabetic coma is caused by:
A. Ketosis
B. Hyperglycemia with hyper-osmolar ketosis
C. Hyperkalemia
D. Simple hyperglycemia

35. The skin pigmentation in bronze diabetes is due to:
A. Hemosiderin
B. Lipofuschin
C. Melanin
D. Ceroids

36. 'Kala Azar' is treated with compound of:
A. Gold
B. Bismuth
C. Antimony
D. Mercury

37. The following drug may lead to occurrence of Parkinsonism:
A. Bromocriptine
B. Levodopa
C. Methyl dopa
D. Carbidopa

38. Metabolic acidosis occur in:
A. Hyperaldosteronism
B. Excessive liquor ingestion
C. Milk - alkali syndrome
D. Diarrhoea

39. "Peu-de orange" may be seen in:
A. G-6-P-D deficiency
B. Alcoholism
C. Hurler's syndrome
D. Hunter's syndrome

40. "Casal's Necklace" and "Crazy pavement" is seen in"
A. Beri-Beri
B. Scabies
C. Pityriasis rosea
D. Pellagra

41. The vitamin contraindicated in therapy with levodopa is:'
A. B_2
B. Pyridoxine
C. Folic acid
D. Ascorbic acid

42. In metabolic acidosis, respiration is:
A. Deep and slow
B. Deep and sighing
C. Slow and superficial
D. Cheyne Stokes type

43. For excessive sweating, the intravenous fluid of choice is:
A. Dextrose saline
B. Ringer lactate
C. Dextran
D. Plasma

44. The worst complication of high altitude is:
A. Hypoxia
B. Pulmonary oedema
C. Polycythemia
D. Fits

45. The commonest cause of stroke in an elderly is:
A. Thrombosis
B. Embolism
C. Atrial fibrillation
D. Berry aneurysm rupture

46. Best treatment of diabetic ketoacidosis is:
A. 2 hourly insulin
B. 6 hourly insulin
C. Slow infusion with insulin
D. Large bolus of insulin subcutaneously

47. The commonest cause of pulmonary embolism:
A. Superficial cause of pulmonary embolism
B. Deep vein thrombosis
C. Pelvic vein thrombosis
D. Heart failure

48. Major criteria of rheumatic fever includes:
A. Erythema nodosum
B. Subcutaneous nodules
C. ↑ ASO titre
D. Fever

49. Sinus bradycardia is seen in:
A. Hypothyroidism
B. 1st degree block
C. Grave's disease
D. Adrenalectomy

50. 4th Heart sound is Heard in:
A. Early systole
B. Early diastole
C. Late systole
D. Late diastole

51. Enzyme raised within hours of MI & lasts 2-3 days is:
A. LDH
B. CPK
C. AST
D. ALT

52. In hypoparathyroidism:
A. Ionic Ca^{2+} levels are ↓
B. Kidney stones
C. Urinary Ca_2+ ↓
D. Total serum calcium is normal

53. All serum proteins are reduced in nephritic syndrome except:
A. Albumin
B. Transferrin
C. Ceruloplasmin
D. Fibrinogen

54. X - linked recessive disease is characterized by:
A. Vertical transmission
B. 50 % female carriers if male is affected
C. 50 % male affected if female is diseased
D. 50 % male carriers if female is diseased

55. Muscles not usually involved in polymyositis are:
A. Limb muscles
B. Ocular muscles
C. Pharyngeal muscles
D. Jaw muscles

56. Rx of choice in a case of acute MI with arrythmias is:
A. Procainamide
B. Lignocaine
C. Quinidin
D. Digoxin

57. Ectopic ACTH is most commonly produced by:
A. Lung carcinoma
B. Carcinoma breast
C. Ca prostate
D. Adrenal tumors

58. Myaesthenia gravis is associated with:
A. Hyperparathyroidism
B. Thymoma
C. Ca lung
D. Thyroid carcinoma

59. A negative Montoux test is of significance in one of the following conditions:
A. Pulmonary TB
B. Silicosis
C. Sarcoidosis .
D. Wegner's granulomatosis

60. All may be seen during fasting except:

A. Hypoglycemia
B. Hypercholesteroleamia
C. Hyperlipidemia
D. Keto acidosis

61. Rubella leads to following except:

A. PS pulmonary stenosis
B. ASD atrial septal defect
C. VSD ventricular septal defect
D. PDA patent ductus arteriosus

62. Following are the causes of microcytic hypochromic anemia except:

A. Iron deficiency
B. Thalassemia
C. Hypothyroidism
D. Sideroblastic anemia

63. Dawn phenomenon refers to:

A. Early morning hypoglycemia
B. Non-ketotic hypercalcaemia
C. After breakfast hypercalcaemia
D. Recurrent hypoglycemia

64. Exposure to nickel causes:

A. Ca lung
B. Ca nasopharynx
C. Ca ethmoid sinus
D. Ca larynx

65. Which muscle is most commonly involved in thyrotoxicosis:

A. Inferior rectus
B. Inferior oblique
C. Superior rectus
D. Superior oblique

66. Asthma mediator is a form of—

A. PGA_2
B. Prostacyclin
C. Leukotriene
D. Thromboxanes

67. Respiratory alkalosis occurs in:
A. Diabetic ketoacidosis
B. Pyloric stenosis
C. Primary aldosteronism
D. Excessive ventilatıon

68. Most common cause of hypercalcemic crisis is:
A. Parathyroid adenoma
B. CA Breast
C. Parathyroid hyperplasia
D. Pagets disease

69. A common cause of Cushing's syndrome is:
A. Pituitary adenoma
B. Ectopic ACTH productivity by CA
C. Adrenal Koch's
D. None of the above

70. The normal adult CSF pressure is:
A. 1-2 mm Hg
B. 6-12 mm Hg
C. 15-30 mm Hg
D. 735 mm Hg

71. Respiratory acidosis is characterized by:
A. ↓ plasma HCO3 and ↓ pCO_2
B. ↑pCO_2 and ↓ pH
C. ↓ pH and ↓ PCO_2
D. ↑pCO_2 and ↑ pH

72. Least common site for infective endocarditis:
A. ASD
B. VSD
C. Aortic Stenosis
D. Mitral stenosis

73. Autoimmune hemolytic anemia is most common in which type of Leukemia:
A. AML
B. CLL
C. Multiple myeloma
D. Sickle cell anemia

74. Perioral rash, gonadal atrophy, pigmentation in skin creases and neuritis are seen in deficiency of:
A. Zn
B. Mg
C. Selenium
D. Cobalt

75. Motor neuron disease is:
A. Involvement of anterior and lateral columns of spinal cord
B. Sensory involvement
C. Intellectual impairment
D. Ocular motility impaired

76. Commonest complication of mumps is:
A. Meningoencephalitis
B. Orchitis
C. Nerve deafness
D. Polyarthritis

77. Pulsus bisferiens is best felt in:
A. Carotid
B. Femoral
C. Radial
D. Brachial

78. Immediate treatment of peripheral circulatory failure in dengue shock syndrome is:
A. I/V high dose of dexamethasone
B. I/V crystalloid infusion
C. I/V dextrose saline
D. Dopamine + dobutamine

79. Least common site for vegetation is:
A. MS
B. AS
C. MR
D. ASD

80. Arterial blood gas analysis in carbon monoxide poisoning is:
A. PO_2 normal, O_2 saturation less
B. PO_2 less , O_2 saturation normal
C. PO_2, , O_2 saturation both decreased
D. PO_2, O_2 saturation both normal

81. Commonest chromosomal syndrome is:
A. Trisomy 13
B. Trisomy 17
C. Trisomy 21
D. Fragile x syndrome

82. What is the major change in blood vessels in hypertension:
A. Hyaline arteriosclerosis
B. Atherosclerosis
C. Multiple small aneurysms
D. Fibrinoid necrosis

83. Embolism of posterior cerebral artery leads to memory impairment because of damage to:
A. Hippocampal gyrus
B. Angular gyrus
C. Premarginal area
D. Superior temporal gyrus

84. Auto immune destruction of platelets seen in:
A. Rheumatoid arthritis
B. SLE
C. Reiter's disease
D. Polyarteritis nodosa

85. Bronchiectasis is commonest in:
A. Right middle lobe
B. Right upper lobe
C. Left lower lobe
D. Left upper lobe

86. Antihypertensive agent of choice in diabetic patient with proteinuria;
A. Enalapril
B. Clonidine
C. Alpha methyldopa
D. Propranolol

87. Endocarditis is commonest in:
A. MR
B. AS
C. Venous bypass graft
D. PDA

88. Diagnostic of RHD is:
A. Aschoff's nodule
B. MacCallum patch
C. Bread butter pericarditis
D. Shaggy vegetations

89. Tertiary parathyroidism is due to:
A. Autonomy in functioning
B. CRF
C. Adenoma
D. Malabsorption syndrome

90. Vitamin B_{12} deficiency causes:
A. Haemorrhage
B. CNS affected
C. Fits
D. Depression

91. In zinc deficiency, which of the following is not seen:
A. Acrodermatitis
B. Hypogonadism
C. Decreased wound healing
D. Goitre

92. Least common site for vegetation is:
A. MS
B. AS
C. MR
D. ASD

93. Endocarditis is commonest in:
A. MR
B. LDH
C. Venous bypass graft
D. PDA

94. Characteristic of Rheumatic / Infective endocarditis vegetations do not include:
A. Friable large vegetations on valve leaflets
B. Valve perforation
C. Myocardial absorption
D. LA thrombus

95. Region of spine most commonly affected in rheumatoid arthritis:
A. Cervical
B. Thoracic
C. Lumbar
D. Sacral

96. Which is not seen in myasthenia gravis:
A. Proximal involvement
B. ↑ In symptoms on exertion
C. Remissions occur
D. Absent DTR

97. Earliest sensation lost in diabetic neuropathy:
A. Pain
B. Temperature
C. Vibration
D. Weakness of small muscles of hand

98. Following are associated with malignancy except:
A. Down syndrome
B. Fragile X-syndrome
C. Bloom syndrome
D. Fanconi anemia

99. Acute attack of migraine is best abolished by:
A. Ergotamine
B. Sumitriptan
C. Propranolol
D. Amitriptyline

100. Alcohol damage is detected by:
A. GGT
B. SGOT
C. SGPT
D. Alk. Phosphatase

101. Weight gain is seen in following except:
A. Pheochromocytoma
B. Cushing syndrome
C. Hypothyroidism
D. Hypersecretion of insulin

102. Least common cause of infective endocarditis:
A. ASD
B. MVP
C. PDA
D. VSD

103. PCT proximal convoluteo tubular necrosis is seen in:
A. Phenol poisoning
B. Arsenic poisoning
C. Aconite poisoning
D. Lead poisoning

104. Most common presentation of primary Hyperparathyroidism is:
A. Gall stones
B. Subtle neurological and Psychiatric symptoms
C. Abdominal pain
D. Recurrent abortion

105. Most characteristic CNS lesion of HIV is:
A. Perivascular Giant cells
B. Vasculitis
C. Spongiform degeneration
D. Microglial nodules

106. Hypokalemia occurs in:
A. Meningitis
B. Hepatitis
C. Osteomyelitis
D. Bronchiolitis

107. Side effect of Zidovudine in AIDS patients is:
A. Megaloblastic anemia
B. Hyperuricemia
C. Nephrocalcinosis
D. Pancreatitis

108. Type I (IDDM) DM patient (42 years male) presenting with unilateral offensive discharge per nose. O / E, black mass is seen; the diagnosis is:
A. Inferior Turbinate atrophy
B. Mucormycosis
C. Midline lethal granuloma

D. Angiofibroma

109. To differentiate, proximal from distal renal tubular acidosis, what is used:

A. Urine pH
B. Urine aminoacids
C. Urine glucose
D. HCO_3 - levels

110. Interferon is not used in?

A. CML
B. Polymyositis
C. Hairy cell leukaemia
D. Chronic Hepatitis C infection

111. Hodgkin's lymphoma with best prognosis is:

A. Nodular sclerosing
B. Lymphocyte predominant
C. Lymphocyte depleted
D. Mixed cellularity

112. In nephritic syndrome, levels of following serum proteins decrease except:

A. Albumin
B. Fibrinogen
C. Transferrin
D. Ceruloplasmin

Answer key to general medicine

1	C	2	D	3	A	4	B
5	A	6	C	7	C	8	B
9	C	10	D	11	A	12	C
13	C	14	A	15	B	16	C
17	E	18	C	19	A	20	B
21	B	22	D	23	C	24	C
25	D	26	A	27	C	28	A
29	C	30	B	31	A	32	A
33	B	34	B	35	A	36	C
37	C	38	D	39	C	40	D
41	B	42	B	43	B	44	B
45	A	46	C	47	B	48	B
49	A	50	D	51	B	52	A
53	D	54	D	55	B	56	B
57	A	58	B	59	C	60	C
61	A	62	D	63	C	64	B
65	B	66	C	67	D	68	C
69	A	70	B	71	B	72	A
73	B	74	A	75	A	76	B
77	A	78	C	79	D	80	A
81	C	82	A	83	A	84	B
85	C	86	A	87	A	88	A
89	A	90	B	91	D	92	D
93	A	94	C	95	A	96	D
97	C	98	B	99	B	100	A
101	A	102	A	103	A	104	B
105	D	106	A	107	A	108	B
109	A	110	B	111	B	112	B

Reader's Notes

7

Oral Pathology

1. **Oral radiographs of a patient with scleroderma would show:**
   A. A "sun-ray" appearance of the bone
   B. An obscure lamina dura
   C. An abnormal widening of the periodontal ligament
   D. Vertical bone loss

2. **Which of the following soft tissue tumors is most likely to be found over the mental foramen in an edentulous patient?**
   A. Traumatic neuroma
   B. Neurilemoma (Schwannoma)
   C. Neurofibroma
   D. Neuroblastoma

3. **All of the following conditions demonstrate pigmentation of the intraoral mucous membranes except:**
   A. Addison's disease
   B. Albright syndrome
   C. Cushing syndrome
   D. Peutz-Jeghers syndrome

4. **Which cyst listed below is found in place of a tooth rather than directly associated with one?**
   A. Residual cyst
   B. Traumatic bone cyst

C. Primordial cyst
D. Periodontal cyst

5. **The etiology of verruciform xanthoma is:**
A. Bacterial
B. Viral
C. Fungal
D. Unknown

6. **All of the following are characteristics of Sjogren's syndrome except:**
A. Rheumatoid arthritis
B. Nephrosclerosis
C. Xerostomia (dry mouth)
D. Keratoconjunctivitis sicca (dryness of the eyes)

7. **Traumatic bone cysts are non-cysts often found in:**
A. Infants
B. Teenagers
C. Middle aged adults
D. Elderly people

8. **Which odontogenic tumor listed below has a high rate of recurrence if it is inadequately treated?**
A. Odonotogenic myxoma
B. Odontogenic fibroma
C. Squamous cell carcinoma
D. Pleomorphic adenoma

9. **Which of the following odontogenic cysts is always associated with the crown of an unerupted or developing tooth?**
A. Lateral periodontal cyst
B. Dentigerous cyst
C. Odontogenic keratocyst
D. Lateral Periodontal cyst

10. **The most common site in the oral cavity for a lymphangioma is the:**
A. Palate
B. Tonsils
C. Floor of the mouth
D. Tongue

11. The most common site for pyogenic granuloma to occur is:
A. The palate
B. The mucogingival junction
C. The interdental gingiva
D. The tongue

12. Which of the following tumors is also called the Pindborg tumor?
A. Adenomatoid odontogenic tumor
B. Calcifying epithelial odontogenic tumor
C. Squamous odontogenic tumor
D. Pleomorphic adenoma

13. The most frequently encountered intraoral benign neoplasm of connective tissue origin is:
A. A papilloma
B. A fibroma
C. A lipoma
D. A nodular melanoma

14. Which odontogenic tumor listed below usually affects males under the age of 25 years old?
A. Benign cementoblastoma
B. Gigantiform cementoma
C. Ameloblastoma
D. Squamous cell carcinoma

15. A dental granuloma and a radicular cyst can be differentiated:
A. Based on symptoms
B. Radiographically
C. Histologically
D. By an Electric Pulp Tester

16. The leukemic cells of more than 95% of patients having chronic myelogenous leukemia (CML) have a (an):
A. Missing chromosome
B. Extra chromosome
C. Philadelphia chromosome
D. New York chromosome

17. Which of the following is most often caused by retained foreign material (i.e., bone fragment etc.)?
A. Pyogenic granuloma
B. Pregnancy tumor
C. Epulis ganulomatosum
D. Fibroma

18. Which cyst listed below is extraosseous soft tissue cyst?
A. Median alveolar cyst
B. Globulomaxillary cyst
C. Nasiolabial cyst
D. Nasopalatine cyst

19. All of the statements concerning cherubism are true except:
A. It is an autosomal dominant inherited disease
B. The expansion of the jaw gives the children a very rounded face reminding one of cherubs in paintings
C. Histologically, the lesions bear a close resemblance to those seen in central giant cell granulomas
D. The treatment is radiation therapy

20. An enamel defect resulting from the incomplete formation of the enamel matrix is called:
A. Enamel pearls
B. Hypercementosis
C. Enamel hypoplasia
D. Dentinal dysplasia

21. The permanent mandibular lateral incisor typically erupts around what age?
A. 5 years old
B. 7 years old
C. 10 years old
D. 12 years old

22. The abnormal or pathological wearing away of tooth substance is referred to as:
A. Erosion
B. Attrition
C. Abrasion
D. Ablation

23. Which type of amelogenesis imperfecta is characterised by having enamel so soft that it can be removed during a prophylaxis?

A. Hypoplastic type
B. Hypocalcified type
C. Hypomaturation type
D. All of the above

24. Which of the following are characteristics of dentin dysplasia:

A. Normal enamel
B. Atypical dentin and Pulpal obliteration
C. Defective root formation
D. A tendency towards multiple periapical radiolucencies and early exfoliation of teeth
E. All of the above

25. All of the following can cause intrinsic staining of teeth except:

A. Dentinogenesis imperfecta
B. Erythroblastosis fetalis
C. Porphyria
D. Fluorosis
E. Diabetes mellitus
F. Pulpal injury
G. Internal resorption
H. Tetrcayclines

26. All of the following statements concerning benign mucous membrane pemphigoid are true except:

A. It is chronic, self-limiting, mucocutaneous disease
B. It is usually limited to the oral and ocular mucous membranes
C. It usually affects women under the age of 20
D. It is more common in the oral cavity than pemphigus, but is associated with much less morbidity and mortality

27. Mucoceles most frequently occur on the:

A. Upper lip
B. Palate
C. Lower lip
D. Gingiva

28. Which of the following infections is the one most likely to result in a chronic suppurative lesion about the jaws?

A. Actinomycosis
B. Blastomycosis
C. Histoplasmosis
D. Botryomycosis

29. The most common tumor of major and minor salivary glands is:

A. Basal cell adenoma
B. Sebaceous adenoma
C. Pleomorphic adenoma
D. Intraductal papilloma

30. The symptoms of hypothyroidism include all of the following except:

A. Feeling run down
B. Depression
C. Increased weight
D. Increased perspiration
E. Dryness and brittleness of hair
F. Dry and itchy skin
G. Constipation
H. Muscle cramps

31. Which of the following soft tissue tumors is mostly likely to be found on the tongue?

A. Traumatic neuroma
B. Neurilemmoma (Schwannoma)
C. Neurofibroma
D. None of the above

32. Which of the following are oral manifestations of patients with cerebral palsy?

A. They have a higher incidence of periodontal disease, caries, bruxism and malocclusion
B. They are prone to gingival hyperplasia if dilantin is used to control seizures
C. They are more susceptible to trauma, particularly to the maxillary anterior teeth
D. All of the above

33. A chronic condition characterized by extreme muscle weakness is called:
A. Myasthenia gravis
B. Myelofibrosis
C. Multiple sclerosis
D. Graves disease

34. Of the following types of the squamous cell carcinomas, which is the least common?
A. Squamous cell carcinoma of the palate
B. Squamous cell carcinoma of the nasopharynx
C. Squamous cell carcinoma of the oropharynx
D. Squamous cell carcinoma of the maxillary sinus

35. The most common site for necrotizing sialometaplasia is:
A. The soft plate
B. The buccal mucosa
C. The hard palate
D. The tongue

36. The peripheral giant cell granuloma always occurs on:
A. The buccal mucosa
B. The gingiva or the alveolar process
C. The lower lip
D. The palate

37. All of the following statements are true concerning Peutz-Jeghers syndrome except:
A. It is an inherited disorder, transmitted as an autosomal dominant trait
B. It is also called Hereditary Intestinal Polyposis Syndrome
C. Multiple intestinal polyps are usually distributed through the entire intestine, especially in the jejunum.
D. Melanin pigmentation of the lip and oral mucosa is usually present a birth.
E. The tongue almost invariably shows this melanin pigmentation
F. When this syndrome is suspected on the basis of oral pigmentations, other conditions to be considered in the differential diagnosis are Addison's disease and Albright's syndrome

38. Which of the following is a characteristic of malignancy?

A. Dysplasia
B. Anaplasia
C. Metaplasia
D. All of the above

39. Primary herpes is most common in:

A. Middle age adults
B. Elderly people
C. Children and young adults
D. Infants

40. The most common viral disease of salivary gland is :

A. Sialolithiasis
B. Mumps
C. Measles
D. Candidiasis

41. A five year-old lacks sweat and sebaceous gland. He has fine, sparse hair and exhibits heat intolerance. His radiographs do not reveal tooth buds of either the primary or permanent dentition. These findings are all consistent with:

A. Pierre Robin syndrome
B. Ectodermal dysplasia
C. Cleidocranial dysostosis
D. Cherubism

42. Which of the following are symptoms of acute fluoride poisoning?

A. Nausea and abdominal pain
B. Excessive salivation
C. Vomiting & Diarrhea
D. Convulsions
E. Hypotension
F. All of the above

43. All of the following statements concerning the peripheral ossifying fibroma are true except:

A. It is most common in elderly people .
B. It usually presents as a well-demarcated focal mass of hyperplastic tissue on the gingiva with sessile or pedunculated base.

C. It is usually the same color as normal mucosa or slightly reddened.
D. It may demonstrate bone radiographically and often demonstrates bone formation histologically

44. The oral traumatic neuroma usually appears as a small nodule or swelling of the mucosa typically:
A. Near the mental foramen
B. On the alveolar ridge in edentulous areas
C. On the lips
D. On the tongue
E. All of the above

45. Which form of ameloblastoma is the more aggressive one and requires more extensive treatment?
A. Solid (multicystic)
B. Unicystic
C. Extraosseous
D. All of the above

46. Which of the following is defined as a persistent velvety red patch that cannot be characterized clinically as any other condition?
A. Leukoedema
B. Psoriasis
C. Erythroplakia
D. White sponge nevus

47. Median rhomboid glossitis frequently affects:
A. Toddlers
B. Infants
C. Middle-aged adults
D. Teenagers

48. Which malignant salivary gland tumor listed below most often occurs in the minor salivary gland of the palate?
A. Adenoid cystic carcinoma
B. Mucoepidermoid carcinoma
C. Pleomorphic adenoma
D. None of the above

49. A persons with mucormycosis generally is treated with:

A. Penicillin
B. Erythromycin
C. Amphotericin B
D. Clindamycin

50. All of the following statements concerning syphilis are true excepts:

A. It is a sexually transmitted disease caused by a bacterium called Treponema palidum (a spirochete).
B. It occurs in 3 stage, viz. primary, secondary and tertiary.
C. First symptom of primary syphilis is chancre.
D. It is usually treated with tetracycline injections.

51. "Burning tongue syndrome" typically affects:

A. Children
B. Teenagers
C. Middle-aged females
D. Middle-aged males

52. All of the following statements concerning the central ossifying fibroma of bone are true except:

A. It is a slow-growing, painless, asymptomatic neoplasm which may occur in either jaw
B. It may occur at any age, but it is far more common in elderly people
C. The displacement of teeth may be an early clinical feature
D. Because of this slow growth, the cortical plates of bone and overlying mucosa and skin are almost always invariably intact.

53. A malignant tumor developing from bone marrow, usually in long bones or the pelvis of adolescent boys is called

A. Myeloma
B. Ewing's sarcoma
C. Osteogenic sarcoma
D. Multiple myeloma

54. A severe bullous form of erythema multiforme is known as:

A. Plummer- Vinson syndrome
B. Peutz- Jeghers syndrome
C. Gardener's syndrome
D. Stevens- Johnson syndrome

55. Which type of acquired nevi listed below is the most common variety seen in the oral cavity?
A. Intradermal Nevus
B. Compound nevus
C. Junctional nevus
D. Blue nevus
E. Intramucosal nevus

56. An acute condition characterized by pronounced leukopenia with a severe reduction in the number of polymorphonuclear leukocytes is called:
A. Infectious mononucleosis
B. Agranulocytosis
C. Sickle-cell anemia
D. Porphyria

57. Which virus listed below can cause herpes zoster lesions along sensory nerve roots in later life?
A. Pox virus
B. Epstein - Barr virus
C. Varicella virus
D. Mumps virus

58. The treatment of choice for Sjogren syndrome is:
A. Radiation
B. Surgical excision
C. Chemotherapy
D. None of the above

59. All ɔf the following are oral or para-oral presentations of herpes simplex except:
A. Acute herpetic gingivostomatitis
B. Herpes digitalis
C. Recurrent herpetic stomatitis
D. Herpes labialis

60. Cementomas (periapical cemental dyplasia) occur most frequently in the:
A. Mandible
B. Maxilla
C. Zygoma
D. Clavicle

61. Which of the following odontogenic tumors have a mixed origin (ectodermal- mesodermal) ?
A. Ameloblastic fibroma
B. Ameloblastic fibro-odontoma
C. Ameloblastic odontoma
D. All of the above

62. Which neoplasm listed below has strong evidence of a viral etiology?
A. Ewing's sarcoma
B. Burkitt's lymphoma
C. Liposarcoma
D. Osteoid osteoma

63. The central giant cell granuloma occurs predominantly in:
A. Infants
B. Children or young adults
C. Middle aged adults
D. Elderly people

64. Oral lesions are most likely to be observed in:
A. Myelogenous leukemia
B. Lymphocytic leukemia
C. Monocytic leukemia
D. Myelo-monocytic leukemia

65. An inability to absorb adequate amounts of vitamin B_{12} from the digestive tract may result in:
A. Thalassemia
B. Pernicious anemia
C. Aplastic anemia
D. None of the above

66. There is increasing evidence that Mikukicz's disease is closely related to:
A. Pierre-Robin syndrome
B. Sjogren's syndrome
C. Goltz-Gorlin syndrome
D. Apert syndrome

67. Recurrent aphthous ulcers:
A. Are caused by the Epstein-Barr virus
B. Are caused by the Herpes Simplex virus

C. Appear to be associated with stress
D. Are caused by a Poxvirus

68. Occlusal radiographs are useful in locating:
A. The hyoid bone
B. The mental foramen
C. Sialoliths in Wharton's duct
D. Sialoliths in Stensen's duct

69. A chronic skin disease that is characterized by the formation of vesicles and bullae is called:
A. Lichen planus
B. Candidiasis
C. White sponge nevus
D. Pemphigus

70. Hairy tongue is a condition characterized by hypertrophy of the:
A. Filiform papillae
B. Fungiform papillae
C. Circumvallate papillae
D. Foliate papillae

71. The characteristic lesion of erythema multiforme is:
A. Melanin pigmentation
B. A chancre
C. The "bull's-eye- shaped" lesion
D. A blister

72. A poorly differentiated squamous carcinoma involving lymphoid tissues in the region of the tonsils and nasopharynx is called:
A. A lipoma
B. A lymphoepithelioma
C. A lymphoma
D. A nasopharyngioma

73. The most common form of fibrous dysplasia is:
A. Monostotic
B. Polyostotic
C. Polyostotic with endocrine involvement (Albright's syndrome)
D. All of the above.

74. Which of the following is also known as Rendu-Osler-Weber disease?
A. Hereditary hemorrhagic telangiectasia
B. Encephalotrigeminal angiomatosis
C. Juvenile nasopharyngeal angiofibroma
D. Hereditary intestinal polyposis

75. All of the following statements are true concerning the aneurysmal bone cyst except:
A. It is an uncommon expansile osteolytic lesion of bone consisting of a proliferation of vascular tissue that forms a lining around blood filled cystic lesions
B. Most aneurysmal bone cysts occur in patients under 20 years of age, and it is uncommon after the age of 30
C. It commonly involves the jaws
D. The lesions are usually tender or painful particularly upon motion of the bone affected
E. Upon entering the lesion surgically, excessive bleeding is encountered

76. The most common form of malignant melanoma is
A. Superficial spreading
B. Nodular
C. Acrolentiginous
D. Lentigo maligna

77. Which type of a cancer listed below occurs most frequently in the oral cavity?
A. Basal cell carcinoma
B. Squamous cell carcinoma
C. Angiosarcoma
D. Pindborg tumor

78. The etiology of leukemia is:
A. Viral
B. Bacterial
C. Fungal
D. Unknown

79. An unusual phenomenon, with arises as a result of damage to the auriculotemporal nerve and subsequent reinnervation of the sweat glands by parasympathetic salivary fibers is called:
A. Postherpetic neuralgia

B. Orolingual paresthesia
C. Frey's syndrome
D. Glossopharyngeal neuralgia

80. The multiple endocrine neoplasia syndromes are a group of syndromes characterized by:
A. Tumors of the CNS
B. Tumors of the skin
C. Tumors of the various endocrine glands
D. Tumors of the salivary glands

81. A condition characterized by hemorrhages in the skin and mucous membranes that results in the appearance of purplish spots or patches is called:
A. Addison's disease
B. Purpura
C. Aplastic anemia
D. Hemophilia

82. Lateral clefting of the lip results from the failure of:
A. The maxillary processes to merge
B. The palatine processes to merge
C. The maxillary and frontonasal processes to merge
D. None of the above

83. A periapical abscess usually arises as a result of:
A. Orthodontics
B. Trauma
C. Infection of the pulp of a tooth
D. Periodontal disease

84. All of the following statements concerning eosinophilic granuloma are true except:
A. It tends to start between the age of 50 and 70
B. It affects males more than females
C. It usually affects the bones but also affects the lungs
D. Clinically, the lesions may present no physical signs or symptoms.

85. Which of the following terms refers to a small section of tissue that is removed for examination?
A. Excisional biopsy
B. Incisional biopsy

C. FNAC
D. Neither of the above

86. All of the following statements concerning craniofacial fibrous dysplasia are true except:
A. This condition frequently causes expansion and deformity of the jaw bones, as well as displacement of the teeth.
B. There is a characteristic thickening at the base of the skull, which can be seen radiographically.
C. Radiographically, the lesion is usually radiopaque, not well-circumscribed, and may have a "ground-glass" appearance.
D. The treatment of choice is radiation therapy
E. It is also referred to as "monostotic" fibrous dysplasia of the jaw

87. The most common site for carcinoma of the tongue is the:
A. Dorsum
B. Tip
C. Lateral border
D. Sulcus terminalis

88. A form of leukemia in which the abnormal cells are thought to be the precursors of lymphoblasts, myeloblasts, monoblasts is called:
A. Aleukemic leukemia
B. Subleukemic leukemia
C. Stem cell leukemia
D. None of the above

89. Excessive formation of cementum on the surface of the root is referred to as:
A. Cemental pearls
B. Hypercementosis
C. Secondary cementum
D. Condensing osteitis

90. The nevoid basal cell carcinoma syndrome may present which of the following abnormalities?
A. Cutaneous anomalies
B. Dental and osseous anomalies
C. Ophthalmologic abnormalities
D. Neurologic anomalies

E. Sexual abnormalities
F. All of the above

91. All of the statements concerning chronic leukemia are true except:
A. It has an abrupt onset
B. The skin is frequently involved in chronic leukemia and may manifest as petechiae or ecchymoses.
C. Massive splenomegaly is characteristic of chronic myelogenous leukemia.
D. Lymph node enlargement is the main pathologic finding in chronic lymphocytic leukemia

92. The term iatrogenic refers to:
A. A disease or condition of unknown cause or origin
B. A condition caused by medical personnel or procedures
C. A tissue or an organ transferred into a new position within the body of the same individual
D. Any of the above

93. All of the following statements concerning Addison's disease are true except:
A. It is a rare endocrine disorder which occurs when the adrenal glands do not produce enough cortisol.
B. It is sometimes called chronic adrenal insufficiency or hypocorticolism.
C. It most commonly affects teenagers
D. It afflicts men and women equally
E. It is characterized by weight loss, muscles weakness, low blood pressure, and darkening of the skin in both exposed and unexposed parts of the body.

94. After the initial primary attack during the early childhood period, the herpes simplex virus remains inactive most commonly in the
A. Geniculate ganglion
B. Ciliary ganglion
C. Trigeminal ganglion
D. Pterygopalatine ganglion

95. All of the following statements concerning developmental salivary gland defects are true except:
A. They are very common

B. They are asymptomatic
C. They are next to impossible to palpate manually
D. They are discovered only during radiographic examination of the area

96. All of the following statements concerning malignant melanoma are true except:
A. It is relatively benign form of skin cancer
B. Currently about 1 in 100 persons in the United States can except to develop this cancer in a lifetime.
C. Without treatment, it has the tendency to become widely metastatic and result in the demise of the patient
D. There are four general clinical types of melanoma i.e. superficial spreading, nodular acrolentiginous and lentigo maligna

97. Kaposi's sarcoma is an oral manifestation of:
A. Diabetes
B. Hypothyroidism
C. AIDS
D. Lichen planus

98. All of the following statements concerning amelogenesis imperfecta are true except:
A. It is an inherited condition which is transmitted as a dominant trait
B. It only effects the permanent teeth
C. It causes the enamel of the teeth to be soft and thin
D. The teeth appear yellow, because the dentin is visible through the thin enamel
E. The teeth are easily damaged and susceptible to decay

99. An incisional biopsy is indicated for which of the following lesions?
A. A 5 cm papillary fibroma of the gingiva
B. A 2 cm exostosis of the hard palate.
C. A 2 cm area of Fordyce's disease of the cheek
D. A 3 cm hemangioma of the tongue
E. A 3 cm area of leukoplakia of the soft palate

100. All of the following metabolic conditions are associated with chronic salivary gland enlargement except:
A. Diabetes mellitus

B. Chronic alcoholism
C. Malnutrition (including anorexia and bulimia)
D. Hypothyroidism

101. Which of the following is one of the most important substances that influences the rate of healing of wounds in the oral cavity?
A. Fat
B. Protein
C. Iron
D. Calcium

102. Actinic cheilitis is caused by:
A. A virus
B. Stress
C. Chronic and excessive exposure to the ultraviolet radiation in sunlight
D. Certain medications

103. Osteogenesis imperfecta is caused by a genetic defect that affects the body's production of:
A. Viamin K
B. Collagen
C. Reticulin
D. Elastin

104. All of the following statements concerning condensing osteitis are true except:
A. It most often occurs in young patients
B. The mandibular second molar is the tooth most commonly involved
C. It is most often seen associated with a long -standing periapical infection
D. There may be no signs or symptoms of the disease other than mild pain associated with an infected pulp.

105. Condylar hyperplasia is:
A. A common, bilateral enlargement of the condyle
B. A rare, bilateral enlargement of the condyle
C. A common, unilateral enlargement of the condyle
D. A rare, unilateral enlargement of the condyle

106. All of the following are characterized by granulomatous inflammation except:
A. Sarcoidosis
B. Tuberculosis
C. Pneumonia
D. Histoplasmosis
E. Tertiary syphilis

107. All of the following statements concerning an osteosarcoma are true except:
A. It is a malignant bone tumor composed of anaplastic tissue derived from mesenchyme.
B. Its peak incidence is after epiphyseal fusion, particularly the years between 50 and 60.
C. This tumor seems to arise in the long bones, which show the greatest longitudinal growth.
D. Joint involvement is rare

108. A severe hemolytic disease of the fetus / newborn caused by the production of maternal antibodies for fetal red blood cells is called:
A. Sickle- cell anemia
B. Erythroblastosis fetalis
C. Erythrocyanosis
D. Aplastic anemia

109. The fusion of the alveolar bone to a tooth is known as:
A. Hypercementosis
B. Gomphosis
C. Ankylosis
D. Gemination

110. In an OPG of a 14-year-old patient, a large radiolucent area on the left side of the mandible apical to the premolars and first molar is seen. No clinical symptoms are present. Teeth are not carious and respond normally to vitality tests. Medical history is unremarkable. Upon opening in to the area, no fluid or tissue is evident. What is the most probable diagnosis?
A. Dentigerous cyst
B. Traumatic bone cyst

C. Primordial cyst
D. Residual cyst

111. All of the following statements concerning polycythemia vera are true except:
A. It is characterized by excessive erythrocyte production
B. It usually occurs within the age range of 10-35, with 20 being the mean age of onset
C. Polycythemia vera is considered to be one of the chronic myeloproliferative disorders
D. Clinical features include headaches, weakness, weight loss, and pruritus
E. Hemorrhage and thrombosis may be evident at any time

112. A patient is observed to have a drooping mouth on one side and a watering eye. She complains of having a loss of taste sensation on the anterior portion of her tongue. This patient is most likely suffering from:
A. Cerebral palsy
B. Bell's palsy
C. Tic douloureux
D. Multiple sclerosis

113. When using the TNM method in assessing the prognosis and therapy of malignant neoplasms, the N represents:
A. The presence of Nikolsky's sign
B. The presence of nodules
C. The presence of regional lymph node involvement
D. The presence of erythroplakia.

114. All of the following statements concerning Plummer-Vinson syndrome are true except:
A. It is a rare disorder associated with severe and chronic iron-deficiency anemia
B. It occurs chiefly in adolescent teenagers
C. Systemic symptoms include weakness, pallor, difficulty in swallowing and difficulty in breathing
D. Oral symptoms include angular stomatitis and a smooth, red painful tongue with atrophy of the papillae

115. All of the following statements concerning acute leukemia are true except:

A. It has an insidious onset

B. Acute myelogenous leukemia is more common in adults

C. Acute Lymphocytic Leukemia is largely confined to children.

D. Symptoms include severe anemia, hemorrhages, and slight enlargement of the lymph nodes or the spleen

116. All of the following are histological characteristics of malignancy except:

A. Abnormal mitosis

B. Metaplasia

C. Pleomorphism

D. Hyperchromatism

E. Anaplasia

F. Increased nuclear-cytoplasmic ratio

117. The leukemic cells of more than 95% of patients having chronic myelogenous leukemia (CML) have a (an):

A. Missing chromosome

B. Extra chromosome

C. Philadelphia chromosome

D. New York chromosome

118. Benign migratory glossitis is also known as:

A. Fissured tongue

B. Macroglossia

C. Geographic tongue

D. Hairy tongue

119. The general characteristics listed below describe malignant neoplasm except ?

A. Invasion

B. Movable

C. Rapid growth

D. Metastasis

E. Not well- differentiated (or anaplastic)

120. All of the following cysts are congenital except:

A. Thyroglossal duct cyst

B. Branchiogenic cyst

C. Globulomaxillary cyst
D. Dermoid cyst

121. All of the following are dental manifestations of hypoparathyroidism except:
A. Delayed eruption of teeth
B. Small tooth crowns with short crown/root ratio
C. Blunted root apices
D. Enamel hypoplasia

122. All of the following statements concerning metastatic tumors of the jaws are true except:
A. They may be completely asymptomatic
B. The patient is usually aware of slight discomfort or pain
C. The maxilla is affected far more frequently than the mandible
D. The molar region is predominantly involved

123. All of the following diseases have traditionally been grouped under the generic term Histiocytosis X except:
A. Eosinophilic granuloma
B. Tay-Sachs disease
C. Hand Schuller-Christian disease
D. Letterer- Siwe disease

124. All of the following statements concerning verrucous carcinoma are true except:
A. It is rare form of squamous cell carcinoma that occurs in either the oral or laryngeal cavity
B. There is a characteristic whitish, cauliflower, or coral appearance to the mass
C. Typically, the lesion develops on the vocal cords of an elderly male who has been a heavy cigarette smoker
D. It is known for its slow growth pattern and well-developed hyperkeratotic epithelial boundaries
E. It usually shows rapid metastasis

125. A malignancy of plasma cells is called:
A. Histoplasmosis
B. Multiple myeloma
C. Osteomalacia
D. Amyloidosis

126. Oncocytomas are true tumors that may occur:
A. In the kidney
B. In the salivary glands
C. In endocrine gland
D. All of the above

127. Which of the following are thought to be predisposing factors to the development of angular cheilitis (perleche):
A. Intraoral infection by Candida albicans
B. Loss of intermaxillary distance (decreased vertical dimension)
C. Trauma to the commissure induced by prolonged dental treatment
D. Vitamin deficiencies (particularly riboflavin or thiamine)
E. All of the above

128. A condition that mimics leukoplakia in that it seems to be a white patch is called
A. Leukemia
B. Leukemoid
C. Leukoedema
D. Leukochloroma

129. The inflammation or infection of the bone marrow and adjacent bone is called
A. Osteopetrosis
B. Osteoporosis
C. Osteomyelitis
D. Osteonecrosis

130. Which type of hepatitis is also know as "Serum Hepatitis"?
A. Hepatitis A
B. Hepatitis B
C. Hepatitis AB
D. Hepatitis C

131. The cause of infectious mononucleosis is:
A. The pox virus
B. The Epstein- Barr virus
C. The rubella virus
D. The paramyxovirus

132. An uncommon hereditary disorder characterized principally by the overgrowth and denseness of bones is called:
A. Osteopetrosis
B. Osteogenesis imperfecta
C. Achondroplasia
D. Fibrous dysplasia

133. In the African form of Burkitt's lymphoma:
A. The patients are generally older than in the non- African form
B. The patients are generally younger than in the non-African form
C. There is no gender predilection
D. It presents most often as an abdominal mass

134. Mandibular tori most often appear:
A. In the retromolar pad region
B. On the lingual surface of the mandible, most often in the premolar region
C. On the lingual surface of the mandible, inferior to the mylohyoid ridge
D. Along the midline of the hard palate

135. Follicular and dentigerous cysts that contain keratinizing material are known as:
A. Residual cysts
B. Traumatic bone cysts
C. Keratocysts
D. Granulomas

136. In most cases, what is the proper treatment for an eruption cyst?
A. Incise and drain
B. Prescribe antibiotics
C. No treatment is necessary
D. Extract the tooth associated with the eruption cyst

137. Which of the following may occur at any age and presents as a single or multiple small, flat brown asymptomatic lesions occurring mostly on the lower lip?
A. Blue nevus

B. Compound nevus
C. Focal melanosis
D. Lipoma

138. The most common location for an intraoral congenital nevi (birthmark) is the
A. Buccal mucosa
B. Tongue
C. Hard palate
D. Alveolar mucosa

139. All of the following statements concerning acromegaly are true except:
A. It is a hormonal disorder that results when the pituitary gland produces excess ACTH.
B. It most commonly affects middle-aged adults and can result in serious illness and premature death.
C. Soft tissue swelling of the hands and feet is often an early feature, with patients noticing a change in ring or shoe size.
D. Gradually, body changes alter the patient's facial features (i.e., the brow and lower jaw protrude, the nasal bone enlarges ,and spacing of the teeth increases)

140. The erythrocyte sedimentation rate (ESR) is a nonspecific test that monitors
A. Bleeding rate
B. The progression of disease
C. Prothrombin time
D. Platelet function

141. The most common primary malignant tumor of bone is:
A. An osteosarcoma
B. A chondrosarcoma
C. Ewing's sarcoma
D. A myeloma

142. Which of the following types of skin cancer is considered to be the most severe?
A. Basal cell carcinoma
B. Squamous cell carcinoma
C. Malignant melanoma
D. Fibroma

143. All of the following cysts occur with in bone except:
A. The nasopalatine cyst
B. The median palatal cyst
C. The nasiolabial cyst
D. The globulomaxillary cyst

144. All of the following are characteristics of Gardner's syndrome except:
A. This syndrome is inherited in a dominant manner
B. Thousands of polyps develop in the colon, as well as the stomach and duodenum
C. This syndrome is also associated with bony tumors in the jaw and skull
D. The polyps rarely undergo malignant transformation

145. Xerostomia is caused by:
A. Sialadenitis
B. Sjogren's syndrome
C. Medications
D. Cancer therapy
E. Nerve damage
F. Conditions such as Alzheimer's disease or stroke, bone marrow transplants, endocrine disorders, stress, anxiety, depression and nutritional deficiencies
G. All of the above

146. An increased serum alkaline phosphatase level is clinically significant and aids in the diagnosis of
A. Hyperparathyroidism
B. Paget's disease of bone
C. Myasthenia gravis
D. Prostate cancer

147. Hypophosphatasia is one of several disorders that resembles:
A. Acromegaly
B. Paget' disease
C. Osteogenesis imperfecta
D. Ewing's sarcoma

148. Ludwig's angina refers to cellulitis of the floor of the mouth, in which the infection spreads to the:
A. Submental space

B. Sublingual space
C. Submandibular space
D. All of the above

149. All of the following statements concerning white sponge nevus are true except:
A. It is an autosomal dominant condition
B. It is also called familial white folded dysplasia
C. It is characterized by soft, white, or opalescent, thickened and corrugated folds of mucous membrane
D. The treatment for white sponge nevus is surgical excision and radiation

150. The most common form of recurrent aphthous stomatitis is:
A. Recurrent aphthous minor
B. Recurrent aphthous major
C. Recurrent herpetiform
D. Herpetic lesions

151. What is the most probable diagnosis for a lesion that presents as a translucent, bluish, well- rounded, smooth surfaced and protrudes from one side of the floor of the mouth?
A. A mucocele
B. Squamous cell carcinoma
C. A ranula
D. A lymphangioma

152. Which of the of the following cysts is most commonly found in relation to a developing third molar?
A. Lateral periodontal cysts
B. Dentigerous cyst
C. Fissural cyst
D. Primordial cyst
E. Traumatic cysts
F. Residual cyst
G. Gingival cyst

153. A developmental abnormality characterized by the total absence of teeth is called:
A. Hypodontia
B. Anodontia

C. Diphyodontia
D. Hypsodontia

154. Which of the following bone lesions is most likely to be fatal?
A. Osteochondroma
B. Paget's disease
C. Giant cell tumor
D. Multiple myeloma
E. Odontogenic myxoma

155. Which form of hepatitis is caused by an RNA enterovirus and is usually transmitted by the fecal - oral route?
A. Hepatitis A
B. Hepatitis B
C. Hepatitis C
D. Hepatitis E

156. The etiology of verruca vulgaris is:
A. Fungal
B. Bacterial
C. Viral
D. Parasitic

157. All of the following tests can be used to diagnose herpetic lesions except
A. The Tzanck smear
B. Fluorescent staining
C. An arthrogram
D. Isolation in tissue culture
E. Antibody titers
F. Biopsy

158. Which term listed below is a development defect characterized by an overgrowth of tissue not normal to the organ in which it arises?
A. Teratoma
B. Choristoma
C. Hamartoma
D. Lipoma

159. An acute infectious disease caused by a group a coxsackie virus is called:
A. Herpes zoster

B. Chickenpox
C. Herpangina
D. Herpes labialis

160. All of the following are clinical features of benign salivary gland tumors.except:
A. Mucosa is normal
B. Painless
C. Nodular
D. Movable
E. Fixed
F. Firm
G. Slow-growing

161. All of the followings statements concerning oral candidiasis are true except:
A. It is also called "thrush"
B. It is a bacterial infection of the mouth
C. It is most often caused by Candida albicans
D. The most common symptoms of oral candidiasis are discomfort and burning of the mouth and throat and an altered taste
E. Antibiotics prescribed for a dental infection may cause oral candidiasis

162. Warthin's tumor is almost exclusively seen in the:
A. Submandibular gland
B. Sublingual gland
C. Parotid gland
D. Minor salivary glands

163. All of the following statements concerning osteomalacia are true except:
A. Osteomalacia means hardening of the bones
B. The signs and symptoms include pain in the arm, legs, spine, and pelvis
C. It is the adult form of Rickets
D. One of the most common causes is a problem of fat malabsorption called steatorrhea.

164. The symptoms of hyperthyroidism include all of the following except:
A. Nervousness
B. Irritability
C. Increased perspiration
D. Constipation
E. Fine brittle hair
F. Muscular weakness
G. Weight loss despite a good appetite

165. All of the following cysts are developmental (or fissural except:
A. Nasopalatine cyst
B. Nasolabial cyst
C. Globulomaxillary cyst
D. Branchiogenic cyst
E. Median palatal cyst
F. Median alveolar cyst

166. Inflammatory papillary hyperplasia is found on the:
A. Soft palate
B. Buccal mucosa
C. Hard palate
D. Tongue

167. All of the following are clinical features of malignant salivary gland tumors except:
A. Mucosa is ulcerated
B. Painless
C. Nodular
D. Firm
E. Fixed
F. Rapid growth

168. A white patch on the oral mucosa that cannot be rubbed off and cannot be assigned to any other disease is most probably:
A. Candidiasis
B. Lichen planus
C. Leukoplakia
D. Erythroplakia

169. Acinic cell carcinoma is a malignant salivary gland tumor that is most likely to be associated with the:
A. Submandibular gland
B. Parotid gland
C. Sublingual gland
D. Minor gland of the palate

170. The term used to describe permanent incisors which may be characteristic of congenital syphilis is:
A. Blandi's incisors
B. Turner's incisors
C. Franklin's incisors
D. Hutchinson's incisors

Answer key to oral pathology

1	C	2	A	3	C	4	C
5	D	6	B	7	B	8	A
9	B	10	D	11	C	12	B
13	B	14	A	15	C	16	C
17	C	18	C	19	D	20	C
21	B	22	C	23	B	24	E
25	E	26	C	27	C	28	A
29	C	30	D	31	B	32	D
33	A	34	B	35	C	36	B
37	E	38	D	39	C	40	B
41	B	42	F	43	A	44	B
45	A	46	C	47	C	48	A
49	C	50	D	51	C	52	B
53	B	54	D	55	E	56	B
57	C	58	D	59	B	60	A
61	D	62	B	63	B	64	C
65	B	66	B	67	C	68	C
69	D	70	A	71	C	72	B
73	A	74	A	75	C	76	A
77	B	78	D	79	C	80	C
81	B	82	C	83	C	84	A
85	B	86	D	87	C	88	C
89	B	90	F	91	A	92	B

93	C	94	C	95	A	96	A
97	C	98	B	99	E	100	D
101	B	102	C	103	B	104	B
105	D	106	C	107	B	108	B
109	C	110	B	111	B	112	B
113	C	114	B	115	A	116	B
117	C	118	C	119	B	120	C
121	B	122	C	123	B	124	E
125	B	126	D	127	E	128	C
129	C	130	B	131	B	132	A
133	B	134	B	135	C	136	C
137	C	138	C	139	A	140	B
141	A	142	C	143	C	144	D
145	G	146	B	147	C	148	D
149	D	150	A	151	C	152	B
153	B	154	D	155	A	156	C*
157	C	158	B	159	C	160	E
161	B	162	C	163	A	164	D
165	D	166	C	167	B	168	C
169	B	170	D				

Reader's Notes

8

Periodontics

1. **The primary reason for splinting teeth is:**
   A. As a preventive measure
   B. For esthetics
   C. To immobilize excessively mobile teeth for patient comfort
   D. To aid a patient in home care

2. **All of the following are advantages of placing a periodontal dressing after surgical procedures except:**
   A. Protects the surgical wound
   B. Minimizes patient discomfort
   C. Enhances the healing rate to the tissues
   D. Helps maintain tissue placement
   E. Helps to prevent postoperative bleeding

3. **Which focal sign of acute inflammation listed below is caused by increased capillary permeability?**
   A. Redness (Rubor)
   B. Heat (Calor)
   C. Swelling (Tumor)
   D. Pain (Dolor)

4. **Which of the following vitamins functions in collagen formation?**
   A. B
   B. C
   C. D
   D. A

5. Most root amputations involve the:
A. Mandibular first and second premolars
B. Maxillary first and second molars
C. Maxillary canines
D. Maxillary and mandibular third molars

6. Which of the following are important factors that must be evaluated before performing a laterally repositioned flap?
A. The presence of bone on the facial surface of the donor tooth
B. The thickness of the gingiva at the donor site
C. The width of attached gingiva at the donor site
D. All of the above

7. Cervical line contours are closely related to the attachment of the gingiva at the neck of the tooth. The greatest contour of the cervical lines and gingival attachments occurs on
A. The distal surface of anterior teeth
B. The distal surface of posterior teeth
C. The mesial surface of anterior teeth
D. The mesial surface of posterior teeth

8. The alveolar process is that part of the maxilla and mandible that houses the teeth. It consists of two main parts. Which part is a thin layer of lamellar bone that surrounds the root to the tooth and is where the periodontal ligament fibers attach?
A. Alveolar bone proper
B. Supporting alveolar bone

9. The air syringe is used during scaling to locate the epithelial attachment. When the explorer is used to detect subgingival calculus it should be grasped firmly.
A. The first statement is true, the second is false
B. The first statement is false; the second is true
C. Both statements are true
D. Both statements are false

10. Which of the following are objectives of gingival curettage?
A. To eliminate or reduce inflammation (edema)
B. To remove chronically inflamed tissues
C. To reduce pocket depth and promote better tissue architecture
D. All of the above

11. The effectiveness of tooth brushing is best measured by:
A. The amount and location of plaque
B. The caries experience
C. The tooth brushing frequency
D. The condition of the toothbrush

12. Which of the following home care aids consists of a plastic handle that will receive round polished toothpicks and permits the patient to cleanse the teeth at gingival margins, where accessible, and in the areas of difficult access?
A. Dental floss
B. Perio Aid
C. Stim-U- Dent
D. Proxa brush

13. Which of the following is the main function of cementum?
A. Compensation for tooth wear
B. Reparative
C. To attach the principle fibers of the periodontal ligament to the tooth
D. Protection

14. When probing, the tip of the periodontal probe should always be kept in contact with the tooth. Four measurements are recorded for each tooth.
A. Both statements are true
B. Both statements are false
C. The first statement is true, the second is second is false
D. The first statement is false, the second is second is true

15. The characteristic cell components of chronic inflammation include all of the following except:
A. Lymphocytes
B. Plasma cell
C. Polymorphonuclear leukocytes
D. Macrophages

16. The acquired pellicle could become stained by all of the following except:
A. Chromogenic bacteria
B. Cariogenic bacteria

C. Food
D. Chemicals

17. The main goal of osseous recontouring (surgery) is:
A. To cure periodontal disease
B. To eliminate the existing microflora
C. To eliminate periodontal pockets
D. To change the existing microflora

18. Which graft listed below is one in which the transplant is connective tissue without an epithelial covering?
A. Free gingival graft
B. Free mucosal autograft
C. Neither of the above
D. Both of the above

19. The narrowest band of attached gingiva is found:
A. On the lingual surfaces of maxillary incisors and the facial surfaces of maxillary first molars
B. On the facial surfaces of mandibular second bicuspids and the lingual surface of canines
C. On the facial surfaces of the mandibular canines and first bicuspids and the lingual surfaces of the mandibular incisors
D. None of the above

20. Parts of the free gingiva include all of the following except:
A. Gingival margin
B. Free gingival groove
C. Mucogingival junction
D. Gingival sulcus
E. Interdental (interproximal) gingiva

21. What should be done if a patient experience sensitivity while being scaled with an ultrasonic scaling device?
A. Proceed to another tooth and often return to the sensitive tooth later in the appointment
B. Make necessary adjustments to the water spray
C. Use less pressure
D. All of the above

22. Which of the following instruments is best for performing root planing procedures?
A. An ultrasonic instrument

B. A hoe
C. A periodontal curette
D. Periodontal files

23. Periodontal disease in multiple sites in patients who continue to demonstrate attachment loss after apparently appropriate periodontal treatment is referred to as?
A. Gingivitis
B. Localized juvenile periodontitis
C. Refractory periodontitis
D. Rapidly progressive periodontitis

24. In a healthy sulcus, which bacteria below are most abundant?
A. Actinobacillus actinomycetemcomitans and Bacteroides forsythus
B. Streptococcus species and Actinomyces species
C. Treponema species and Capnocytophaga species
D. Prevotella intermedia and Prophyromonas gingivalis

25. Water irrigation devices have been shown to:
A. Produce a transient bacteremia in patients with gingival inflammation
B. Stimulate a new epithelial attachment
C. Remove acquired tooth pellicle
D. Cause no harm to the gingival tissues

26. Which of the following brushing techniques emphasizes placing the bristles of the toothbrush at a 45° angle on the tooth and pointing apically so that the bristles enter the gingival sulcus?
A. Charter's technique
B. Stillman technique
C. Roll technique
D. Bass technique (Sulcular)

27. All of the following will reduce the abrasive action of a polishing agent except?
A. Using an agent with nice large particles
B. Using an agent containing particles that are dull and round
C. Applying the polishing agent with firm pressure and increasing to a heavy constant pressure
D. Polishing at a low speed with light pressure

28. All of the following are indications for the use of an apically respositioned flap except:
A. Moderate or deep pockets
B. Patients at risk for root caries
C. Furcation -involved teeth
D. Crown Lengthening

29. Which cells listed below are the first ones to emigrate into gingival sulcus as a result of inflammation in the initial lesion of gingivitis?
A. Mast cells
B. Lymphocytes
C. Polymorphonuclear neutrophils PMNS's
D. Plasma cells

30. The most common clinical sign of occlusal trauma is:
A. Caries
B. Migration of teeth
C. Periodontal disease
D. Tooth mobility

31. Which of the following conditions predisposes a patient to the development of inflammatory periodontal disease or exacerbation of an existing disease?
A. Pregnancy
B. Neutropenia
C. Agranulocytosis
D. Leukemias
E. All of the above

32. A variation of the laterally repositioned flap is called
A. A coronally repositioned flap
B. A double papilla flap
C. Apically repositioned flap
E. Nine of the above

33. Which group listed below of the principal fibers of the periodontal ligament runs perpendicular from the alveolar bone to the cementum and resists lateral forces?
A. Alveolar crest
B. Horizontal crest
C. Oblique

D. Apical
E. Interradicular

34. Of the choices listed below, which one describes the boundaries that define the attached gingiva?
A. From the gingival margin to the interdental groove
B. From the free gingival groove to the gingival margin
C. From the mucogingival junction to the free gingival groove
D. From the epithelial attachment to the cementoenamel junction

35. Which of the following are indications for the use of ultrasonic scaling devices?
A. Supragingival calculus removal
B. Subgingival debridement
C. Initial debridement of a patient with ANUG
D. Gross scaling prior to extractions
E. Removal of orthodontic cement, bonding material, and overhanging restorations
F. All of the above

36. Name the type of curettage that is performed when the soft tissue wall of a pocket is removed by the offset cutting edge of a curet during a root planing procedure.
A. Non-definitive curettage
B. Coincidental curettage
C. Closed sub gingival curettage
D. Open sub gingival curettage

37. The most accepted theory as to the cause of root sensitivity is the
A. Baeyer's theory
B. Chemo-isosmotic theory
C. Hydrodynamic theory
D. Quantum theory

38. Which of the following is a constituent of gram-negative microogranisms and has been suggested as an important agent in the pathogenesis of inflammatory periodontal disease?
A. Exotoxin
B. Endotoxin
C. Plaque
D. Carbohydrates

39. Pseudopocketing is a condition in which pocketing occurs without:
A. Bleeding
B. Exudate
C. Attachment loss
D. Inflammation

40. Which of the following is a condition in which there is expansion of the marginal tissue coronally rather than an apical movement of the epithelial attachment?
A. The periodontal pocket
B. The gingival pocket
C. An infrabony pocket
D. All of the above

41. Which of the following refers to an excessive occlusal force being applied to a tooth or teeth with normal supporting structures (no periodontal disease)?
A. Primary occlusal trauma
B. Secondary occlusal trauma
C. Tertiary occlusal trauma
D. None of the above

42. What should be done if the periodontal probe comes into contact with an obstacle once it has been inserted into the gingival sulcus
A. Remove the probe and then reinsert it in another area
B. Push the probe beyond the obstacle
C. Attempt the move past the obstacle and then continue to move the probe apically
D. Record the measurement where the probe stopped
E. Remove the probe and reinsert a much thinner one.

43. A modified Widman flap is:
A. A partial - thickness flap
B. A full - thickness flap
C. An epithelial graft
D. None of the above

44. All of the following statements concerning B cells are true, except:
A. They mature in the bone marrow and migrate to lymphoid organs

B. They are found in the germinal centers of the spleen and lymph nodes
C. They are progenitors of plasma cells
D. Are involved in humoral (antibody-mediated) and cell-mediated immunity
E. They function to search out, identify, and bind with specific antigens

45. There are various distal flap approaches used for retromolar reduction. The simplest is the:
A. Gingivectomy
B. Gingivoplasty
C. Distal wedge
D. None of the above

46. When measuring the pocket depth with a periodontal probe it may not stop at the bottom or base of the pocket. How far it reaches will depend on which of the following factors?
A. Size of the probe
B. The force exerted
C. The dimensions of the pocket
D. Access to the pocket
E. Degree to the pocket
F. The presence of deposits
G. The accuracy of the examiner in reading the probed measurements
H. All of the above

47. The periodontal ligament is composed primary of:
A. Elastic fibers
B. Reticulin fibers
C. Collagen fibers
D. Spindle fibers

48. Which of the following cells may be found in the periodontal ligament?
A. Fibroblasts
B. Osteoblasts
C. Cementoblasts
D. Macrophages
E. All of the above

49. Which of the following are possible uses of the periodontal file?
A. Calculus removal where access is limited
B. Incision placement
C. Final smoothing of the tooth surface
D. Curettage

50. Which of the following is most significant in regard to the prognosis of a periodontally involved tooth?
A. Pocket depth
B. Attachment loss
C. Anatomical crown length
D. Bleeding upon probing

51. Which of the following is a progressive proliferation of the gingiva, particularly the collagenous elements?
A. Inflammatory gingival enlargement
B. Hereditary gingivofibromatosis
C. Both of the above
D. Neither of the above

52. All of the following statements concerning calculus are true, except:
A. It is calcified or mineralized bacterial plaque
B. It forms on natural teeth, dentures and other dental prostheses
C. The surface is very rough and is covered by a layer of bacterial plaque
D. Inorganic material makes up about 10-15% of the composition while organic material and water make up about 70-90% of the composition
E. Its main role in periodontal disease is to serve as a collection site for more bacteria

53. Which of the following is the key etiologic agent in initiation of gingivitis and periodontal diseases?
A. Calculus
B. Plaque
C. Tooth brush abrasion
D. Saliva

54. All of the following types of oral mucosa are nonkeratinized except.
A. Buccal mucosa
B. Inferior surface of the tongue
C. The soft palate
D. The hard palate
E. Floor of the mouth

55. The free gingival graft is most commonly used for which purpose listed below
A. To halt gingival recession
B. For crown lengthening
C. To increase the width of gingiva either on the facial or lingual surfaces of the teeth
D. None of the above

56. Which of the following has been shown to be the most effective antimicrobial agent for reducing plaque and gingivitis long-term?
A. Stannous fluoride
B. Phenolic compounds
C. Chlorhexidine
D. Quaternary ammonium compounds

57. The junctional epithelium in health is:
A. A collar-like band of stratified columnar epithelium 2-5 cells thick near the sulcus and 1-2 cells thick at the apical end
B. A collar-like band of stratified squamous epithelium 10-20 cells thick near the sulcus and 2-3 cells thick at the apical end
C. A collar-like band of simple columnar epithelium 5-10 cells thick near the sulcus and 20-25 cells thick at the apical end
D. A collar-like band of pseudostratified columnar epithelium 2-5 cells thick near the sulcus and 10-15 cells thick at the apical end

58. Which of the following signs and symptoms are typical of a perioendo abscess?
A. Radiographic involvement of the periodontium and periapex
B. Significant probing depths
C. Percussion sensitivity
D. Pulpal sensitivity
E. All of the above

59. Which surgical procedure below is directed towards reshaping the gingiva and papilla of a tooth for correction of deformities and to provide the gingiva with normal and functional form?

A. Gingivoplasty
B. Gingivectomy
C. Free mucosal graft
D. None of the above

60. How should a periodontal probe be adapted in an interproximal area?

A. It should be parallel to the long axis of the tooth at the point angle
B. It should be parallel to the long axis of the tooth at the contact area
C. It should touch the contact area the tip should angle slightly beneath and beyond the contact area
D. It should be perpendicular to the long axis of the tooth, in front of the contact area

61. The periodontal ligament fibers are anchored into cementum and bone by

A. Purkinje's fibers
B. Sharpey's fibers
C. Spindle fibers
D. Gray fibers

62. Surrounding each tooth is a specialized epithelium known as

A. Connective tissue attachment
B. Periodontal ligament attachment
C. Junctional epithelium
D. Nasmyth's membrane

63. How an instrument shank is designed influences the intended use of the instrument. It is recommended that an instrument with a rigid shank be used for removal of heavy calculus deposits.

A. Both statements are true
B. Both statement are false
C. The first is true, the second is false
D. The first is false, the second is true

64. While scaling subgingivally, the tip of the curet breaks off. All of the following are appropriate actions to take to try and remove this tip, except:
A. Use a push stroke to force the tip out of the sulcus
B. Gently examine the gingival sulcus
C. Take a periapical radiograph of the area
D. Place the patient in an upright position

65. In health, the crest of the alveolar bone lies at a level approximately
A. 3-4 mm below the level of the CEJ's of adjacent teeth
B. 1-2 mm below the level of the CEJ's of adjacent teeth
C. 4-5 mm above the level of the CEJ's of adjacent teeth
D. 2-3 mm above the level of the CEJ's of adjacent teeth

66. Which of the following needs to be evident in order to make a diagnosis of periodontitis?
A. Bleeding
B. Pocket depths of 5 mm or more
C. Radiographic evidence of bone loss
D. A change in tissue color and tone

67. All of the following are considered to be the basic principles of flap management except:
A. Conserve the attached gingiva so that after healing there is adequate width of gingiva
B. Make the flap uniformly thick so that it is not very flexible and can be easily sutured to place
C. Avoid flap necrosis (by avoiding desiccation or maltreating the flap or injuring the blood supply)
D. Design the flap sufficiently long and deep to permit it to be retracted fully and with ease
E. Avoid excessive use of relieving incisions coupled with narrow two- three-or four- toot flaps

68. Which of the following etiologic factors is the most common cause of gingival recession?
A. Gingival inflammation
B. Tooth brush injury (abrasion)
C. Faulty tooth alignment
D. Anatomic abnormalities
E. Deleterious habits

69. All of the following statements concerning the periodontal ligament are true, except:

A. It is highly vascular and cellular connective tissue that surrounds the roots of the teeth and bridges the cementum with the alveolar bone

B. It is shaped like an hour glass with the narrowest portion at the middle of the root

C. The average thickness in the adult is 2.0 mm and it increases with age

D. It acts as a cushion by ameliorating the impact of the forces generated during mastication on the alveolar bone.

70. Infrabony pockets (or defects) are generally classified by:

A. The number of bony walls that were destroyed by periodontal disease

B. The number of bony walls left surrounding the tooth

C. The number of bony walls that will remain after surgery

D. Periodontal probe readings

71. Which of the following is the objective of instrument sharpening ?

A. To produce a "wire edge" on the cutting edge

B. To sharpen infrequently to extend the life of the instrument

C. To produce a sharp cutting edge without changing the original design of the instrument

D. To round the cutting edge slightly to prevent tissue trauma

72. Which of the following is true of hoes:

A. They are not designed for removal of heavy calculus

B. It is impossible to adapt them to curved tooth surfaces

C. They are only able to be adapted to facial mesial surfaces

D. Sharpening is not possible

73. The frequency of maintenance visits for a patient who has had pervious periodontal treatment should be dependent upon which factor listed below?

A. On whether or not the patient feels that frequent visits will help maintain his/her periodontium.

B. On the appearance and clinical condition of the gingival tissues.

C. On the amount of attachment loss prior to the periodontal treatment.

D. On the presence of inadequate amount of plaque.

74. Which of the following is the most common error when performing periodontal probing?
A. Using the wrong type probe
B. Incorrectly reading the periodontal probe
C. Excessively angling the probe when inserting it interproximally beyond the long axis of the tooth
D. Forgetting to also probe the lingual of every tooth

75. Gingival change evident during pregnancy probably result from the effect of which of the following?
A. Estrogen
B. Progesterone
C. Histamine
D. None of the above

76. What is guided tissue regeneration?
A. A soft tissue graft used to correct mucogingival junction involvement
B. Placement of a membrane (such as Gore-Tex) over a bony defect
C. A free gingival graft used to increase the amount of attached gingiva
D. Placement of an autograft to treat a bony defect

77. Which of the following is the main objective of root planing?
A. To remove chronically inflamed tissues
B. To change the bacterial microflora
C. To prove optimally smooth root surfaces
D. To eliminate pockets

78. When extensive scaling and root planing must be performed, the best approach would be
A. A series of appointments set up to scale and root plane a segment or quadrant of teeth at a time (thoroughly and completely)
B. Gross debridement (sub and supragingival) of the entire mouth, following by a series of appointments for fine scaling and polishing

79. Which of the following is the primary purpose of a night guard that is worn for the treatment of periodontal trauma?
A. To stabilize the dentition

B. To provide patient comfort
C. To modify the nature of the habit (bruxism) or redirect the forces into non-traumatic pattern
D. To act as a splint after periodontal surgery

80. A bone grafting procedure is least likely to be successful in a:
A. One-walled defect
B. Two-walled defect
C. Three-walled defect
D. Through - and - through furcation defect

81. All of the following are goals that a clinician strives to attain by performing flap procedures except:
A. Pocket elimination
B. Regrowth of alveolar bone and reattachment of connective tissue at more coronal levels
C. To cure periodontal disease
D. Establishment or retention of gingival of adequate width
E. Establishment of an adequate soft and hard tissue contour

82. Bruxism is a pathologic manifestation of:
A. Erosion
B. Abrasion
C. Attrition
D. Resorption

83. Which immunoglobulin listed below is most abundant in the gingival exudate common in gingivitis:?
A. IgA
B. IgG
C. IgD
D. IgE

84. The primary reason for the failure of a free gingival graft is:
A. Infection
B. Edema
C. Disruption of the vascular supply before engraftment
D. None of the above

85. Which group of gingival fibers listed below resist rotational forces that are applied to a tooth?
A. Transseptal fibers

B. Dentogingival fibers
C. Alveologingival fibers
D. Circumferential fibers
E. Dentoperiosteal fibers

86. The periodontium includes:
A. The gingiva
B. The periodontal ligament
C. The cementum
D. The alveolar and supporting bone
E. All of the above

87. Which of the following cells participates in the early phase of inflammation for example, the early lesion of gingivitis?
A. Eosinophils
B. Kupffer's cells
C. Mast cells
D. Epithelioid cells

88. All of the following are examples of an endogenous intrinsic stain except?
A. Tobacco stain
B. Tetracycline
C. Amelogenesis imperfecta
D. Systemic fluoride

89. Which of the following are specific contraindications to the selection of gingival curettage as a definitive surgical procedure?
A. Gingival tissues that are firm and fibrotic
B. When the lateral gingival wall is extremely thin
C. Wide or tortuous infrabony pockets
D. In bi- and trifurcation involvement
E. All of the above

90. All of the following bacteria have been found to be the chief periodontal pathogens except:
A. Prophyromonas gingivalis
B. Bacteroides forsythus
C. Eubacterium
D. Campylobacter rectus

91. The normal, healthy mouth consists mainly of:
A. Obligate anaerobes
B. Facultative anaerobes
C. Acidogenic bacteria
D. All of the above

92. Bone destruction in the furcation has been such that a probe can be passed through the furcation from the buccal to the lingual and vice versa . This furcation involvement would be classified as
A. Type I
B. Type II
C. Type III
D. None of the above.

93. Which of the following are contraindications to selective grinding in the natural dentition?
A. When pulp chambers are large
B. In the presence of tooth sensitivity
C. When major occlusal discrepancies may require orthodontics or reconstruction
D. In patients who are poor candidates for full month reconstruction because of psychologic factors
E. All of the above

94. Toothbrush trauma (abrasion) usually occurs on which teeth listed below?
A. Centrals and laterals
B. Canines and premolars
C. Second and third molars
D. First and second molars

95. In acute gingivitis:
A. Gram-negative anaerobic organisms predominate
B. Gram-negative aerobic organisms predominate
C. Gram-positive organisms predominate
D. Spirochetes predominate

96. Which factor below has been shown to be a prime etiologic factor in inflammatory periodontal disease?
A. Open or loose contacts
B. Food impaction

C. Calculus
D. Poorly designed fitting prosthesis

97. Young plaque is dominated by:
A. Gram-positive cocci
B. Gram-positive rods
C. Gram-negative rods
D. Filaments

98. Which of the following statements are true concerning supragingival and subgingival plaque?
A. Subgingival plaque is attached or loosely adherent; supragingival plaque is attached or tooth associated
B. Subgingival plaque is dominated by gram-negative rods; supragingival plaque is dominated by gram-positive cocci
C. Subgingival plaque has more anaerobes than supragingival plaque
D. All of the above statements are true concerning supragingival and subgingival plaque

99. What is the term used to describe a stain which originates from a source outside the tooth and remains on the exterior surface of the tooth?
A. Exogenous intrinsic
B. Endogenous extrinsic
C. Exogenous extrinsic
D. Endogenous intrinsic

100. All corners of a periodontal flap should be:
A. Sharp
B. Rounded
C. It doesn't matter whether the corners of a periodontal flap are sharp or rounded
D. None of the above

101. Gingival fibers are found within the:
A. Attached gingiva
B. Free gingiva
C. Mucogingival junction
D. Attached and free gingiva

102. Which of the following instruments are designed primarily for the removal of subgingival calculus deposits in all tooth surfaces?

A. Gracey curets
B. Universal curets
C. Chisel scalers
D. Sickle scalers

103. All of these bacteria have been found to be the principal bacteria associated with acute necrotizing ulcerative gingivitis (ANUG) except?

A. Prevotella intermedia
B. Spirochetes
C. Fusobacterium species
D. Porphyromonas gingivalis

104. Which of the following are clinical criteria used for diagnosing gingivitis?

A. Color of gingiva
B. Contour of gingiva
C. Size of gingiva
D. Bacterial plaque and calculus
E. All of the above

105. The base of the pocket (epithelial attachment) is coronal to the crest of the alveolar bone in a?

A. Infrabony pocket
B. Suprabony pocket
C. Both of the above
D. Neither of the above

106. When evaluating an osseous defect, the only way to determine the number of walls left surrounding the tooth is by:

A. Periodontal probing
B. Radiographs
C. Exploratory surgery
D. Testing for mobility

107. Which of the following is the best way to distinguish between a periodontal abscess and a periapical (pulpal) lesion?

A. Radiograph
B. Pulp testing

C. Hot and cold tests
D. Asking the patient the nature of the pain

108. The most important aspect of Phase I (initial therapy) of periodontal treatment planning is:
A. Extraction of hopeless teeth
B. Oral Hygiene Instructions
C. Occlusal adjustment
D. Splinting

109. The reshaping or recontouring of nonsupportive bone is called:
A. Ostectomy
B. Osteoplasty
C. both of the above
D. None of the above

110. The vascular phase of acute inflammation involves all of the following cells except:
A. Platelets
B. Tissue mast cells
C. Eosinophils
D. Basophils

111. Which of the following describe how an ultrasonic scaling device removes calculus deposits:
A. Blunt, shearing action of the tip
B. Vibratory action of the tip
C. Pressure of the water
D. High frequency sound

112. Which structure listed below is the inner layer of cells of the junctional epithelium and attaches the gingiva to the tooth?
A. Mucogingival junction
B. Free gingival groove
C. Epithelial attachment
D. Gingival pocket

113. All of the following statements are true concerning desquamative gingivitis, except:
A. It is a chronic gingival disease characterized by erythematous erosive, vesiculobullous and /or desquamative involvement of the free and attached gingiva

B. The majority of patients are males between the age of 20 and 30
C. While many diseases and conditions have been associated with this gingival disease, the majority are dermatologic
D. Topical corticosteroids (Triamcinolone, e.g., kenalog in Orabase) are effective in treating the oral lesions

114. An exploratory stroke is used to remove calculus. A waling stroke is utilized during periodontal probing.
A. Both statements are true
B. Both statements are false
C. The first statement is true, the second is false
D. The first statement is false, the second is true

115. Which of the following are considered to be pedicle grafts?
A. Apically repositioned flaps
B. Laterally repositioned flaps
C. Coronally repositioned flaps
D. All of the above

116. Which type of cementum is found on the apical third of the root?
A. Cellular
B. Acellular

117. Which statement below is true?
A. Periodontitis is the same as gingivitis
B. Periodontitis usually does not begin as gingivitis
C. Periodontitis always begins as gingivitis
D. All of the above.

118. All of the following bacteria have been found to be the principle bacteria associated with juvenile periodontitis, except:
A. Actinobacillus actiomycetemcomitans (AA)
B. Capnocytophaga species
C. Wolinella recta
D. Prevotella intermedia
E. Eikenella corrodens

119. All of the following bacteria have been found to be principle bacteria associated with rapidly progressive periodontitis, except:
A. Porphyromonas gingivalis

B. Actinobacillus actinomycetemcomitans (AA)
C. Capnocytophaga species
D. Prevotella intermedia
E. Fusobacterium nucleatum
F. Eikenella corrodens
G. Campylobacter rectus

120. All of the following statement concerning bacterial plaque are true, except:

A. It is the key etiologic agent in the initiation of gingivitis and periodontal disease
B. It is an accumulation of a mixed bacterial community in a dextran matrix
C. It forms on a cleaned tooth within minutes
D. It is composed of solids (80%; 95% of which are bacteria) and water (20%)
E. There are two categories: supragingival and subgingival plaque
F. Different bacteria may be found in plaque (cocci, rods and filaments) and their proportions change with time, diet and location.

Answer key to periodontics

1	C	2	C	3	C	4	B
5	B	6	D	7	C	8	A
9	D	10	D	11	A	12	B
13	C	14	C	15	C	16	B
17	C	18	B	19	C	20	C
21	D	22	C	23	C	24	B
25	A	26	D	27	A	28	B
29	C	30	D	31	E	32	B
33	B	34	C	35	F	36	B
37	C	38	B	39	C	40	B
41	A	42	C	43	B	44	D
45	C	46	H	47	C	48	E
49	A	50	B	51	B	52	D
53	B	54	D	55	C	56	C
57	B	58	E	59	A	60	C
61	B	62	C	63	A	64	A
65	B	66	C	67	B	68	B
69	C	70	B	71	C	72	B
73	B	74	C	75	B	76	B
77	C	78	A	79	C	80	D
81	C	82	C	83	B	84	C
85	D	86	E	87	C	88	A
89	E	90	B	91	D	92	C
93	E	94	B	95	C	96	C
97	A	98	D	99	C	100	B
101	B	102	B	103	D	104	E
105	B	106	C	107	B	108	B
109	B	110	C	111	B	112	C
113	B	114	D	115	D	116	A
117	C	118	C	119	C	120	D

Reader's Notes

9

Orthodontics, Pedodontics and Endodontics

1. **Which of the following is most important to the orthodontist with regard to the time treatment should begin?**
   A. The chronologic age of the patient
   B. The physiologic age of the patient
   C. Dental age of the patient
   D. None of the above

2. **Continuous heavy orthodontic forces may cause:**
   A. The PDL to become crushed
   B. Resorption of cementum
   C. Resorption of the alveolar bone
   D. All of the above

3. **Which cusp listed below of the maxillary first permanent molar serves as a reference point in identifying Angle's Class I, II and III occlusions?**
   A. Distobuccal
   B. Mesiobuccal
   C. Mesiolingual
   D. Distolingual

4. Which space maintainer is most often used when the primary first molar needs to be prematurely extracted?

A. "Band and loop" space maintainer
B. "Distal shoe" space maintainer
C. "Lingual arch" appliance
D. "Nance" appliance

5. A child with a pulpally involved primary tooth comes into your office. Which of the following ideally is the best space maintainer for this child?

A. A "band and loop" space maintainer
B. A "distal shoe" space maintainer
C. The pulpally involved primary tooth
D. A "lingual arch" space maintainer

6. Displacement of a tooth from the socket in the direction of eruption is referred to as:

A. Tipping
B. Translation
C. Extrusion
D. Intrusion
E. Torque
F. Rotation

7. Which of the following determines the effect of a facebow headgear on the molars to which it is attached?

A. The relation of the outer bow to the center of resistance of the tooth
B. The direction of pull of the headgear strap
C. The length and position of the outer bow in relation to the inner bow
D. All of the above

8. Serial extraction procedures involve:

A. The orderly removal of selected permanent teeth only in a predetermined sequence
B. The orderly removal of selected primary teeth only in a predetermined sequence
C. The orderly removal of selected primary and permanent teeth in a predetermined sequence
D. The orderly removal of selected wisdom teeth only

9. Which appliance listed below is probably the most widely used today by orthodontists?
A. The universal appliance
B. The edgewise appliance
C. Begg's appliance
D. Removal appliance
E. Neither of the above

10. Which of the following alloys are used for archwires in orthodontics?
A. Stainless steel
B. Chromium-cobalt
C. Nickle—Titanium
D. All of the above

11. Which of the following are common characteristics of a Class II, Division 2 malocclusion?
A. The maxillary centrals are near normal anteroposteriorly or slightly in linguoversion
B. The maxillary lateral incisors are usually labiomesially flared and overlap the central incisors
C. Impinging overbite
D. All of the above

12. Conditions that may complicate molar uprighting include:
A. A high mandibular plane and open bite
B. Poor crown-to-root ratio and/or short roots
C. A severe lingual inclination of the tooth in addition to the mesial tipping
D. Occlusal plane disharmony (i.e. extruded maxillary and mandibular molars)
E. All of the above

13. A seven year old child with an otherwise good occlusion has a lingually locked maxillary permanent central incisor. There is sufficient overbite. What should be done?
A. Wait until all permanent teeth have erupted
B. Surgically reposition the central incisor
C. Correct the condition immediately with a simple appliance
D. None of the above

14. A diastema between erupting permanent maxillary incisors may indicate which of the following?
A. A normal stage of development before eruption of canines
B. It may be related to tooth size discrepancy or a mesiodens
C. It may indicate an abnormal frenum attachment
D. All of the above

15. A steep mandibular plane angle correlates with a:
A. Short anterior facial vertical dimensions and anterior open bite malocclusion
B. Long anterior facial vertical dimensions and anterior open bite malocclusion
C. Short anterior facial vertical dimensions and anterior deep bite malocclusion
D. Long anterior facial vertical dimensions and anterior deep bite malocclusion

16. A 13-year old patient has all teeth present and normal occlusion, molar root apices are not totally closed. The mandibular left first molar has been extracted. The ideal treatment at this time is what?
A. Place a fixed bridge
B. Place a space maintainer
C. Place a removable partial denture
D. Do nothing and observe

17. In a young child, which structure listed below grows in height and length to accommodate the developing dentition?
A. The tuberosity
B. The ramus
C. The condyles
D. The alveolar process

18. Class III malocclusion is also referred to as:
A. Retrognathism
B. Prognathism
C. Proclination
D. Neither of the above

19. A severe malocclusion may compromise which of the following aspects of oral function?
A. Mastication

B. Sw·llowing
C. Speech
D. All of the above

20. Displaced teeth related to functional shifts are usually seen in which two of the following circumstances?
A. Posterior crossbite after prolonged thumb sucking
B. Class II, Division I malocclusion
C. Anterior crossbite in mildly prognathic children
D. An anterior open bite after prolonged thumb sucking

21. An appropriate candidate for post-orthodontic circumferential supracrestal fibrotomy is:
A. An intruded mandibular second molar
B. A rotated maxillary lateral incisor
C. An extruded maxillary second premolar
D. A mandibular first molar that is in crossbite

22. The flat bones of the skull and part of the clavicle are formed by:
A. Intramembranous ossification
B. Endochondral ossification
C. Erythropoiesis
D. Epiphyseal formation

23. Relative to the primary mandibular canines, the permanent mandibular canines erupt:
A. Lingually
B. Facially
C. Distally
D. Mesially

24. Class I malocclusions share what basic characteristic?
A. The midface is concave
B. A harmonious skeletal profile
C. The midface is convex
D. None of the above

25. Which of the following are uses of cephalometrics in orthodontics?
A. Diagnosis
B. Analysis of treatment results

C. Longitudinal study of growth
D. All of the above

26. An anterior crossbite in the primary dentition is often indicative of which two of the following?
A. Impacted permanent maxillary canines
B. A skeletal growth problem
C. A developing Class II malocclusion
D. A developing Class III malocclusion

27. Bone deposition in which region listed below is responsible for the lengthening of the maxillary arch?
A. Palate
B. Tuberosity
C. Incisor
D. Zygomatic

28. In which direction do the permanent teeth move during eruption?
A. Mesially and occlusally
B. Occlusally and buccally
C. Buccally and mesially
D. Occlusally and lingually

29. Malocclusion is most often:
A. Acquired from a friend
B. Hereditary
C. Caused by antibiotics
D. Caused by bad habits

30. Ectopic eruption of a permanent maxillary first molar is frequently treated by:
A. Disking the distal of the primary first molar
B. An appliance incorporating a finger spring to move the primary second molar mesially
C. A brass wire placed between the primary second molar and permanent first molar
D. Extraction of the primary second molar

31. Which of the following statements are true concerning a mixed dentition analysis?
A. It is used to predict the amount of crowding after the permanent teeth come in

B. It is performed during the mixed dentition
C. It is performed with a boley gauge, study models and prediction table
D. All of the above statements are true

32. Which of the following is the most common removable retainer used in orthodontics?
A. Tooth positioner
B. Hawley retainer
C. Functional retainer
D. Anterior spring retainer

33. All of the following are fixed orthodontic appliances except:
A. Lingual archwire
B. Palate-separating devices
C. Lip bumpers
D. Edgewise mechanisms
E. Light-wire appliances

34. Which of the following is the best method for tipping proximally maxillary and mandibular anterior teeth?
A. Finger springs
B. Z-springs
C. Canine retractors
D. All are equally efficient

35. Class II malocclusion is also referred to as:
A. Retrognathism
B. Prognathism
C. Both of the above
D. Neither of the above

36. A major site of growth of the mandible is the:
A. Angle
B. Condyle
C. Ramus
D. Chin

37. Which of the following are true concerning a posterior crossbite in the mixed dentition?
A. It should be corrected as soon as possible
B. It should be thoroughly diagnosed as to whether it is of a dental, functional or skeletal origin

C. May be corrected with palatal expansion
D. May be associated with a mandibular shift
E. All of the above are true

38. "Primate spaces" in the primary dentition are found in which two locations?
A. In the maxillary arch, the primate space is located between the central incisors and lateral incisors
B. In the maxillary arch, the primate space is located between the lateral incisors and canines
C. In the mandibular arch, the primate space is located between the canines and first molars
D. In the mandibular arch, the primate space is located the lateral incisors and canines

39. In most Class II, Division I malocclusions, the body of the mandible and its superimposed dental arch are in a:
A. Mesial relationship to the maxilla and the maxillary incisors are usually in a labial axial inclination
B. Distal relationship to the maxilla and the maxillary incisors are usually in a lingual axial inclination
C. Mesial relationship to the maxilla and the maxillary incisors are usually in a lingual axial inclination
D. Distal relationship to the maxilla and the maxillary incisors are usually in a labial axial inclination

40. Which of the following would be indicative of maxillary retrognathism?
A. An SNB angle of approximately 82°
B. An SNA angle greater than 82°
C. An SNA angle less than 82°
D. An SNB angle less than 70°

41. There are many reasons why cross bites occur. Which one of the following is not one of them?
A. Jaw size
B. Heredity
C. Faulty restorations
D. Mouth breathing
E. Prolonged retention of primary teeth

42. Hyaline cartilage differs from bone in that hyaline cartilage may grow:
A. By appositional growth
B. By interstitial growth
C. Both of the above
D. Neither of the above

43. Which of the following theories most likely explains why there is a strong tendency for mandibular crowding in the late teens and early twenties?
A. Lack of leeway space
B. Pressure from third molars
C. Late mandibular growth
D. Late maxillary growth

44. The most commonly impacted teeth are:
A. Maxillary canines
B. Maxillary central incisors
C. Mandibular first premolars
D. Mandibular lateral incisors

45. Which of the following is the difference in the total of the mesiodistal widths between the primary canine, first molar and second molar, and the permanent canine, first premolar and second premolar?
A. Primate space
B. Leeway space
C. Moyer's space
D. Anatomic space

46. Which of the following facial profiles is usually accompanied by a Class II malocclusion?
A. An orthognathic profile
B. A retrognathic profile
C. A prognathic profile
D. None of the above

47. Which type of malocclusion listed below is most often associated with mouth breathing?
A. Dental open bite
B. Skeletal open bite

C. Dental cross bite
D. Skeletal cross bite

48. Which of the following types of headgear produces a distal and upward force on the maxillary teeth and maxilla?
A. Straight pull headgear
B. Reverse-pull headgear
C. Cervical-pull headgear
D. High-pull headgear

49. Which of the following is usually used as an etching agent before direct bonding of orthodontic bracket?
A. 10-15% unbuffered phosphoric acid
B. 35-50% unbuffered phosphoric acid
C. 75-85% unbuffered phosphoric acid
D. 100% unbuffered phosphoric acid

50. The most rapid losses in the perimeter of the arch usually are due to a:
A. Distal tipping and rotation of the permanent second molar after removal of the permanent third molar
B. Mesial tipping and rotation of the permanent first molar after removal of the primary second molar
C. Mesial tipping and rotation of the permanent canine after removal of the primary lateral incisor
D. Distal tipping and rotation of the permanent second premolar after removal of the permanent first molar

51. The rational for retention in orthodontics is to:
A. Allow for reorganization of the gingival and periodontal tissues
B. Minimize changes due to growth
C. Permit neuromuscular adaptation to the corrected tooth position
D. Maintain teeth in a stable conditions
E. All of the above

52. The time required to upright a molar can vary from:
A. 2-3 weeks
B. 1-2 months
C. 6-12 months
D. 2-3 years

53. A phase of dentition during which some of the teeth present in the oral cavity are permanent and some are primary is referred to as what?
A. Intermediate dentition
B. Succedaneous dentition
C. Mixed dentition
D. Non-succedaneous dentition

54. The existence of a forward shift of the mandible during closure is found in:
A. "True" Class III malocclusions
B. "Pseudo" Class III malocclusions
C. Class II div 2 malocclusion
D. Class II div 1 malocclusion

55. The most common site for a supernumerary tooth is:
A. Distal to the mandibular third molar (distomolar)
B. Between the maxillary premolars
C. Between the mandibular central incisors
D. Between the maxillary central incisors (mesiodens)

56. Which of the following can cause an open bite?
A. Tongue-thrusting
B. Thumb-sucking
C. Genetics
D. Speech impediments (i.e. lisping)
E. All of the above

57. Which of the following is the normal relationship of the primary molars in the deciduous dentition?
A. Distal step
B. Flush terminal plane
C. Mesial step
D. None of the above

58. Root fractures in which part of the tooth are more likely to undergo repair?
A. Coronal
B. Mid-root
C. Apical third of the root
D. Vertical fracture of tooth

59. The management of a child who must undergo dental extractions is based on which of the following factors?
A. The age and maturity of the child
B. The past medical and dental experiences that might influence the behavior of the child
C. The physical status of the child
D. The length of time and amount of manipulation necessary to accomplish the surgery
E. All of the above

60. Which of the following is a hereditary dental defect in which the enamel of the teeth is soft and undercalcified in context, yet normal in quantity?
A. Enamel hypoplasia
B. Enamel hypocalcification
C. Enamel hypomaturation
D. Fluorosis

61. What is the most reliable method to determine the pulp vitality in the case of a recently traumatized primary tooth?
A. Radiograph
B. Electric pulp test
C. Thorough intraoral examination
D. There is no reliable method

62. The pH of acidulated phosphate fluoride gels is in which of the following ranges?
A. 1 to 4
B. 4 to 7
C. 7 to 10
D. 10 to 12

63. Which pulpotomy technique listed below is recommended in the treatment of a permanent tooth with a carious exposure which also has immature root development?
A. Calcium hydroxide technique
B. Formocresol technique
C. Indirect pulp capping
D. Apexification

64. All of the following procedures have proved beneficial in treating a mentally retarded child except:
A. Speak slowly and in very simple terms
B. Listen carefully to the patient
C. Schedule long appointments
D. Ask the patient if there are any questions about anything you will be doing

65. Discolored primary teeth that are symptom-free and show no radiographic changes are best treated by:
A. No treatment
B. Extirpation of the pulp tissue followed by the placement of ZOE paste in the root canal space
C. Extraction
D. Pulpotomy

66. A condition characterized by an attention span that is less than expected for the age of the child, hyperactivity and impulsive behavior is called:
A. Epilepsy
B. Cerebral palsy
C. Attention deficit disorder
D. Muscular dystrophy

67. The hallmarks of cellulitis include:
A. Warmth
B. Erythema
C. Edema
D. Pain (tenderness)
E. All of the above

68. Which of the following is a primary center of calcification of a Tooth?
A. Ridges
B. Lobes
C. Grooves
D. Pearls

69. Ordinarily, a 6-year-old child would have what teeth clinically visible in the mouth?
A. All (20) primary teeth and 4 permanent first molars
B. 18 primary teeth and 2 permanent mandibular central incisors

C. 18 primary teeth, 2 permanent mandibular central incisors, and 4 permanent first molars
D. 16 primary teeth and 4 mandibular incisors

70. Which of the following drugs is widely used for pediatric sedation?
A. Meperidine
B. Chloral hydrate
C. Barbiturates
D. None of the above

71. Which of the following statements are true concerning cystic fibrosis?
A. Cystic fibrosis is an inherited disease of the exocrine glands, affecting approximately 30,000 children and adults.
B. Cystic fibrosis causes the body to produce an abnormally thick, sticky mucus, due to a faulty transport of sodium and chloride within cells lining organs such as the lungs and pancreas
C. Cystic fibrosis has a variety of symptoms. The most common of which are: a very salty tasting skin; persistent coughing, wheezing or pneumonia; excessive appetite but poor weight gain; and bulky stools
D. An individual must inherit a defective copy of the CF gene-one from each parent to have cystic fibrosis
E. All of the above statements are true

72. All of the following statements concerning dental fluorosis are true except:
A. It is a diffuse, symmetric, hypomineralization disorder of ameloblasts
B. It is reversible
C. It only occurs with exposure to fluoride when enamel is developing (calcification period)
D. It is a toxic manifestation of chronic (low-dose, long-term) fluoride intake

73. Amelogenesis imperfecta is a condition in which:
A. The teeth have short roots and tend to wear rapidly
B. The teeth develop abnormally and many teeth are missing
C. The teeth are covered with thin, malformed enamel

D. Tooth buds are joined together during development and appear as macrodonts

74. All of the following statements concerning recurrent aphthous ulcers (canker sores) are true except:

A. They occur in women more than men
B. They may occur at any age, but usually first appear between the ages of 10 to 40
C. The cause is a coxsackie virus
D. They appear to be associated with stress
E. They usually appear on nonkeratinized oral mucosa including the inner surface of the cheeks and lips, tongue, soft palate and the base of the gingivae

75. An outstanding oral manifestation of both ectodermal dysplasia and cleidocranial dysplasia is:

A. Oversized crowns
B. Elongated roots
C. Enlarged mandible
D. Retained primary teeth

76. All of the following instances, except one, may make the use of a rubber dam impractical. Which is the exception?

A. The presence of fixed orthodontic appliances
B. A patient with congested nasal passages or other nasal obstruction
C. A very nervous or anxious patient
D. A recently erupted tooth that will not retain a clamp

77. The teeth joined together by cementum is diagnosed as:

A. Gemination
B. Fusion
C. Concresence
D. Dens in dente

78. Which of the following is true concerning a young epileptic who has a grand mal seizure in the dental office?

A. It is generally fatal
B. It is best treated by injecting insulin
C. They generally recover if restrained from self-injury and oxygen is maintained
D. It can be prevented with antibiotics

79. Type 1 diabetes:

A. It also called juvenile-onset or insulin dependent diabetes
B. Is the type of diabetes in which the body completely stops producing any insulin
C. Affects young adults
D. Is characterized by all of the above

80. Morphologically, the primary maxillary second molar strikingly resembles which tooth listed below?

A. Permanent maxillary third molar
B. Permanent maxillary second molar
C. Permanent maxillary first molar
D. Permanent mandibular second molar

81. If a child in your office requires antibiotic prophylaxis to prevent bacterial endocarditis, which regimen below is correct?

A. Amoxicillin 100 mg/kg 1 hr prior to dental appointment
B. Amoxicillin 75 mg/kg 2 hrs prior to dental appointment
C. Amoxicillin 50 mg/kg 1 hr prior to dental appointment
D. Amoxicillin 25 mg/kg 2 hr prior to dental appointment

82. The phenomenon of "strawberry tongue" is associated with:

A. Herpangina
B. Scarlet fever
C. Diphtheria
D. Mumps

83. Which of the following are true comparing the normal child periodontium to a normal adult periodontium?

A. There is greater blood and lymph supply
B. The alveolar crest is flatter
C. Gingival pocket depths are larger
D. Attached gingiva is not as wide
E. All of the above

84. Panoramic radiographs are excellent in demonstrating which of the following in a young patient?

A. Supernumerary teeth / Congenitally missing teeth
B. Axial inclinations of teeth / Apical development of the permanent teeth
C. Impacted teeth / Pathological lesions in the jaw

D. View of the mandibular condyles
E. All of the above

85. A veau's Class I cleft palate involves what structures?
A. Hard and soft palates
B. Soft palate only
C. Alveolar process only
D. Hard palate only

86. Cretinism is a deficiency disease, caused by the congenital absence of:
A. Insulin
B. Thyroxine
C. Calcitonin
D. Epinephrine

87. "Koplik's spots" are associated with:
A. Smallpox (Variola)
B. German measles (Rubella)
C. Mumps
D. Measles (Rubeola)

88. What is the minimum number of lobes from which any tooth may develop?
A. Two
B. Three
C. Four
D. Five

89. The permanent mandibular first molar has a morphology that closely resembles which primary tooth listed below?
A. Primary mandibular first molar
B. Primary mandibular second molar
C. Primary maxillary first molar
D. Primary maxillary second molar

90. Emergency treatment in the dental office for a child who has accidentally ingested a large amount of fluoride would include which of the following:
A. Induce vomiting mechanically or with the help of lpecac syrup
B. Have patient drink large quantities of sodium bicarbonate
C. Have patients drink large quantities of milk

D. Crush ammonia vaparole under the patient's nose to keep the patient awake and conscious
E. Only a & c.

91. A child 19 months old will have how many teeth?
A. Four
B. Eight
C. Twelve
D. Sixteen
E. Twenty

92. Which of the following is the most common congenitally missing primary tooth?
A. Primary mandibular canine
B. Primary maxillary lateral incisor
C. Primary maxillary canine
D. Primary mandibular first molar

93. The primary mandibular second molar in a four year old has a large carious lesion with pulpal involvement. Radiographically there is periapical pathology on the distal root. There is furcation involvement and slight mobility. The treatment of choice is:
A. Direct pulp capping
B. Pulpotomy
C. Pulpectomy
D. Extraction

94. Upon oral examination, a three-year-old child is found to have intensely inflamed gingiva, a soar throat, fever, lymphadenopathy, and small fluid-filled vesicles on the mucosa of the lips, tongue and gingiva. The diagnosis is probably:
A. Chicken pox
B. Primary (acute) herpetic gingivostomatitis
C. Scarlet fever
D. Acute necrotizing ulcerative gingivitis (ANUG)

95. Which type of leukemia below is the most common pediatric cancer?
A. Acute myeloid leukemia
B. Chronic myelocytic leukemia

C. Acute lymphocytic leukemia
D. Chronic lymphocytic leukemia

96. What is the most effective method of reducing the dental caries problem in the general population?
A. School water fluoridation
B. Fluoridation of the communal water supply
C. Fluoride rinses at home
D. Frequent dental visits
E. Patient education

97. When placing a Class II amalgam in a primary tooth, the width of the isthmus should be:
A. About one-half the intercuspal width
B. About one-third the intercuspal width
C. About two-third the intercuspal width
D. About three-quarters the intercuspal width

98. Nursing-bottle caries is a widespread caries destruction of the deciduous teeth, which of the deciduous teeth are most commonly affected?
A. Mandibular incisors
B. Maxillary first molars
C. Mandibular first molars
D. Maxillary incisors

99. Gingivostomatitis is a condition that is:
A. Common particularly among elderly people
B. Common particularly among middle-aged adults
C. Common particularly among children
D. Uncommon

100. At the age of six years a child's head is what percentage of its adult size?
A. 30%
B. 50%
C. 80%
D. 90%

101. All of the following statements are true, except:
A. The primary teeth are darker in color than the permanent teeth

B. The pulp cavities are proportionately larger in the primary teeth
C. In general, the crowns of primary teeth are more bulbous and constricted than the permanent counterpart
D. The crown surfaces of all primary teeth are much smoother than the permanent teeth (in other words, there is less evidence of pits and grooves)

102. Preventive dentistry for adolescents may include which of the following?
A. Frequent dental office visits
B. Fluoride rinses at home
C. Fluoride tray applications
D. Brushing and flossing
E. Sealants
F. Fluoride tablets
G. All the above

103. All of the following statements are true except:
A. The occlusal anatomy of primary teeth is not as defined as that of permanent teeth therefore amalgam preps can be more conservative
B. Enamel and dentin are thicker in primary teeth, therefore amalgam preparations are deeper
C. The pulpal horns of primary teeth are longer and pointed, therefore amalgam preps must be conservative to avoid a pulpal exposure
D. Primary molars have an exaggerated cervical bulge that makes matrix adoption much more difficult

104. Which of the following is the first deciduous (primary) tooth to erupt?
A. Mandibular central
B. Mandibular first molar
C. Maxillary central
D. Maxillary first molar

105. Listed below are the usual events in the histogenesis of a tooth. Place them in their correct sequence (from what happens first to what happens last)
1. Deposition of the first layer of dentin

2. Differentiation of odontoblasts
3. Deposition of the first layer of enamel
4. Elongation of the inner enamel epithelial cells of the enamel organ
   A. 3,2,4,1
   B. 1,2,4,3
   C. 2,1,3,4
   D. 4,3,2,1

106. Which primary mandibular tooth listed below does not resemble any other primary or permanent tooth?
A. Primary mandibular canine
B. Primary mandibular lateral incisor
C. Primary mandibular first molar
D. Primary mandibular second molar

107. When do the permanent teeth begin to calcify?
A. At birth
B. One month
C. Four months
D. One year

108. Which stage in the life cycle of a tooth listed below includes final shaping of the tooth?
A. Initiation (Bud stage)
B. Proliferation (Cap stage)
C. Differentiation (Bell stage)
D. Apposition

109. Which of the following is the most frequently utilized route of administration for sedation in pediatric patients?
A. Oral
B. Inhalation
C. IV
D. IM

110. Which of the following cause delayed exfoliation of the primary teeth and delayed eruption of the permanent teeth?
A. Hypothyroidism
B. Hypopituitarism
C. Hypoparathyroidism
D. All of the above

111. The primary central incisors are usually exfoliated between what ages?
A. 6-8 years old
B. 7-9 years old
C. 9-10 years old
D. 10-12 years old

112. The primary maxillary canine differs from the permanent maxillary canine in which way listed below?
A. The cusp on the primary canine is much shorter and rounded
B. The mesial cusp ridge is longer than the distal cusp ridge
C. The mesial cusp ridge is shorter than the distal cusp ridge
D. None of the above

113. The greatest concentration of fluoride ions exists just beneath the enamel surface. During a routine prophylaxis it is possible that the use of abrasive polishing agents may remove the fluoride-rich layer of enamel.
A. Both statements are true
B. The first statements is true and the second statements false
C. The first statements is false and the second statement is true
D. Both statements are false

114. Which treatment listed below is the proper one for a Class II fracture of a permanent tooth with an immature apex?
A. Pulpectomy
B. Apply calcium hydroxide to exposed dentin and restore tooth with a permanent restoration
C. Pulpotomy
D. Observe

115. All of the following are dental characteristics of a Down syndrome child except:
A. A prominent thickened tongue
B. A high rate of caries
C. Delayed eruption of teeth
D. A high prevalence of malocclusion
E. Enamel dysplasia

116. The primary maxillary canine typically erupts around what age?
A. 7 months old

B. 10 months old
C. 18 months old
D. 24 months old

117. All of the following are the major features of Apert syndrome except:
A. Prematurely fused cranial sutures
B. A retruded midface
C. Fused fingers
D. Blindness
E. Fused toes

118. When treating a child who is obviously afraid, the dentist should:
A. Use restraint
B. Use the hand-over-mouth technique (HOME)
C. Permit the child to express his fear
D. Avoid all references to the child's fear

119. In most cases, the proper treatment for intruded primary anterior teeth is:
A. Repositioning
B. Extraction
C. Intermaxillary fixation
D. Administer no treatment

120. Which of the following are primary goals of indirect pulp capping?
A. To preserve the pulp vitality
B. To prevent pulp exposure
C. To save tooth structure
D. To arrest caries
E. To promote the formation of reparative dentin
F. All of the above

121. The process of shaping a patient's behaviour through appropriately timed feedback is called:
A. Tell-show-do
B. Voice control
C. Positive reinforcement
D. Distraction
E. Nonverbal communication

122. When operative or surgical procedures are performed on the mandibular primary or permanent teeth, which nerve listed below must be blocked?

A. Posterior superior alveolar nerve
B. Lingual nerve
C. Inferior alveolar nerve
D. Long buccal nerve

123. Which primary molar listed below is the most atypical of all the molars, primary and permanent, and appears to be intermediate in form and development between a premolar and a molar?

A. Primary mandibular first molar
B. Primary maxillary first molar
C. Primary mandibular second molar
D. Primary maxillary second molar

124. Which of the following is a beneficial effect of fluoride?

A. Interferes with plaque formation on teeth
B. Has antibacterial qualities
C. Remineralization is enhanced
D. Decreased enamel solubility
E. Inhibits glycolysis
F. All of the above

125. All of the following fluoride therapies should be recommended to a 13-year-old child who is prone to decay and lives in a community where the water is fluoridated at an appropriate level except?

A. Professionally applied fluoride every six months
B. Fluoride toothpaste
C. A low concentration fluoride mouth rinse
D. A high concentration fluoride mouth rinse

126. A simple fracture of the crown of a tooth involving little or no dentin would be classified as what?

A. Ellis Class I fracture
B. Ellis Class II fracture
C. Ellis Class III fracture
D. Ellis Class IV fracture

127. Which of the following are true concerning over-retained primary teeth in the mixed dentition?
A. They may prevent normal eruption of permanent teeth
B. This may be caused by abnormal root resorption of primary teeth
C. They are often treated by extraction
D. All of the above

128. All of the following are contraindications of performing a direct pulp cap on a primary tooth except:
A. Spontaneous pain from the tooth
B. A pinpoint exposure with little or no hemorrhaging (bleeding)
C. A large exposure
D. Excessive hemorrhaging (bleeding)
E. Radiographic evidence of internal resorption

129. Which of the following is the main advantage of using 8% solution of stannous fluoride instead of a 2% solution of sodium fluoride for a topical fluoride treatment?
A. Will not stain
B. Better taste
C. Stable when kept in a polyethylene container
D. A single treatment may be given

130. Which pulpotomy technique listed below is recommended in the treatment of primary teeth with a carious exposure?
A. Calcium hydroxide technique
B. Formocresol technique
C. Zinc oxide eugenol technique
D. None of the above

131. The most common benign tumor of infants is:
A. A lymphangioma
B. A hemangioma
C. A neurofibroma
D. A pyogenic granuloma

132. All of the following are factors to consider when deciding whether a fluoride supplement should be prescribed to a child except:
A. The amount of fluoride in the child's drinking water

B. The age of the child
C. The type of topical fluoride applied professionally in the office
D. How responsible is the person who will be administering the supplement, whether it be the patient or the patient's parents

133. All of the following teeth are non-succedaneous, except:
A. The permanent maxillary and mandibular premolars
B. The permanent maxillary and mandibular first molars
C. The permanent maxillary and mandibular second molars
D. The permanent maxillary and mandibular third molars

134. An outstanding oral manifestation of achondroplasia is:
A. Rampant caries
B. Periodontal disease
C. Overcrowding of teeth
D. Supernumerary teeth

135. All of the following statements are true except:
A. Compared to the permanent maxillary central incisors, the incisal edge of the primary maxillary central incisors is straighter
B. No mamelons are present on the primary maxillary central incisors. There are mamelons present on the permanent maxillary central incisors
C. The crown of the primary maxillary central incisors is smaller Mesiodistally than the permanent maxillary central incisors
D. The crown of the primary maxillary central incisors has a shorter length inciso-cervically than the permanent maxillary central incisors

136. Interproximal caries on primary teeth may result in:
A. Eventual loss of the primary tooth
B. Loss of tooth structure
C. Arch length loss
D. All of the above

137. The most common of the craniofacial malformations is:
A. Bifid tongue
B. Macroglossia

C. Cleft palate and cleft lip
D. Anodontia

138. The sum of the mediodistal widths of the primary molars in any one quadrant is:
A. 5-10 mm greater than the permanent teeth that succeed them (premolars)
B. 2-5 mm less than the permanent teeth that succeed them (premolars)
C. 2-5 mm greater than the permanent teeth that succeed them (premolars)
D. 5-10 mm less than the permanent teeth that succeed them (premolars)

139. All of the following statements concerning acute necrotizing ulcerative gingivitis are true except:
A. It is also called Vincent's infection or "trench mouth"
B. It is a gingival disease characterized by painful hyperemic gingiva, punched out erosions of the interproximal papilla, covered by a gray pseudomembrane with an accompanying fetid odor
C. Risks include poor oral hygiene, poor nutrition, smoking, and emotional stress
D. It is usually affects children between the age of 5 to 10 years old

140. Which of the following is the most important technique of behavioral management in the pediatric dental patient?
A. Tell-show-do
B. Voice control
C. Positive reinforcement
D. Distraction
E. Nonverbal communication

141. Which primary mandibular molar has a prominent transverse ridge that unites the mesiobuccal and the mesiolingual cusps?
A. Primary mandibular first molar
B. Primary mandibular second molar
C. Both of the above
D. None of the above

142. A child eleven years old traumatized a permanent maxillary central incisor some time ago. The tooth in now painful and there is evidence of swelling. A periapical x-ray discloses a pathosis associated with the apex. The suggested treatment is:
A. Pulpotomy
B. Extraction
C. Pulpectomy
D. Observation

143. A 15-year -old female has lived in a non-fluoridated area all of her life. Which of the following is most likely to occur in this female when she moves to a community where the drinking water naturally contains 6 ppm of fluoride?
A. 50% reduction in dental caries
B. Moderate dental fluorosis
C. An increase in the amount of fluoride stored in her bones
D. Gastrointestinal problems

144. When preparing a primary tooth for a stainless steel crown, the cusps are reduced:
A. Approximately 1 to 1.5 mm
B. Approximately 5 to 6.5 mm
C. Approximately 10 mm
D. Approximately 15 mm

145. When do the primary teeth begin to form in utero?
A. One week
B. Three weeks
C. Six weeks
D. Ten weeks

146. Which two structures listed below join to form Hertwigs epithelial root sheath?
A. Stratum intermedium
B. Inner enamel epithelium
C. Stellate reticulum
D. Outer enamel epithelium
E. Stratum basale

147. Which two of the following decrease with age in the dental pulp?
A. Number of collagen fibers

B. Number of reticulin fibers
C. The size of the pulp
D. Calcifications within the pulp

148. No endodontic cases lend themselves to successful treatment without some degree of:
A. Irrigation
B. Debridement
C. Obturation
D. Medication

149. Which of the following irrigants is the most widely used in endodontics?
A. Sodium hypochlorite
B. Urea peroxide
C. Hydrogen peroxide
D. Saline

150. Which of the following appears to be the ideal storage media for a tooth that has been traumatically avulsed and will be out of its socket for more than an hour?
A. Soda
B. Sodium hypochlorite
C. Milk
D. Hydrogen peroxide

151. Which of the following are useful diagnostic aids that can be used to determine if a tooth has a vertical crown-root fracture?
A. Fiberoptic light for transillumination
B. Wedging the tooth in question and then taking an x-ray
C. Persistent periodontal defects in an otherwise healthy tooth
D. Having a patient bite forcefully on a bite stick
E. All of the above

152. Which of the following is generally believed to be the cause of internal resorption of a tooth?
A. Orthodontic treatment
B. Tooth fracture
C. The presence of a chronic pulpitis
D. Periodontal disease

153. Which of the following intracanal instruments is designed for the removal of pulp tissue, cotton pellet absorbent points and other soft materials, but not for canal enlargement?
A. Files
B. Reamers
C. Broaches
D. None of the above

154. Which of the following canals in a maxillary first molar is usually the most difficult to locate?
A. Palatal
B. Distobuccal
C. Mesiobuccal
D. All of the canals are relatively easy to find

155. The primary function of root canal sealers is:
A. To act as a lubricant, facilitating placement of the gutta-percha
B. To form a bond between the filling material and the dentin walls
C. To fill in the discrepancies between the filling material and the dentin walls
D. To exert antibacterial activity

156. Which material listed below has historically been the retrofilling material of choice?
A. Composite
B. Zinc-free amalgam
C. Gutta-percha
D. Methyl methacrylate

157. Which of the following will have a pulp chamber that will be triangular?
A. Permanent mandibular second premolars
B. Permanent mandibular molars
C. Permanent maxillary molars
D. Permanent maxillary lateral incisors

158. Which condition below is an apical lesion that develops as an acute exacerbation of a chronic apical abscess (also called a suppurative apical periodontitis)?
A. Cyst
B. Phoenix abscess

C. Granuloma
D. None of the above

159. Which of the following flap designs is preferred when performing endodontic surgery in the maxillary anterior region?
A. Vertical (single or double) flap
B. Scalloped (Leubke-Ochsenbein) flap
C. Curved (semilunar flap)
D. Palatal flap

160. Which condition listed below is the result of a pulpal infection that extends through the apical foramen to the periapical tissues?
A. Periodontal abscess
B. Gingival abscess
C. Periapical abscess
D. All of the above

161. Which mandibular premolar presents with more variations in root canal anatomy?
A. First premolar
B. Second premolar
C. Both of the above
D. None of the above

162. An apicoectomy is a resection:
A. Of the most coronal portion of the root
B. Of the coronal portion of the pulp horn
C. Of the most apical portion of the root
D. Of the entire pulp horn

163. Which of the following are chelating agents?
A. EDTA
B. RC-Prep
C. EDTAC
D. All of the above

164. According to the buccal object rule, when the x-ray tube is repositioned either at a more mesial or at a more distal angulation and a film is exposed, the root or canal farther from the film (the buccal) will
A. More in the opposite direction that the cone is directed

B. Move in the direction that the cone is directed
C. Not move at all
D. Moves up and down

165. Which of the following criteria must be met before a canal is considered ready to fill with gutta-percha?
A. The canal must be prepared in a manner that ensures optimum debridement and access to the apical area so that the filling material can be condensed to obliterate the entire preparation
B. The tooth must be asymptomatic
C. At the time of fill, the canal must be dry
D. If a bacteriologic culture test is being used, a negative culture must be obtained
E. All of the above

166. Anatomically, the dental pulp is divided into two portions, the coronal and radicular pulp. Which portion is located in the pulp chamber and pulp horns?
A. Coronal pulp
B. Radicular pulp
C. Pulp canal
D. Pulp cells

167. Which of the following are contraindications to the use of the electric pulp tester?
A. Inability to dry the tooth
B. Teeth that have crowns or are heavily restored
C. Tooth traumatized recently
D. Anesthetized teeth
E. Patient in severe pain
F. All of the above

168. Which tooth below will almost always have two canals?
A. Maxillary first premolar
B. Maxillary second premolar
C. Mandibular first premolar
D. Mandibular second premolar

169. Which of the following methods for using endodontic instruments involves no rotation of the instrument

whatsoever and relies on hard tissue removal on the outstroke only?

A. Filing
B. Reaming
C. Circumferential filing
D. All of the above

170. In all of the following conditions, the pulps of the involved teeth are likely to be non-vital except?

A. Apical scar
B. Radicular cyst
C. Traumatic bone cyst
D. Chronic dental abscess
E. Chronic periapical granuloma

171. In all of the following conditions, the pulps of the involved teeth are likely to be vital except?

A. Cementoma
B. Radicular cyst
C. Traumatic bone cyst
D. Globulomaxillary cyst

172. Which tooth listed below requires endodontic treatment most frequently?

A. Maxillary second molar
B. Mandibular first molar
C. Mandibular second bicuspid
D. Maxillary first bicuspid

173. Which of the following is the main function of the dental pulp?

A. Nutritive
B. Sensory
C. Protective
D. Formative

174. Which of the following is the procedures of choice when a broken endodontic instrument protrudes past the apex of a tooth?

A. Extract the tooth
B. The broken instrument is surgically removed, and then the entire canal is filled with gutta-percha

C. Fill the tooth with gutta-percha and observe
D. None of the above

175. Wearing gloves when using the electric pulp tester to test the vitality of a tooth may lead to a:
A. False-positive response
B. False-negative response
C. Both of the above
D. None of the above

176. Gutta-percha is freely soluble in which solvents listed below?
A. Alcohol
B. Chloroform
C. Xylol
D. Eugenol

177. The chronic apical abscess (CAA) is generally:
A. Very painful
B. Asymptomatic
C. Mildly painful
D. None of the above

178. Which of the following are contraindications to endodontic therapy?
A. A non-restorable tooth
B. A tooth with insufficient periodontal support
C. A tooth with a vertical root fracture
D. All of the above

179. Which two of the following situations offer better success for pulp capping?
A. Accidental exposure of the pulp
B. Pulp of a middle-aged person
C. Carious exposure of the pulp
D. Pulp of a young child

180. Which of the following is the most commonly used bleaching agent for endodontically treated teeth?
A. Ether
B. Superoxol
C. Chloroform
D. Sodium hypochlorite

181. Which condition listed below is characterized by pain that is spontaneous and has periods of cessation (intermittent in nature)?
A. Reversible pulpitis
B. Irreversible pulpitis
C. Chronic alveolar abscess
D. None of the above

182. The root canal for a mandibular canine is:
A. Wide Mesiodistally but thin labiolingually
B. Thin Mesiodistally but wide labiolingually
C. The same width Mesiodistally and labiolingually
D. Circular

183. Which type of external root resorption listed below may occur from combined injury to the PDL and cementum complicated by bacteria from an infected root canal space?
A. Surface resorption
B. Inflammatory resorption
C. Replacement resorption
D. None of the above

184. All of the following cells would be found in a hyperemic pulp after an exposure during caries removal, except:
A. Plasma cells
B. Lymphocytes
C. Goblet cells
D. Mast cells
E. Neutrophils (PMNs)

185. Which tooth listed below may have a pulp chamber that is somewhat triangular as opposed to oval?
A. Maxillary central incisor
B. Mandibular central incisor
C. Maxillary lateral incisor
D. Mandibular lateral incisor

186. Which of the following are considered to be the two objective of the access opening?
A. To provide patient comfort
B. To provide direct access to the apical portion of the canal
C. To facilitate visualization (location) of the canal
D. To remove all old restorative materials from the tooth

187. The earliest and most common symptom of an acute pulpitis is:
A. A dull throbbing sensation
B. Pain upon chewing
C. Thermal sensitivity
D. Discomfort, particularly on palpation

188. Which of the following teeth most often refer pain to the temporal region?
A. Mandibular molars
B. Maxillary incisors
C. Maxillary second premolars
D. Maxillary molars

189. The most common cause of acute osteomyelitis of the jaws is:
A. Unknown
B. Iatrogenic
C. Dental infection
D. Radiation

190. Which of the following are the two basic reasons for the use of post when restoring an endodontically treated tooth?
A. To strengthen the root
B. To retain the restoration
C. To protect the remaining tooth structure
D. To help in the fabrication of a crown

191. The most widely used material for apexification procedures is:
A. Gutta-percha
B. Calcium hydroxide
C. Zinc oxide
D. Eugenol

192. Which tooth listed below is most likely to have a curved root?
A. Maxillary central incisor
B. Maxillary lateral incisor
C. Maxillary canine
D. Mandibular central incisor

193. Which of the following factors are important to the success of intentional replantation?

A. A short extraoral time period (to maintain the viability of the periodontal ligament)
B. A healthy periodontium
C. A skillful extraction technique
D. All of the above

194. If an electric pulp tester is used to test a hyperemic tooth, the useful response will be which of the following?

A. The tooth will respond to less current than normal
B. The tooth will respond immediately to any current
C. The tooth will respond to higher current than normal
D. The tooth will not respond to any current

195. Which of the following are indications for performing a pulpotomy?

A. Treatment of pulp exposures in deciduous teeth
B. Treatment of pulp exposures in permanent teeth with undeveloped root apices
C. An alternative to extraction when endodontic therapy is unavailable
D. Temporary emergency treatment for an acute pulpitis
E. All of the above

196. When symptoms and clinical tests show the presence of pulpal pathosis in a posterior tooth and the radiograph shows no decay or restoration in any proximity to the pulp, this is virtually pathognomonic of:

A. Condensing osteitis
B. A vertical fracture of the tooth
C. Periodontal abscess
D. Secondary occlusal trauma

197. Avulsed primary/deciduous teeth:

A. Should be cleaned very well and replanted if within five hours of the injury
B. Are usually not replanted
C. Should be replanted immediately
D. Should have a pulpotomy performed on them prior to replantation

198. A reaming action produces a canal that is relatively:
A. Square in shape
B. Irregular in shape
C. Round in shape
D. Triangular in shape

199. When fitting the master cone in a properly prepared canal, the cone must:
A. Be 2 mm from the apex
B. Be within 1 mm of the working length and have a slight resistance to dislodgement
C. Fit to the exact apex
D. Be at least 1 mm past the apex

200. In most cases where there is endodontic-periodontic therapy indicated on a tooth, which is performed first?
A. Endodontic therapy
B. Periodontic therapy
C. Both should go simultaneously
D. None of the above

201. Orthodontic appliances can:
A. Cause irritation to the gingiva
B. Act as plaque harbors
C. Make proper oral hygiene difficult to perform
D. All of the above

Answer key to orthodontics, pedodontics, endodontics

1	B	2	D	3	B	4	A
5	C	6	C	7	D	8	C
9	B	10	D	11	D	12	E
13	C	14	D	15	B	16	B
17	D	18	B	19	D	20	A, C
21	B	22	A	23	B	24	B
25	D	26	D, B	27	B	28	B
29	B	30	C	31	D	32	B
33	C	34	A	35	A	36	B
37	E	38	B, C	39	D	40	C
41	C	42	B	43	C	44	A
45	B	46	B	47	B	48	D
49	B	50	B	51	E	52	C
53	C	54	B	55	D	56	E
57	B	58	C	59	E	60	B
61	D	62	A	63	A	64	C
65	A	66	C	67	E	68	B
69	A	70	B	71	E	72	B
73	C	74	C	75	D	76	C
77	C	78	C	79	D	80	C
81	C	82	B	83	E	84	E
85	B	86	B	87	D	88	C
89	B	90	E	91	D	92	B
93	C	94	B	95	C	96	B
97	B	98	D	99	C	100	D
101	A	102	G	103	B	104	A
105	A	106	C	107	A	108	C
109	B	110	D	111	A	112	B
113	C	114	B	115	B	116	C
117	D	118	C	119	D	120	F
121	C	122	C	123	B	124	F
125	D	126	A	127	D	128	B
129	D	130	B	131	B	132	C
133	A	134	C	135	C	136	D
137	C	138	C	139	D	140	A
141	A	142	C	143	C	144	A
145	C	146	B, D	147	B, C	148	B

149	A	150	C	151	E	152	C
153	C	154	C	155	C	156	B
157	C	158	B	159	B	160	C
161	A	162	C	163	D	164	B
165	E	166	A	167	F	168	A
169	A	170	C	171	B	172	B
173	D	174	B	175	B	176	B, C
177	B	178	D	179	A, D	180	B
181	B	182	B	183	B	184	C
185	A	186	B, C	187	C	188	C
189	C	190	B, C	191	B	192	B
193	D	194	A	195	E	196	B
197	B	198	C	199	B	200	A
201	D						

Reader's Notes

10

Prosthodontics

1. **The size of posterior teeth for a removable partial denture is determined primarily by which two of the following?**
   A. The useful posterior tooth space
   B. The lip line of the patient
   C. The age of the patient
   D. The characteristics of the denture-supporting tissues
   E. The facebow transfer

2. **A device that relieves the abutment teeth, to which a fixed or removable partial denture is attached, of all or part of the forces generated by occlusal function is called a:**
   A. Pontic
   B. Stressbreaker
   C. Major connector
   D. Minor connector

3. **Custom trays are an important part of rubber base impression technique since elastomers are**
   A. More accurate in uniform, thin layers 0.5 to 1.0 mm thick
   B. More accurate in uniform, thin layers 1.0 to 1.5 mm thick
   C. More accurate in uniform, thin layers 2.0 to 4.0 mm thick
   D. More accurate in uniform, thin layers 5.0 to 6.0 mm thick

4. **Which of the following are functions of the reciprocal clasp arm of a removable partial denture?**
   A. Reciprocation

B. Stabilization
C. Auxiliary indirect retention (bracing)
D. All of the above

5. Inflammatory papillary hyperplasia frequently is observed
A. On the dorsum of the tongue
B. Under ill-fitting maxillary dentures, especially those having a relief chamber
C. On the gingiva of a pregnant patient
D. About the anterior part of a complete maxillary denture when a patient has natural anterior mandibular teeth but no posterior replacement.

6. After taking an alginate impression you notice that the impression material appears grainy. Which of the following could be the cause?/
A. Improper mixing
B. Prolonged mixing
C. Water/powder ratio too low
D. All of the above

7. The periodontium remains much healthier when crown margins are placed
A. Above the gingival crest
B. At the gingival crest
C. Below the gingival crest
D. Anywhere

8. A bony extension of the medical pterygoid plate of the sphenoid bone is called the:
A. Hamulus
B. Hamular notch
C. Maxillary tuberosity
D. Fovea palatini

9. The finish line of choice when fabricating either a porcelain jacket crown or an all - ceramic crown is:
A. Shoulder
B. Bevel
C. Chamfer
D. Shoulder with a bevel

10. The absolute maximum number of posterior teeth, which can be safely replaced with a fixed bridge is:
A. One
B. Two
C. Three
D. Four

11. How would you classify a removable partial denture in which a portion of the functional load is carried by the ridge at one end of the denture base segment while the other end of the base segment is supported by natural teeth?
A. A tooth borne removable partial denture
B. A bilateral distal extension removable partial denture
C. A unilateral distal extension removable partial denture
D. None of the above

12. Which of the following marginal designs is theoretically the best finishing margin for cast gold restorations, allowing burnishing and adaptation of the gold to the tooth?
A. Shoulder
B. Shoulder with a bevel
C. Chamfer
D. Bevel or feathered edge

13. A good temporary restoration for a tooth prepared for a crown should
A. Provide pulpal protection
B. Be able to be easily cleaned
C. Have non-impinging margins
D. All of the above

14. Paget's disease is often discovered in the dental office because:
A. These patients will have rampant caries due to xerostomia
B. The patient's dentures do not fit due to widening of the alveolar ridges
C. These patients will have multiple fractured restorations due to bruxims
D. These patients often have a sore tongue

15. The principal difference between dental plaster and dental stone powders is:
A. Color

B. Shelf life
C. Particle size and shape
D. Chemical formula

16. Dental stone is produced by:
A. Heating gypsum in an open kettle
B. Heating gypsum under pressure with water vapor in an autoclave
C. Heating gypsum in a 30% solution of calcium chloride
D. None of the above

17. Which of the following are indications for porcelain veneers?
A. Coverage of labial surface defects, e.g. hypoplasia of the enamel
B. Masking of discolored teeth, e.g. tetracycline staining, discoloration following loss of vitality
C. Repair of structural damage, e.g. fractured incisal edges
D. Reduction of spacing in cases when orthodontics would be inappropriate
E. All of the above

18. High-gold noble alloys, which are used in fabricating metal-ceramic restorations, are:
A. 50% gold, platinum
B. 75% gold, platinum, and palladium
C. 98% gold, platinum, and palladium
D. 100% gold, platinum, and palladium

19. A wrought-wire clasp
A. Is less flexible than a cast clasp
B. Is not as tough as cast clasp
C. Has a tensile strength that is at least 25% greater than that of the cast alloy from which it was made
D. Is not as adjustable as cast clasp

20. In the early stages of lateral movements, the condyle appears to rotate with a slight lateral Shift in the direction of the movement. This movement is called the Bennett movement. This Bennett movement refers to the
A. Nonworking side condyle only
B. Working side condyle only
C. Both the nonworking and working side condyles
D. None of the above

21 Which muscle listed below moves the disc of the TMJ forward (protrusion of mandible) ?

A. Masseter
B. Medial pterygoid
C. Lateral pterygoid
D. Temporalis

22. Which of the following is not an advantage of using polysulfide rubber impression materials?

A. Superior strength in a deep sulcus
B. Dimensionally stable after one pour
C. Have a short setting time
D. Pouring may be delayed for one hour if necessary
E. The finish line can be easily read
F. Have a good tear resistance
G. Compatible with all die materials and may be electroplated
H. Long working time and shelf life

23. Which of the following are considered to be the basic principles for occlusal adjustment?

A. The maximum distribution of occlusal stresses in centric relation
B. The forces of occlusion should be borne as much as possible by the long axis of the teeth
C. When there is surface-to-surface contact of flat cusps, it should be changed to a point-to-surface contact
D. Once centric occlusion is established, never take the teeth out of centric occlusion
E. All of the above

24. All of the following are considered to be standard components used to describe color except:

A. Chroma
B. Hue
C. Intensity
D. Value

25. Which of the following is not associated with diabetes?

A. Delayed healing
B. Rapidly periodontal disease with marked alveolar bone loss
C. Mucosal bleeding
D. Increased calculus formation
E. A predilection for periapical abscesses

26. The compensating curve is defined as:

A. The amount of separation between the mandible and maxilla when the mandible and its supporting muscles are in a resting position
B. The anteroposterior and lateral curvature in a alignment of the occluding surfaces and incisal edges of artificial teeth which is used to develop a balanced occlusion
C. The angle made by the slopes of a cusp with a perpendicular line bisecting the cusp, measured Mesiodistally or buccolingually
D. None of the above

27. Which of the following constituents of alginate power (irreversible hydrocolloid) functions as a plasticizer?

A. Trisodium phosphate
B. Zinc oxide
C. Calcium sulfate
D. Potassium titanium fluoride

28. All of the following statements concerning pontics are true except:.

A. With regard to the ease of cleaning and good tissue health proper pontic design is more important than the choice of material used in fabricating the pontic
B. The contour and nature of the pontic contact with the ridge is very important
C. The area of contact between the pontic and the ridge should be small
D. The portion of the pontic approximating the ridge should be as concave as possible
E. The pontic should exert no pressure on the ridge (passive contact with no blanching of the tissue)

29. Soldering flux is composed of:

A. Chromium, graphite and silica
B. Boric acid, silica and chromium
C. Graphite sodium pyroborate and boric acid
D. Sodium pyroborate, boric aid and silica

30. Which of the following statements concerning centric relation are true ?

A. The mandible cannot be forced into centric relation from the rest position because the patient reflex neuromuscular defense would resist the applied force

B. The mandible should be relaxed and gently guided into centric relation

C. In fixed and removable prosthodontics, centric relation should be established prior to designing the frame works

D. All of the above statements are true

31. All of the following are advantage of reversible hydrocolloid impression materials except

A. No custom trays required

B. Some moisture can be tolerated in the sulcus

C. Clean and easy placement

D. Easy to pour

E. Can be poured whenever you want

F. Inexpensive

G. Excellent shelf life *(3.5 years)*

32. When treatment planning for fixed prosthodontics, all of the following information can be obtained by studying diagnostic casts *except*

A. The length of the abutment teeth can be accurately gauged

B. The true inclination of the abutment teeth will be evident

C. The presence of periodontal pockets and the crown-to-root ratio of potential abutment teeth

D. Mesiodistal drifting rotation and faciolingual displacement of potential abutment teeth can be clearly seen

33. The partially edentulous arch which is bilateral without any distal abutments would be classified as :

A. Kennedy Class I

B. Kennedy Class II

C. Kennedy Class III

D. Kennedy Class IV

34. Which of the following is not a characteristic of polyether impression material

A. Have a clean, pleasant taste and odor

B. Slow setting
C. Dimensionally stable if more than one cast is poured
D. Excellent dimensionally stability when dry

35. Prior to fabricating removable partial denture for a patient surveying the diagnostic casts will enable the dentist to determine
A. Areas that can be used for support
B. A path of travel for insertion and removal of the denture
C. The crown to root ratio of potential abutment teeth
D. The periodontal health of potential abutment teeth

36. A wrought-wire of a given composition is:
A. Generally inferior in mechanical properties to a casting of the same composition
B. Generally has the same mechanical properties as a casting of the same composition
C. Generally superior in mechanical properties to a casting of the same composition
D. None of the above

37. Anterior guidance is the result of :
A. Horizontal overlap
B. Vertical overlap
C. Horizontal and vertical overlap
D. Cusp heights

38. Conventional feldspathic porcelain is composed of :
A. Silica
B. Alumina
C. Potash and soda
D. All of the above

39. Which of the following are function of the posterior palatal seal ?
A. Completes the border seal of the maxillary denture
B. Prevents impaction of food beneath the tissue surface of the denture
C. Improves the physiologic retention of the denture
D. Compensates for shrinkage of the denture resin during processing
E. All of the above

40. "T" and "D" sounds are formed by:

A. The tongue protruding slightly between the maxillary and mandibular anterior teeth
B. Contact of the tip of the tongue with the anterior palate and lingual surfaces of the maxillary anterior teeth
C. The lips only
D. None of the above

41. The ease and accuracy in border molding depends on which of the following

A. An accurately fitting custom tray
B. Control of bulk and temperature of the modeling compound
C. The tray being thoroughly cured
D. All of the above

42. Which of the following are indications for fixed bridgework or important considerations to think about when contemplating the fabrication of fixed bridge work for a patient?

A. A limited number of edentulous areas which would not otherwise be more satisfactorily restored with removable partial denture
B. The need to prevent the over-eruption of opposing teeth and the drifting of teeth neighboring the edentulous space
C. The presence of suitable abutment teeth, favorable crown/root ratio, adequate alveolar support, absence of apical pathology etc.
D. Esthetics
E. Patient motivation including time availability
F. Clinical and technical ability
G. All of the above

43. Which of the following elastomeric impression materials has the longest working and setting times?

A. Polyester
B. Polysulfide
C. Condensation silicone
D. Addition silicone

44. Which of the following elastomeric impression materials has very poor dimensional stability?

A. Polyether

B. Polysulfide
C. Condensation silicone
D. Addition silicone

45. The preparation for a full gold crown involves circumferential and occlusal reduction of between:
A. 0.5 and 1.0 mm
B. 2.0 and 2.5 mm
C. 3.0 and 3.5 mm
D. 4.0 and 4.5 mm

46. In casting the metal substructure for a metal-ceramic crown it is necessary to use which type of investment?
A. Gypsum-bonded investment
B. Phosphate-bonded investment
C. Silica-bonded investment
D. Any of the above

47. The principal component of dental plaster is:
A. Alpha hemihydrates
B. Beta-hemihydrates
C. Delta-hemihydrates
D. None of the above

48. Which of the following statements is correct in reference to polysulfide rubber base impression materials?
A. A decrease in temperature or humidity will accelerate the setting time of this material
B. An increase in temperature or humidity will accelerate the setting time of this material
C. Temperature and humidity have no effect the setting time of this material
D. All of the above

49. As the width of a claps increases, its flexibility
A. Increases
B. Decreases
C. Stays the same
D. First increases and then decreases

50. Claps that originated from above the survey line usually form an occlusal rest and angle downward across the clinical crown

until the tip is located in a prescribed amount of undercut are:

A. Suprabulge retainers
B. Infrabulge retainers
C. Bar clasps
D. Roach clasps

51. **Decreased vertical dimension of occlusion refers to an occluding vertical dimension that results in**

A. A loss of interocclusal distance when the mandible is in the rest position *(decreased freeway space)*
B. An excessive interocclusal distance when the mandible is in the rest position (Increased freeway space)
C. An increase in leeway space
D. None of the above

52. **Which of the following statements concerning the altered cast technique are true ?**

A. The purpose of this technique is two fold :
To record the form of the edentulous segment without tissue displacement
To accurately relate the edentulous segment to the teeth via the framework
B. The technique helps to obtain soft tissue support to aid abutments in resisting functional streses
C. This technique is a secondary impression system which utilizes the metal framework to hold customized impression trays for the edentulous areas
D. All of the above statements are true

53. **All of the following are advantages of dental porcelain restorations except:**

A. Excellent color and translucency
B. Low thermal and electrical conductivity
C. Low plastic deformation
D. High hardness

54. **During typical empty mouth swallowing, the mandible is braced in:**

A. The intercuspal position (IP)
B. The retruded contact position (RCP)

C. The protruded contact position (PCP)
D. Centric relation (CR)

55. Which teeth on a maxillary complete denture are the most important when considering esthetics?
A. Maxillary laterals
B. Maxillary centrals
C. Maxillary canines
D. Maxillary first premolars

56. Which of the following are the primary requirements for making a centric relation record when fabricating a removable partial denture?
A. To record the correct horizontal relation of the mandible to the maxilla
B. To stabilize the lower record base with equalized vertical pressure
C. To retain the record in an undistorted condition until the casts have been accurately mounted on the articulator or until a previous record can be verified
D. All of the above

57. Remounting and equilibration of complete dentures is carried out to:
A. Compensate for slight errors which may have occurred during the mounting of the casts
B. Correct for minor deficiencies in the setting of the denture teeth
C. Correct for tooth movement which may have occurred during processing of the dentures
D. All of the above

58. All of the following are disadvantages to immediate denture therapy. Which one is considered to be the major disadvantages to immediate denture therapy?
A. Increased post-insertion care
B. Increased post-insertion soreness
C. Not being able to have an anterior tooth try in to evaluate esthetics
D. Greater complexity of clinical procedures
E. A higher cost of treatment

59. An articulator which has the condylar elements on the lower member of the articulator and the condylar path elements on the upper member is called the

A. Arcon articulator
B. Non-arcon articulator
C. Hinge articulator
D. Free plane articulator

60. The first step in the treatment of abused tissues in a patient with existing dentures is to:

A. Fabricate a new set of dentures
B. Reline the dentures
C. Educate the patient
D. Excise the abused tissues

61. The primary reason for choosing a ¾ crown over a full cast crown is:

A. The preparation is easier
B. Tooth structure is spared
C. Less anesthesia is required
D. It's cheaper to make

62. Which of the following best describes the term "quenching"?

A. A metal is elevated to a temperature above room temperature and held there for a length of time
B. A metal is rapidly cooled from an elevated temperature to room temperature or below
C. Softening a metal by controlled heating and cooling
D. None of the above

63. Which of the following indirect retainers will provide the best leverage against lifting of the denture base?

A. To one located the closest to the clasp tips which is located furthest from the edentulous area
B. The one located the farthest from the clasp tips which is located nearest to the edentulous area
C. The one located the furthest from the clasp tips which is located furthest from the edentulous area
D. It doesn't matter

64. Clasps are:
A. Intracoronal retainers
B. Extracoronal retainers
C. May be both
D. Subgingival retainers

65. Condylar guidance is a factor which:
A. Is totally controlled by the dentist
B. Is totally dictated by the patient
C. Is partially dictated by the patient but can be adjusted by the dentist if necessary
D. Can be adjusted by the laboratory technician

66. Frequently overextended areas of the acrylic denture base include:
A. Frenal attachments
B. Distobuccal flange
C. Distolingual flange
D. In the vestibules (mucobuccal area)
E. All of the above

67. Which of the following statements concerning the functionally generated pathway technique are true:
A. A prerequisite for the use of this technique for the restoration of a single tooth is the presence of an optimal occlusion
B. This technique allows the cuspal movements of the dentition to be recorded in wax intra-orally and transferred to the articulator in the form of a static plaster cast
C. This static plaster cast is also called the functional index
D. By registering the pathways of the opposing tooth surfaces during mandibular movements, the technique allows a laboratory technician to provide a restoration with an occlusal surface less likely to incorporate occlusal interferences.
E. All of the above statements concerning the functionally generated pathway are true

68. Posterior teeth that are set edge to edge may cause:
A. Gagging
B. Cheek biting
C. Reduced taste
D. Speech aberrations

69. Bite registration material used to make an accurate interocclusal record should have what important characteristic listed below?

A. Offer a maximum resistance to the patient's jaw closure and have high flow at mixing
B. Offer a maximum resistance to the patient's jaw closure and have low flow at mixing
C. Offer a minimum resistance to the patient's jaw closure and have low flow at mixing
D. Offer a minimum resistance to the patient's jaw closure and have high flow at mixing

70. All of the following statements are true concerning a facebow or a facebow transfer except:

A. The face bow is a caliper like device used to record the patient's maxilla/hinge axis relationship (opening and closing axis)
B. If the transfer is done properly, the arc of closure on the articulator should duplicate that exhibited by the patient
C. The facebow transfer is a maxillo-mandibular record
D. The facebow transfer is used to transfer the maxilla/hinge axis relationship to the articulator during the mounting of the maxillary cast.

71 Factors that may contribute to porosities in a denture include:

A. Insufficient pressure on the flask during processing
B. Insufficient material in the mold
C. A rapid elevation in temperature to 212°F causing vaporization of the liquid
D. All of the above

72. An edentulous patient has slight undercuts in both tuberosities and also in the facial of the anterior maxilla. To construct a satisfactory maxillary complete denture, you should reduce which of the following:

A. All undercuts
B. The anterior undercut only
C. Both tuberosity undercuts
D. None of them

73. The treatment plan for a patient indicates that both mandibular and maxillary immediate dentures are to be fabricated. The ideal way to do this is:
A. Fabricate the maxillary immediate denture first
B. Fabricate the mandibular immediate denture first
C. Fabricate the maxillary and mandibular Immediate dentures at the same time
D. None of the above

74. Balancing side (nonworking side) interferences generally occur on the inner aspects of the:
A. Facial cusps of mandibular molars
B. Facial cusps of maxillary premolars
C. Lingual of mandibular molars
D. Facial cusps of maxillary molars

75. Which of the following elastomeric impression materials has the shortest working and setting times?
A. Polyether
B. Polysulfide
C. Condensation silicone
D. Addition silicone

76. The ideal crown-to-root ratio of a tooth to be utilized as a bridge abutment is
A. 3:1
B. 2:1
C. 1:2
D. 1:1

77. Which of the following is defined as "the vertical distance or space between the incisal and occlusal surfaces of the maxillary and mandibular teeth with the mandible in the physiological test position?
A. Vertical dimension of occlusal (VDO)
B. Vertical dimension of rest (VDR)
C. Interocclusal distance (freeway space)
D. None of the above

78. The setting time of a zinc oxide-eugenol impression paste may be accelerated by
A. Adding a drop of alcohol to the mix

B. Using the frozen-stab method of mixing
C. Adding a drop of water to the mix
D. Decreasing the amount of eugenol

79. The path of insertion for an anterior ¾ crown should:
A. Be perpendicular to the incisal one-half of the labial surface rather than the long axis of the tooth
B. Be parallel to the incisal one-half to two-thirds of the labial surface rather than the long axis of the tooth
C. Be parallel to the long axis of the tooth
D. Be parallel to the cervical one-third of the labial surface rather than the long axis of the tooth

80. Which of the following Kennedy classes of removable partial dentures are tooth borne?
A. Class I
B. Class II
C. Class III
D. Class IV

81. An increase in the temperature of the water used in mixing alginate impression materials will:
A. Shorten the setting time
B. Lengthen the setting time
C. Prevent setting
D. Not effect on the setting time at all

82. All of the following advantages of precision attachment restorations except:
A. They provide retention without an unsightly display of metal
B. They are easy to repair
C. The functional load is dispersed down the long axis of the abutments by virtue of the low central loading at the base of the attachments
D. The restorations permit the patient access to all areas of the tissues when the denture is not in place
E. If both sides of the dental arch have this type of restoration and are joined by a rigid major connector excellent bilateral stabilization is provided to the abutments.

83. All of the following are indications for using a linguoplate as a mandibular major connector except:

A. To avoid a high lingual frenum or when there is no space in the floor of the mouth
B. Mandibular tori that cannot be removed
C. To support periodontically weakened teeth
D. Severe anterior crowding
E. To serve as retention for lower anterior denture teeth when the prognosis for the natural teeth is guarded

84. All of the following statements concerning supporting cusps are true, except:

A. They contact the opposing tooth in the intercuspal position
B. They support the vertical dimension of the face
C. They are nearer the faciolingual center of the tooth than the non-supporting cusps
D. The outer incline has a potential for contact
E. They have narrower and sharper cusp ridges than non-supporting cusps

85. The process by which investment ring is heated in a porcelain furnace to a temperature of 980°C to burn off any remaining impurities prior to adding porcelain is called:

A. Quenching
B. Pickling
C. Degassing
D. Investing

86. All of the following are the theoretical determinants needed for restoring a complete and functional occlusal surface of a tooth, except:

A. The amount of vertical overlap of the anterior teeth
B. The contour of the articular eminence
C. The height of the pulp horn of that particular tooth
D. The amount and direction of lateral shift in the working side condyle
E. The position of the tooth in the arch

87. The first layer of porcelain applied to the metal coping is called the:

A. Opaque porcelain

B. Body porcelain
C. Incisal porcelain
D. None of the above

88. Which of the following statements is true concerning the posterior palatal seal?
A. The outline and depth of the posterior seal is the same for every patient
B. The posterior palatal seal will vary in outline and depth according to the palatal form of the patient
C. A posterior palatal seal is not necessary when fabricating a complete denture on a patient with a flat palate
D. Once the complete denture fits properly, it is okay to remove the posterior palatal seal.

89. The most important benefit of an over denture (root-retained denture) is:
A. The psychological comfort of avoiding the loss of all teeth
B. The continuous functional feedback for the neuromuscular system from proprioceptors in the PDL
C. The preservation of the alveolar ridge
D. The improved support and stability for the denture
E. The increased retention of the denture

90. Which of the following changes are usually evident on the maxillary arch in a patient who wears a complete maxillary denture and lacs posterior occlusion
A. Excessive amount of hyperplasic tissue present on the anterior portion of the maxillary ridge
B. Poor bone structure in the anterior part of the maxilla
C. Fibrous tuberosities
D. All of the above

91. The process of the joining of two metals by the use of a filler material which has a substantially lower fusion temperature than that of the metal parts being joined is called
A. Pickling
B. Soldering
C. Fluxing
D. Casting

92. A patient comes to your office one week after delivery of new dentures She has developed a dispersed pattern of traumatic ulcers over the crest of the mandibular residual ridge. What is the most likely cause of these ulcers?
A. Acrylic resin spicules
B. An inaccurate denture base
C. Premature occlusal contacts
D. Particles of food trapped under the denture base

93. Before an accurate facebow transfer record can be made on a patient, which of the following must be determined?
A. Location of the hinge axis point
B. The inclination of each condyle
C. Vertical dimension of occlusal
D. Centric relation

94. The temporomandibular joint is a:
A. Hinge joint
B. Gliding *(Sliding)* joint
C. Combined hinge and gliding joint
D. Ball and socket joint

95. All new dentures should be evaluated:
A. 3 hours after delivery
B. 12 hours after delivery
C. 24 hours after delivery
D. 48 hours after delivery

96. Where do the occlusal contact possibility occur during protrusive movement
A. On the maxillary mesial inclines and mandibular distal inclines
B. On the maxillary mesial inclines and mandibular mesial inclines
C. On the maxillary distal inclines and mandibular mesial inclines
D. On the maxillary distal inclines and mandibular distal inclines

97. Your are about to take alginate impressions on a patient. What can you do to help prevent the patient from gagging during this procedure?
A. Take your time

B. Work quickly
C. Use warm water to mix the alginate
D. Use cold water to mix the alginate
E. Have the patient breathe through his/her nose
F. Have the patient breathe his/her mouth
G. Recline the patient
H. Seat the patient in an upright position

98. The determinants of occlusion include:
A. The right temporomandibular joint and its suspensor ligaments
B. The left temporomandibular joint and its suspensor ligaments
C. The occlusal surface of the teeth
D. The neuromuscular system
E. All of the above

99. The major weakness of all-ceramic crowns is:
A. Poor esthetics
B. Their inability to flex
C. Their lack of translucency
D. Their high compressive strength

100. In an ideal intercuspal position the mesio buccal cusp of the permanent maxillary second molars oppose what?
A. The distobuccal groove of the mandibular first molar
B. The buccal groove of the mandibular second molar
C. The mesio buccal groove of the mandibular second molar
D. The development groove between the distobuccal and the distal cusp of the mandibular first molar

101. Teeth that appear to be color matched under one type of light appear very different under light source. This phenomenon is called what?
A. Fluorescence
B. Metamerism
C. Opaqueness
D. None of the above

102. In metal-ceramic restorations, where does the failure or fractures usually occur?
A. In the porcelain

B. At the porcelain metal interface
C. In the metal
D. None of the above

103. The primary role of anterior teeth on denture is :
A. To incise food
B. Occlusion
C. Esthetics
D. Stability of the denture

104. The primary dentures support area for a mandibular complete denture is :
A. The labial vestibule
B. The buccal shelf
C. The palatopharyngeal fold
D. The frenulum

105. Endodontically treated teeth that have been restored with a cast and core and crown are subjected to the high incidence of :
A. Periodontal disease
B. Recurrent caries
C. Vertical root fracture
D. The need for an apicoectomy

106. Which of the following best describes Camper's line *(plane)*
A. It is a line *(plane)* which is determined by the occlusal surfaces of the teeth
B. It is a line *(plane)* which extends from the outer canthus of eye to the superior border of the tragus of the ear
C. It is the line *(plane)* running from the inferior border of the ala of the nose to the superior border of the tragus of the ear
D. None of the above

107. Alginate impressions were placed in a bowl of water so that they would not dry up before pouring them up in dental stone. Which of the following was the result of leaving these impressions immersed in water for a few hours?
A. Gelatin
B. Adsorption
C. Syneresis
D. Imbibition

108. Which of the following pontics is primarily used in the nonappearance zone ?

A. The saddle pontic
B. The sanitary pontic
C. The modified ridge lap pontic
D. Ridge lap pontics

109. Which of the following statements concerning selective grinding in complete denture fabrication for centric relation are true?

A. Ideally, selective grinding should result in harmonious cusp-fossa contacts of all upper and lower fossa (and marginal ridges of bicuspids)
B. Only grind cusp tips that interfere in centric, lateral and protrusive movements
C. Neither of the above statements are true
D. Both of the above statements are true

110. What is the recommended treatment for a patient that has lost her four maxillary incisors some time ago and suffered excessive ridge resorption?

A. A conventional six- unit fixed bridge
B. No treatment
C. A removable partial denture
D. A Maryland bridge

111. Which of the following impressions material are very accurate if the model is poured immediately but are dimensionally unstable on storage because they shrink due to the evaporation of ethanol, a by-product of the polymerization process ?

A. Polysulfide
B. Silicones
C. Polyvinyl siloxanes
D. Polyethers

112. All of the following are considered to be the basic rules for occlusal rest design when fabricating a removable partial denture except:

A. The rest should minimize the tilting action of the appliance
B. The rest must be placed so that it will prevent movement of the appliance in an occlusal direction

C. The rest should be placed so that it will prevent movement of the appliance in a cervical direction
D. The rest must have sharp angles to permit maximum retention

113. The function of an indirect retainer is:
A. To prevent horizontal dislodgement of the distal extension base of a removable partial denture
B. To connect the parts of the prosthesis located on one side of the arch with those on the opposite side
C. To prevent vertical dislodgement of the distal extension base of a removable partial denture
D. To link the major connector and other parts of the prosthesis together

114. The fixed vegetable or mineral oil present in a tube of zinc oxide performs what function when it is mixed with eugenol to form ZOE impression paste?
A. Accelerator
B. Plasticizer
C. Filler
D. All of the above

115. Which of the following elastic impression materials have very limited dimensional stability?
A. Irreversible (alginate) & Reversible hydrocolloid (agar-agar)
B. Silicones
C. Polyethers
D. Polyvinyl siloxanes

116. You are ready to place packing cord around a tooth that was prepared for a crown on a patient with hypertension. It is recommended to use a cord impregnated with:
A. Epinephrine
B. Alum (aluminum potassium sulfate)
C. Zinc chloride
D. None of the above

117. Which of the following is the most important reason for treatment of hyperplastic tissue before construction of a complete or removable partial denture?
A. It will make the patient feel better
B. It will make the facebow transfer easier to perform

C. To provide a firm, stable base for the denture
D. The final impression material will flow better

118. A nonrigid connector is comprised of:
A. A key
B. A keyway
C. A key and a keyway
D. None of the above

119. Which of the following cements is indicated when maximum retention is required or when the pulp is of no concern?
A. Zinc polycarboxylate cement
B. Glass ionomer cement
C. Zinc phosphate cement
D. ZOE cement

120. The most rigid palatal major connector is the:
A. Single palatal bar
B. Palatal horseshoe-shaped connector
C. Palatal plate
D. Anterior posterior palatal bar connector

121. The glaze firing:
A. Is the first firing and produces a rough surface
B. Is performed prior to adding body porcelain to ensure a rough surface
C. Is a separate firing and produces a smooth, translucent surface
D. Is performed on the metal coping to clean the surface of any impurities

122. The "Glossary of Prosthodontic Terms" defines balanced occlusion as:
A. An occlusion of the teeth which presents a harmonious relation of the occluding surfaces in centric position within the functional range
B. An occlusion of the teeth which presents a harmonious relation of the occluding surfaces in eccentric positions only within the functional range
C. An occlusion of the teeth which presents a harmonious relation of the occluding surfaces in centric and eccentric positions within the functional range
D. An occlusion of teeth of maximum intercuspation of teeth

123. In the inter cuspal position, the mesiolingual cusp of a permanent maxillary second molar occludes where?
A. Central fossa of the mandibular first molar
B. Central fossa of the mandibular second molar
C. The interproximal marginal ridge areas between the mandibular first and second molars
D. The interproximal marginal ridge areas between the mandibular second and third molars

124. The powder (polymer) used in self-cured or heat-cured acrylic resins is usually
A. Benzoyl peroxide
B. Polymethyl methacrylate (PMMA)
C. Hydroquinone
D. Methyl methacrylate (MMA)

125. When establishing a balanced occlusion, the lingual cusps of maxillary posterior teeth on the balancing side should contact:
A. The central fossae of mandibular posterior teeth
B. The lingual inclines of facial cusps of mandibular posterior teeth
C. The lingual inclines of lingual cusps of mandibular posterior teeth
D. The facial inclines of lingual cusps of mandibular posterior teeth

126. Which method below is the preferred method to preserve the facebow transfer?
A. Taking a plaster index
B. Using 10 X wax
C. Hand mount
D. None of the above

127. An overextended distobuccal corner of a mandibular denture will push against which muscle during function?
A. Zygomaticus
B. Orbicularis oris
C. Temporalis
D. Masseter

128. How will the alveolar ridge respond to a mandibular complete denture base that terminates short of the retromolar pad?
A. Marked ridge resorption will occur
B. The apposition of bone on the ridge will occur
C. The alveolar ridge will not be affected at all
D. It has no concern with bone

129. Which of the following impressions are not elastomers?
A. Alginate
B. Polysulfide
C. Silicones
D. Polyether
E. All of the above

130. Which of the following best describes "strain hardening" or work hardening"?
A. Hardening (or deformation) of a metal at room temperature
B. Hardening (or deformation) of a metal at a very high temperature
C. Softening a metal by controlled heating and cooling
D. Softening a metal at room temperature

131. Epulis fissuratum is caused by:
A. Poor oral hygiene
B. Denture cleaners
C. An ill-fitting denture flange
D. An incorrectly placed posterior palatal seal

132. Dental plaster and stone is vibrated after mixing to:
A. Minimize distortion
B. Reduce setting time
C. Eliminate air bubbles
D. Increase the setting time

133. All surfaces of the metal coping or substructure in a metal-ceramic crown should be:
A. Smooth
B. Well-rounded
C. Convex
D. All of the above

134. All of the following are advantages of using a cast chromium-cobalt alloy for removable partial dentures except:
A. Corrosion resistance
B. High strength
C. High flexibility
D. Low specific gravity

135. Die Stone is classified as which type of gypsum product?
A. Type I
B. Type II
C. Type III
D. Type IV

136. Which of the following is defined as "the quality of a restoration to be firm, steady, constant and not subject to change of position when forces are applied"?
A. Retention
B. Stability
C. Adhesion
D. Reciprocation

137. All of the following are advantages of infrabulge retainers as compared to suprabulge retainers except:
A. More efficient retention
B. Less distortion of coronal contours
C. Less tooth contact
D. Cleaner
E. Less bothersome to vestibular tissues
F. Less prone to caries
G. Esthetically superior in most cases
H. Greater adjustability

138. In a protrusive movement, the condyles of the mandible have moved in a:
A. Backward and upward direction
B. Downward and forward direction
C. Backward and downward direction
D. Forward and backward direction one by one

139. In a posterior fixed bridge, a pontic:
A. Should be in contact in centric occlusion
B. May or may not be in contact in working-side movements

C. Should not be in contact in nonworking side movements
D. All of the above

140. When the mandible is in its physiologic rest or postural position, the contact of teeth is:
A. Maximum
B. Not present
C. Premature
D. Slight

141. Centric occlusion (CO) is a:
A. "Muscle-guided" position
B. "Ligament-guided" position
C. "Tooth-guided" position
D. Bone guided position

142. Occlusion rims are used to:
A. Determine and establish the vertical dimension of occlusion
B. Make maxillo-mandibular jaw records
C. Establish and locate the future position of the artificial teeth
D. All of the above

143. An excessive vertical dimension of occlusion is the usual cause of:
A. Cheek biting
B. Gagging
C. Clicking
D. Reduced taste

144. A patient who wears a complete maxillary denture complains of a burning sensation in the palatal area of his/her mouth. This is indicative of too much pressure being exerted by the denture on the:
A. Incisive foramen
B. Palatal mucosa
C. Hamular notch
D. Posterior palatal seal

145. All of the following are benefits that a patient usually realizes from immediate dentures except:
A. Continuously acceptable esthetics
B. Improved speech adaptation
C. Protection of the extraction sites from trauma

D. Decreased post-delivery soreness
E. Continuously acceptable masticatory function
F. Prevention of tongue enlargement

146. Which component of zinc oxide-eugenol impression paste functions as an accelerator of the setting time?
A. Oil of cloves
B. Resinous balsam
C. Rosin
D. Calcium chloride

147. All of the following statements concerning elastomeric impression materials are true except:
A. All elastomeric impression materials expand slightly during setting
B. Elastomeric impression materials are unable to displace both oral fluids and gingival tissues
C. The prepared teeth should be free of surface moisture but not bone dry prior to taking an impression with elastomeric impression materials.
D. Compared to hydrocolloids, elastomeric impression materials are easier to prepare, are much more resistant to tearing on removal and have a superior dimensional stability.

148. Xerostomia can be caused by:
A. Medications (i.e. antihypertensives and antidepressants)
B. Cancer therapy (i.e. chemotherapeutic drugs and radiation treatment)
C. Sjogren's syndrome
D. Trauma to the head and neck causing nerve damage
E. Conditions such as bone marrow transplants, endocrine, disorders, stress, anxiety, depression and nutritional deficiencies
F. All of the above

149. Surgical removal of a maxillary torus is indicated when?
A. The torus impinges on the soft palate
B. The torus is so large that it fills the vault and prevents the formation of an adequate denture base
C. The torus is undercut
D. The torus extends so far posteriorly that it interferes with the posterior palatal seal

E. When it is psychologically disturbing to the patient who suffers from cancerphobia
F. All of the above

150. A reverse ¾ crown is most frequently fabricated for a:
A. Maxillary premolar
B. Mandibular premolar
C. Mandibular molar
D. Maxillary molar

151. When casting conventional gold alloys, which type of dental investment should be used?
A. Phosphate-bonded investment
B. Gypsum-bonded investment
C. Silica-bonded investment
D. None of the above

152. All of the following are indications for electrosurgery except:
A. To remove hyperplastic gingival tissue where it has proliferated into preparations or over crown margins
B. In place of gingival retraction cord where substantial attached gingiva is present
C. Where attached gingival tissues are thin or where an underlying dehiscence is suspected
D. For crown lengthening procedures prior to fabricating a provisional crown

153. What is the general rule for sprue pin diameter when using a centrifugal type of casting machine?
A. The diameter of the sprue pin should be equal to or greater than the thickest portion of the pattern
B. The diameter of the sprue pin should be equal to or smaller than the thickest portion of the pattern
C. The diameter of the sprue pin should be equal to or greater than the thinnest portion of the pattern
D. The diameter of the sprue pin should be equal to or smaller than the thinnest portion of the pattern

154. The major connector is:
A. The connecting tong between the denture and other units of the prosthesis
B. The part of the denture base which extends from the necks of the teeth to the border of the denture

C. The unit of a partial denture that connects the parts of the prosthesis located on one side of the arch with those on the opposite side
D. None of the above

155. Which component of the chromium alloys used to fabricate the framework for removable partial dentures increases the ductility of the alloy?
A. Chromium
B. Cobalt
C. Nickel
D. Copper

156. A definitive evaluation of existing occlusal disharmonies can only be made after:
A. Evaluating the full mouth radiographs
B. A periodontal evaluation
C. Mounting diagnostic casts
D. A full mouth scaling and polishing

157. The cingulum rest is usually confined to preparation on:
A. Maxillary lateral incisors
B. Maxillary canines
C. Mandibular lateral incisors
D. Mandibular canines

158. Prolonged sensitivity to heat, cold, and pressure after cementation of a crown or a fixed bridge is usually related to:
A. Recurrent decay
B. A periodontal problem
C. Occlusal trauma
D. An open margin

159. Which teeth listed below should ideally provide the predominant guidance through the full range of movement in lateral mandibular excursions?
A. Premolars
B. First molars
C. Incisors
D. Canines

160. When border molding a mandibular custom tray that will be used for a final denture impression:

A. The distofacial extension is determined by the position and action of the temporalis muscle and the distolingual extension is limited by the action of the superior constrictor muscle
B. The distofacial extension is determined by the position and action of the masseter muscle and the distolingual extension is limited by the action of the superior constrictor muscle
C. The distofacial extension is determined by the position and action of the mylohyoid muscle and the distolingual extension is limited by the action of the inferior constrictor muscle
D. The distofacial extension is determined by the position and action of the genioglossus muscle and the distolingual extension is limited by action of the inferior constrictor muscle

161. In the intercuspal position, the distobuccal cusp of a permanent mandibular first molar occludes where?

A. The interproximal marginal ridge area between the maxillary second bicuspid and first molar
B. Central fossa of the maxillary first molar
C. Central fossa of the maxillary second molar
D. The interproximal marginal ridge area between the maxillary first molar and second molar.

162. In the mesial rest, guide plane and 1-bar design, reciprocation is achieved by:

A. Rigid plating
B. Minor connectors
C. Guide planes extended around the vertical line of abutments
D. Contact areas of proximal teeth
E. Reciprocal clasp arms
F. All of the above

163. Which mandibular major connector listed below is more popular?

A. Lingual bar
B. Labial bar
C. Lingual plate
D. All of the above

164. In an ideal intercuspal position, the mesiolingual cusps of permanent mandibular molars oppose:

A. The opposing central fossae
B. The lingual embrasure between their class counterpart and the tooth distal to it
C. The opposing distal marginal ridge
D. The lingual embrasure between their class counterpart and the tooth mesial to it

165. When posterior teeth are in a normal ideal relationship, which of the following cusps are considered to be supporting cusps?

A. Maxillary lingual cusps
B. Maxillary buccal cusps
C. Mandibular lingual cusps
D. Mandibular buccal cusps

166. In an ideal intercuspal position, the facial cusps tips of permanent maxillary premolars oppose:

A. The facial embrasure between their class counterpart and the tooth mesial to it
B. The facial embrasure between their class counterpart and the tooth distal to it
C. The opposing central fossae
D. The opposing mesial marginal ridge

167. Reducing occlusal interferences (selective grinding) should usually be done:

A. After a fixed bridge or a partial denture is delivered to a patient
B. Before constructing a fixed bridge or a partial denture for a patient
C. After a fixed bridge but before a partial denture is delivered to a patient
D. After a partial denture but before a fixed bridge is delivered to a patient

168. After border molding the mandibular custom tray, it is important to check for dislodgement in order to detect areas of:

A. Underextension of the tray
B. Overextension of the tray
C. Thickness of the tray
D. None of the above

169. In dentistry, the most frequently used polymer system is:
A. Bis-GMA
B. Polyether
C. Methyl methacrylate
D. Polyvinyl

170. Immediate dentures should be scheduled for relines at:
A. 1 month and 3 months post extraction
B. 4 months and 7 months post extraction
C. 5 months and 10 months post extraction
D. 1 year and 2 years post extraction

171. A generalized speech difficulty with complete dentures is usually caused by which two of the following?
A. Faulty tooth position
B. Excess vertical dimension of occlusion
C. Faulty palatal contours
D. Faulty occlusion

172. Which of the following components found in alginate powder controls the setting time of alginate?
A. Sodium alginate
B. Sodium phosphate
C. Calcium ions
D. Calcium alginate

173. Latex gloves should not be worn when mixing which of the following elastomeric impression materials by hand?
A. Polyether
B. Polysulfide
C. Condensation silicone
D. Addition silicone

174. Overbite is:
A. The horizontal projection of the maxillary anterior teeth beyond the mandibular anterior teeth
B. The vertical overlapping of the maxillary anterior teeth over the mandibular anterior teeth
C. A malocclusion in which the anterior teeth do not close or come together
D. A malocclusion where some of the maxillary teeth are inside of the mandibular teeth .

Answer key to prosthodontics

1	A, D	2	B	3	C	4	D
5	B	6	D	7	A	8	A
9	A	10	C	11	C	12	D
13	D	14	B	15	C	16	B
17	E	18	C	19	C	20	B
21	C	22	C	23	E	24	C
25	C	26	B	27	B	28	D
29	D	30	D	31	E	32	C
33	A	34	B	35	B	36	C
37	C	38	D	39	E	40	B
41	D	42	G	43	B	44	C
45	A	46	B	47	B	48	B
49	B	50	A	51	B	52	D
53	C	54	A	55	B	56	D
57	D	58	C	59	A	60	C
61	B	62	B	63	B	64	B
65	B	66	E	67	E	68	B
69	C	70	C	71	D	72	C
73	C	74	A	75	A	76	C
77	C	78	C	79	B	80	C, D
81	A	82	B	83	D	84	E
85	C	86	C	87	A	88	B
89	C	90	D	91	B	92	C
93	A	94	C	95	C	96	C
97	B, C, E, H	98	E	99	B	100	B
101	B	102	A	103	C	104	B
105	C	106	C	107	D	108	B
109	D	110	C	111	B	112	D
113	C	114	B	115	A	116	B
117	C	118	C	119	C	120	D
121	C	122	C	123	B	124	B
125	B	126	A	127	D	128	A
129	A	130	A	131	C	132	C
133	D	134	C	135	D	136	B
137	E	138	B	139	D	140	B
141	C	142	D	143	C	144	A
145	D	146	D	147	A	148	F

149	F	150	C	151	B	152	C
153	A	154	C	155	C	156	C
157	B	158	C	159	D	160	B
161	B	162	F	163	A	164	D
165	A, D	166	B	167	B	168	B
169	C	170	C	171	A, C	172	B
173	D	174	B				

Reader's Notes

11

Operative Dentistry

1. The optimum fluoride concentration in community drinking water is:
A. 0.1 ppm
B. 0.12 ppm
C. 1.0 ppm
D. 10.0 ppm

2. Which of the following is not an essential factor needed for the initiation of a carious lesion?
A. Susceptible host (tooth)
B. Microflora with cariogenic potential (plaque)
C. Saliva
D. Suitable substrate (dietary carbohydrates)

3. The principal feature of a sealant that is required for success is:
A. High viscosity
B. Adequate retention
C. An added colorant to make the appearance slightly different from the occlusal enamel
D. High strength

4. The outline form of a Class V composite preparation resembles that of a Class V amalgam preparation except for what important feature listed below?
A. No retentive grooves are necessary
B. The internal line angles are much more rounded
C. Pulp protection is not required
D. None of the above

5. Which of the following is formed very rapidly in response to irritants?
A. Primary dentin
B. Secondary dentin
C. Reparative dentin
D. Sclerotic dentin

6. The gypsum bonded investments are used with
A. Type 1 gold allows
B. Type II gold alloys
C. Type III gold alloys
D. All of the above

7. Caries that is often found in older patients and attacks the cementum and radicular (root) dentin is called?
A. Residual caries
B. Secondary (recurrent) caries
C. Root surface (senile) caries
D. None of the above

8. For an efficient four handed dental delivery system, the position of the chairside assistant should be:
A. Lower than the dentist
B. At the same height as the dentist
C. Higher than the dentist
D. None of the above

9. The number one indication for the use of direct filling gold is:
A. The large Class II lesion
B. The small initial Class III lesion
C. The small Class II lesion
D. The large Class III lesion

10. How is high mercury content generally manifested in the clinical amalgam restoration?
A. By tissue irritation adjacent to the restoration
B. By severe marginal breakdown
C. By delayed expansion
D. By increased thermal shock resulting from hot and cold foods.

11. Rapid cooling by immersion in water, of a dental casting from the high temperature at which it has been shaped is referred to as:
A. Annealing
B. Tempering
C. Quenching
D. None of the above

12. High copper and low mercury content of an amalgam restoration will tend to
A. Increase creep
B. Decrease creep
C. Will not effect creep
D. Can either decrease or increase

13. The amount of mercury remaining in dental amalgam after condensation directly affects which of the following?
A. The porosity of the restoration
B. The compressive strength of the restoration
C. The corrosion resistance of the restoration
D. The surface finish of the restoration
E. All of the above

14. Which cement below, when set, has the potential to inhibit the development of recurrent caries at its margin as a result of fluoride release from its surface?
A. Zinc polycarboxylate cement
B. Zinc oxide-eugenol
C. Zinc phosphate cement
D. Glass ionomer cement

15. All of the following are radiographic signs of trauma from occlusion except
A. Hypercementosis
B. Root resorption

C. Periodontal pockets
D. Alternation of the lamina dura
E. Widening of the periodontal ligament space

16. Frequently, the surface of a gold casting is dark due to the formation of a surface oxide film. This surface film is removed by:
A. Quenching
B. Age Hardening
C. Pickling
D. Fusion

17. A short, painful response to cold suggests:
A. Pulpal necrosis
B. Irreversible pulpitis
C. Pulpal hyperemia
D. Acute apical periodontitis

18. A properly acid-etched enamel surface appears:
A. Somewhat yellow in color
B. Identical to unetched enamel
C. Dull white and chalky
D. Slightly gray with a shine

19. The total energy absorbed to the point of fracture is referred to as:
A. Resilience
B. Brittleness
C. Toughness
D. Modulus of elasticity

20. The attraction of unlike molecules is referred to as:
A. Adhesion
B. Cohesion
C. Attraction
D. None of the above

21. Which cement system listed below was the first system developed with a potential for adhesion to tooth structure?
A. Zinc phosphate cement
B. Zinc polycarboxylate cement
C. Zinc oxide-eugenol
D. Calcium hydroxide cement

22. A lesser number of blades on a bur result in
A. More efficient cutting and a smoother surface
B. Less efficient cutting and a rougher surface
C. More efficient cutting but a rougher surface
D. Less efficient cutting but a smoother surface

23. Filled resins *(Composite resin)*
A. Are harder and stronger than unfilled resins
B. Have a lower coefficient of thermal expansion than unfilled resins
C. Are more resistant to abrasion than unfilled resins
D. All of the above

24. Which of the following instruments is designed to most effectively plane the enamel of the facial and lingual walls of a class II amalgam preparation?
A. A gingival margin trimmer
B. A straight chisel
C. An enamel hatchet
D. Spoon excavator

25. Today the most popular way to polymerize matrix monomers is:
A. Self-cured
B. Chemically cured
C. Ultraviolet light-cured
D. Visible light-cured

26. Which of the following are indications for the use of pins
A. A class II amalgam preparation where one or more cusps have been lost or where the outline form otherwise far exceeds that which is considered normal.
B. A very large class III amalgam preparation
C. A class V amalgam preparation which far exceeds minimal dimensions especially in the gingivo-incisal area
D. A preparation for an amalgam buildup over which a cast restoration will be fabricated
E. All of the above

27. All of the following are major parts of a hand - cutting instrument *except*
A. Handle

B. Shank
C. Nib
D. Blade

28. Which of the following statements in reference to amalgam is false?
A. Increased trituration time will increase compressive strength and decrease setting expansion
B. A decrease in particle size will decrease compressive strength and increase setting expansion
C. Increased condensation pressure will increase compressive strength and decrease setting expansion
D. All are false.

29. Essential properties of a Class V cavity prepared for direct filling gold include:
A. Sharp internal line angles
B. Small retentive undercuts placed in the axio-occlusal and axio-gingival line angles
C. Mesial and distal walls that flair and meet the cavosurface at a 90^0 angle
D. An axial wall that is convex and follows the external contour of the tooth, 5 mm into dentin
E. All of the above

30. The selection of a base to be used under a permanent restoration is governed by
A. The design of the cavity
B. The type of permanent restorative material used
C. The proximity of the pulp in relation to the cavity wall
D. All of the above

31. What is the proper amount of time to wait until an amalgam restoration can be finished and polished ?
A. 2 hours
B. 12 hours
C. 24-48 hours
D. Makes no difference

32. Which cavity lining agent below does not provide thermal protection ?
A. Calcium hydroxide

B. Zinc oxide eugenol
C. Copalite
D. All of the above

33. When attempting to isolate an operating field in the oral cavity, which method listed below would be the best to use ?
A. Mouth prop
B. Cotton roll isolation with saliva ejectors
C. Rubber dam
D. All of the above

34. Starting from the lowest to the highest rate, arrange the following materials based on their coefficient of thermal expansion:
- Unfilled resin, 5
- Composite resins, 4
- Amalgam, 3
- Direct gold , 2
- Tooth, 1

A. 3, 4, 5, 2, 1
B. 3, 2 , 1, 5, 4,
C. 5, 4, 3, 2, 1
D. 1, 2, 3, 4, 5

35. Composite filler particles function to do all of the following *except*
A. Increase the coefficient of thermal expansion
B. Increase the tensile strength and compressive strength
C. Reduce the polymerization shrinkage
D. Increase the hardness
E. Improve the wear resistance

36. Which of the statements are true concerning posterior composite restorations
A. Posterior composite restoration are frequently indicated in the treatment of occlusal lesions which allow conservative preparations
B. Posterior composite restoration are contraindicated in patient with heavy occlusion *(bruxims)*
C. Posterior composite restorations are contraindicated in a patient with a carries active mouth

D. Posterior composite restorations may be indicated for the restorations of class II cavities in premolar teeth where the appearances is very important, the cavity margins are in the enamel, and the occlusal contacts are on the enamel
E. All of the above statements are true

37. The one characteristic that is common to all Class II gold inlay preparations is
A. The uniform depth of the pulpal floor
B. The lack of undercuts
C. The placement of a base
D. All of the above

38. Which of the following methods of investing is more dependable in the prevention of surface nodules on a casting?
A. Hand investing
B. Vacuum investing
C. Both produce similar result
D. Hand – cum – vacuum casting

39. The most important design characteristic of a bur blade is :
A. The clearance face
B. The rake face
C. The edge angle
D. The clearance angle
E. The rake angle

40. Silver's major effect in a gold casting alloy is :
A. Corrosion resistance
B. To increase the hardness
C. To offset the color contributions of copper
D. To elevate the melting range

41. The success of pulp capping is recognized by :
A. The symptoms of pulpitis
B. The lack of a vital response after several weeks or months
C. The formation of a complete barrier of dentin at the site of pulpal exposure
D. The patient being able to bite down hard on the tooth.

42. Which tooth below requires special attention when preparing the occlusal aspect for a restoration?
A. Maxillary first bicuspid
B. Mandibular first bicuspid
C. Maxillary second bicuspid
D. Mandibular second bicuspid

43. When is the matrix band removed from the tooth?
A. Prior the final caving of the restoration
B. As soon as the amalgam has been condensed into the prep
C. After the final carving of the restoration
D. None of the above

44. The retention of a pin:
A. Decrease as the diameter of the pin increases
B. Increases as the diameter of the pin increases
C. Increases as the diameter of the pin decreases
D. The retention of a pin has nothing to do with the diameter of the pin

45. When mixing zinc phosphate cement, a cool slab is used to :
A. Accelerate the setting time
B. Create more free zinc oxide in the cement
C. Increase the powder-liquid ratio
D. Increase expansion of the set cement

46. Which preparations listed below has a proximal cavosurface margin that form a 90 angle with the external surface?
A. A conservative class II amalgam
B. A conservative class II inlay
C. Neither of the above
D. Both of the above

47. All of the following statements concerning direct gold are true except:
A. It is most nearly permanent of all restorative materials
B. It provides good adaptation to the cavity walls
C. Its coefficient of thermal expansion is close to that of tooth structure
D. It has a low tensile strength *(edge strength)*
E. It will not corrode

48. Bases are materials that function:
A. As barriers against pulpally irritating agents
B. To provide thermal insulation below a restoration
C. To provide adequate resistance to the compressive forces of mastication
D. All of the above

49. Which class III lesions listed below should not be filled with composite resin
A. Mesial-lingual of canines
B. Distal-lingual of laterals
C. Mesial-lingual of centrals
D. Distal-lingual of canines

50. Zone II of carious dentin is also referred to as :
A. Normal dentin
B. Sub-transparent dentin
C. Transparent dentin
D. Turbid dentin
E. Infected dentin

51. Which rubber dam frame listed below provides more retraction of the tissues
A. Woodbury
B. Young's
C. Both are the same
D. None of the above

52. The main advantage of using an 8% solution of stannous fluoride instead of a 2% solution of sodium fluoride for a topical fluoride treatment is :
A. It will not stain
B. It has a better taste
C. It is stable when kept in a polyethylene container
D. A single treatment may be given

53. The pH of acidulated phosphate fluoride gels is in which of the following ranges?
A. 1 to 4
B. 4 to 7
C. 7 to 10
D. 10 to 12

54. A dental patient may experience a sharp pain when two restorations constructed of dissimilar materials in opposing arches make contact in the wet environment of the oral cavity This clinical phenomenon is commonly known as:

A. Current explosion
B. Voltage flow
C. Electrolyte explosion
D. Galvanic shock

55. Small hybrid size filler particles in composite resins :

A. Result in a composite resin that has better finishing characteristics but a lesser resistance to wear
B. Result in a composite resin that has greater resistance to wear but doesn't finish well
C. Result in a composite resin that has better finishing characteristics and a greater resistance to wear
D. Result in a composite resin that has a lesser resistance to wear and also doesn't finish well

56. Which of the following are advantages of the visible light curing systems compared to the old ultraviolet light curing system ?

A. A greater depth of resin can be cured by visible light
B. The resin can be polymerized through enamel, which is particularly advantageous in class III restorations
C. The intensity of visible light remains relatively constant until the bulb fails completely
D. All of the above

57. A diagonal cut across the cavosurface margin that is flat in one dimension only and curved in other dimensions is called a:

A. Plane
B. Bevel
C. Chamfer
D. Butt

58. Which grasp used with hand instruments allows for the greatest intricacy or delicacy of touch ?

A. The modified pen grasp
B. The inverted pen grasp
C. The palm and thumb grasp
D. The modified palm and thumb grasp

59. All of the following statements concerning the use of base metal casting alloys compared to using noble metal casting alloys for cast restorations are true *except*

A. Base metal alloys are harder to cast and finish
B. Base metal alloys are less dense
C. Base metal alloys are stronger
D. Base metal alloys are more resistant to corrosion

60. Favorable factors for direct pulp capping include:

A. The visual evidence of uninflamed *(pink)* pulp tissue
B. The absence of copious hemorrhage through the exposure
C. No previous symptoms of pulpitis
D. A small non-carious exposure (a mechanical pulp exposure)
E. A clean cavity uncontaminated with saliva
F. All of the above

61. Which of the following cavosurface margins is the only one that is beveled when preparing class II amalgam preparation?

A. The occlusal cavosurface margin
B. The facial cavosurface margin of the proximal box
C. The lingual cavosurface margin of the proximal box
D. The gingival cavosurface margin of the proximal box

62. The outline form of the classical class V amalgam preparation is :

A. Square
B. Deformed trapezoid
C. Triangle
D. Rectangle

63. A short, painful response to cold suggests:

A. Pulpal necrosis
B. Irreversible pulpits
C. Pulpal hyperemia
D. Acute apical periodontitis

64. Which cement listed below is the oldest of the luting cements and thus is the one that has the longest "track record" and serves as the standard to which newer systems can be compared?

A. Glass ionomer cement
B. Zinc polycarboxylate cement

C. Zinc phosphate cement
D. Zinc oxide eugenol

65. The greatest stress to which a material can be subjected such that it will return to his original dimensions when the forces are released is referred to as the.
A. Proportional limit
B. Elastic limit
C. Yield strength
D. Tensile strength

66. Which cement (luting agent) below is also used as a permanent restorative agent ?
A. Zinc polycarboxylate
B. Zinc phosphate
C. Glass ionomer
D. Zinc oxide-eugenol

67. Unfilled resin *(acrylic)* temporaries fabricated for inlays and on lays should have which of the following properties?
A. Restore and maintain proximal contacts
B. Restore and maintain tooth occlusion
C. Restore and maintain tooth contours
D. The margins should be closed and flush with the tooth
E. All of the above

68. All of the following are contraindications to the placement of sealants except
A. Patient behavior does not allow for the maintenance of the dry field necessary for successful application
B. There is a carious lesion on the occlusal surface
C. Children whose teeth have a deep pits and fissures
D. There is a carious lesion on the smooth surface that necessitates preparation of the occlusal surface
E. Tooth has been previously restored
F. Tooth is not fully erupted and a dry field can not be maintained

69. Which of the following instruments is designed for the removal of caries and refinement of the internal parts of a preparations?
A. A hoe
B. A file

C. An excavator
D. A scaler

70. When comparing the physical properties of filled resins to unfilled resin, all of the following are true *except*
A. Filled resins are harder
B. Unfilled resins have a lower coefficient of thermal expansion
C. Filled resins have a higher compressive strength
D. Unfilled resins have a lower modulus of elasticity
E. Filled resin have higher tensile strength

71. The most frequently used pins are :
A. Cemented pins
B. Frictions- locked pins
C. Self-threaded pins
D. All of the above

72. The edge angle of a bur blade is:
A. The angle made between the line connecting the edge of the blade to the axis of the bur and the rake face.
B. The angle formed between the rake face and the clearance face
C. The angle formed between the clearance face and a tangent to the path of rotation.
D. None of the above

73. Which of the following characteristics of amalgam would explain why cold sensitivity is the most common problem encountered after placing a dental amalgam restoration?
A. Its coefficient of thermal expansion
B. Its biocompatibility
C. Its thermal insulation properties
D. Its high edge strength

74. Annealing is the process of heating and cooling a metal to make it:
A. Weaker and more brittle
B. Tougher and less brittle
C. More tarnish resistant
D. Easier to cast and finish

75. If a zinc phosphate cement base is used restoring a tooth, when should the varnish be applied?

A. Prior to placement of the base
B. After placement of the base
C. Makes no difference when the varnish is applied
D. Varnish should not be used in conjunction with zinc phosphate cement

76. Which circumference of the matrix band is always place toward the occlusal surface of the tooth?

A. Smaller
B. Larger
C. Both openings of the band have the same circumference
D. Does not matter

77. Cavity liners are used to:

A. Help retain the restorative material
B. Protect the pulp
C. Add strength to the restorative material
D. Decrease the setting expansion of amalgam

78. The two most frequently quoted disadvantages of using the rubber dam are :

A. Time consumption
B. Patient objection
C. Cost
D. Staff allergies to material

79. Which of the following statements concerning sealants are true:

A. Sealants are highly effectively in preventing pit and fissure caries
B. When sealants are applied correctly, there is a decreased development of new carious lesions and a decreased progression of pre-existing lesions
C. A close correlation exists between the retention of sealants and their effectiveness
D. The effectiveness of sealants appears to be equal whether applied by dentist, dental hygienists or dental assistant, provided that they have received appropriate training
E. Acid-etch resin sealants are classified into three types, based on the method by which they are cured
F. All of the above statements are true

80. All of the following facts concerning fluoride are true *except*.

A. Most fluoride is absorbed in the small intestine and excreted through the kidneys
B. Fluorosis may result from excessive fluoride consumed during the mineralization stage of tooth development and can occur in permanent and deciduous teeth
C. Fluoride passes the placental barrier slowly
D. Fluoride is deposited in calcified tissues *(i.e. bones)*
E. At 1.0 ppm, fluoride is tasteless, colorless and odorless
F. The US Public health Service sets the optimal fluoride level at 1.2 to 2.5 ppm for public water
G. The cariostatic effect of fluoride is produced during the calcification stage of tooth development
H. The uptake of fluoride by the teeth depends on the amount of fluoride ingested (not delivered) and the length of time of exposure.

81. The squeezing of material by external forces is called?

A. Compression
B. Tension
C. Shear
D. Brittleness

82. The most susceptible area of a tooth for the retention of dental plaque is :

A. The cusp tips
B. The proximal surfaces
C. The developmental pits and fissures
D. The buccal and lingual surfaces

83. Pit and fissure caries does not spread laterally to a extent until the

A. Pulp is reached
B. Dentinoenamel junction *(DEJ)* is reached
C. Cementoenamel junction (CEJ) is reached
D. Marginal ridge is reached

84. Enamel is etched with

A. Boric acid
B. Phosphoric acid
C. Acetic acid
D. Nitric acid

85. Crystalline gold is also known as :

A. Mat gold
B. Gold foil
C. Powdered gold
D. Electraloy

86. The softest dental inlay wax is :

A. Type A
B. Type B
C. Type C
D. None of the above

87. With respect to onlay preparations, "shoeing" of a functional cusp is :

A. Sometimes indicated
B. Always indicated
C. Never indicated
D. None of the above

88. The most conservative way to lighten vital teeth is:

A. Bleaching
B. Direct composites
C. Laboratory- fabricated porcelain veneers
D. Full coverage crowns

89. Surrounding the wax pattern with a material which can accurately duplicate its shape and anatomical feature is referred to as :

A. Investing
B. Burnout
C. Casting
D. Picking

90. The outline form a cavity preparation is defined as:

A. That form the cavity takes to resist the forces of mastication
B. That from the cavity takes to resist dislodgement or displacement of the restoration
C. The shape or form of the cavity on the surface of the tooth
D. All of the above

91. A 15-year old female has lived in a non-fluoridated area all of her life. Which of the following is most likely to occur in

this female when she moves to a community where the drinking water naturally contains 6 ppm of fluoride ?

A. A 50% reduction in dental caries
B. Moderate dental fluorosis
C. An increase in the amount of fluoride stored in her bones
D. Gastrointestinal problems

92. After the initial setting period, which of the following cements is the least soluble?

A. Zinc phosphate cement
B. Zinc polycarboxylate cement
C. Glass ionomer cement
D. Zinc eugenol cement

93. Which property of filled resins is primarily to blame for the failure of class II composite restoration?

A. Low flexural strength
B. Low compressive strength
C. Low Tensile strength
D. Low wear resistance

94. Head and neck cancer patients can benefit by using which of the following fluoride types for home-care custom tray use?

A. Stannous fluoride only
B. Acidulated phosphate fluoride only
C. Sodium fluoride and stannous fluoride
D. Sodium fluoride and acidulated phosphate fluoride

95. A necrotic pulp may

A. Have no painful symptoms
B. Not respond to the electric pulp tester at any current level
C. Respond to heat
D. Not respond to acid
E. All of the above

96. If a casting fails to completely seat in a cavity, one should first check for :

A. Undercuts in the tooth preparation
B. Residual temporary cement or other debris in the cavity
C. Premature internal contact
D. Excessively light proximal contacts

97. The mesial and distal walls of a class I amalgam preparation should diverge slightly towards the occlusal surface to :

A. Provide convenience form
B. Provide resistance from
C. Afford support for the mesial and distal marginal ridges
D. Make condensing of the amalgam easier

98. All of the following are disadvantages of cast gold restorations *except*

A. Esthetic
B. Cost
C. Time-consuming
D. Difficulty of technique
E. Gold has a low thermal conductivity
F. The need to use cement, which is the weakest point in the cast gold restoration

99. Match the following four types of ZOE material with their indications for use.

Types of ZOE Materials	Indications for use	Matching
Type I ZOE	Cavity liner	4
Type II ZOE	Temporary cement	1
Type III ZOE	Permanent cement	2
Type IV ZOE	Temporary filling or base	3

100. Which line angle listed below is rounded when preparing a class II amalgam preparation

A. Axiobuccal
B. Axiolingual
C. Axiopulpal
D. None of the above

101. All of the following statements are true regarding glass ionomer restorations *except*

A. Glass ionomer is often the ideal material of choice for restoring root surface carries in patients with high caries activity
B. The best surface finish for a glass ionomer restorations is that obtained against surface matrix

C. Glass ionomer adheres to mineralized tooth issue
D. Glass ionomers are somewhat esthetic and polish much better than composites

102. Pulpal pain, either spontaneous or elicited by an irritant, that lingers more than 10 seconds suggest:
A. Pulpal necrosis
B. Pulpal hyperemia
C. Irreversible pulpits
D. Acute apical periodontitis

103. All of the following statements concerning fluoride are true *except*
A. The substantial reduction in dental decay that have occurred in the young population in the United States are due, for the most part, to the use of systemic and topical fluorides
B. Fluoride reduces caries by increasing the enamel hardness
C. Fluoride converts hydroxyapatite into fluorapatite by the substitution of the OH ion for the fluoride ion
D. The fluoride ion decreases the solubility of the hydroxy-apatite crystal and at the same time increases the size of the crystal itself.

104. All of the following are components of sodium fluoride paste that can be used to treat sensitivity except.
A. Sodium fluoride
B. Kaolin
C. Glycerin
D. Eugenol

105. Which of the following is defined as "that form the cavity preparation takes to aid the operator in preparing, or finishing the restoration"?
A. Retention form
B. Resistance form
C. Convenience form
D. Outline form

106. There is abundant evidence that the initiation of dental caries requires a high proportion of:
A. Staphylococcus aureus within saliva
B. Streptococcus mutans within dental plaque

C. Streptococcus mutans within food
D. Staphylococcus aureus within dental plaque

107. Acute caries is characterized by all of the following except:
A. Most frequently found in children
B. Often multiple, soft in children
C. Slowly progressing
D. Little or no staining

108. Which component of a dentin bonding system listed below functions primarily to remove the smear layer of the dentin?
A. Etchant
B. Conditioner
C. Primer
D. Adhesive

109. The best angle to attach the sprue pin to the proximal wall of a wax pattern is:
A. 20°
B. 45°
C. 90°
D. The angle makes no difference

110. Which of the following are indications for a cast gold onlay?
A. Restoration of large lesions: involving more than one-third intercuspal dimension, extensive loss of supporting structure where at least half of the clinical cusps. Loss of cusp (s) with at least 1 mm of dentin supporting remaining cusps
B. Restoration of ideal occlusion in cases of drifting, hypo- and hyper eruption, etc.
C. Restoration of optimum contour and proximal contact
D. Restoration of brittle teeth (endodontically treated)
E. Restoration of a tooth as an abutment for removable prosthesis, creating ideal guiding planes, rest seals and undercuts
F. Restoration of teeth to meet patient preference for gold
G. All of the above

111. All of the following are advantages or indications for a Class II gold inlay except
A. The desire for permanency
B. A low caries index

C. Less expensive
D. Moderate size lesions with conservative outlines

112. All of the following drugs may be useful in controlling salivary secretions to help in obtaining a dry field except:
A. Atropine
B. Methantheline
C. Diazepam
D. Belladonna derivatives
E. Propantheline bromide

113. Which of the following factors tends to reduce the setting expansion of amalgam.
A. Increasing the amount of mercury in the mix
B. Increasing the silver content of alloy
C. Increasing the trituration time
D. Increasing the zinc content of the alloy

114. Which of the following is the strongest phase of the set amalgam?
A. Gamma
B. Gamma-one
C. Gamma-two
D. They are all the same strength.

115. Why is it important to restore proper proximal contact when restoring teeth?
A. To minimize periodontal pocket formation
B. To maintain the proper height of the interproximal papillae
C. To maintain the mesiodistal dimension of the tooth
D. To minimize food impaction
E. All of the above

116. All of the following are true concerning a Class V amalgam preparation except:
A. The outline form is determined primarily by the location of the free gingival margin
B. The mesial, distal, gingival, and incisal walls of the cavity preparation diverge outward
C. The retention form is provided by the gingival retention groove placed along the incisoaxial line angle
D. A cervical clamp is usually necessary to retract gingival tissues

117. The most ductile and malleable metal is:
A. Silver
B. Gold
C. Copper
D. Platinum

118. In zinc oxide-eugenol (ZOE) cements, the powder is zinc oxide and the liquid is:
A. Phosphate acid
B. Eugenol
C. Zinc polyacrylic acid
D. Saline solution

119. Which restorative material listed below has the lowest thermal conductivity and diffusivity?
A. Amalgam
B. Gold
C. Unfilled resin
D. Filled resin

120. A patient is evaluated about eight months after her sealants were applied. She has lost two out of the four sealants that were placed. Which of the following could be blamed for these sealants being lost?
A. The etchant was not rinsed thoroughly off the tooth surface
B. A dry field was not maintained and the tooth surface was contaminated by saliva after etching
C. A contaminated air supply to air/water syringe
D. The tooth wasn't thoroughly dried prior to application of sealants
E. All of the above.

121. A cavosurface bevel is used when preparing a tooth for a cast gold inlay or onlay. What is the principal reason for its use?
A. To allow room for the cement
B. To improve the marginal adaptation
C. To compensate for shrinkage of the casting gold allow
D. To provide resistance form to the preparation

122. Cavities developing on the proximal surfaces of anterior teeth not involving the incisal edge are classified as:
A. Class I

B. Class II
C. Class III
D. Class IV
E. Class V
F. Class VI

123. Match up the fluoride concentration with the appropriate type of professionally applied topical fluoride.

Topical Fluoride	Concentration	Matching
Sodium fluoride (NaF)	8.0%,	3
Acidulated phosphate fluoride (APF)	2.0%,	1
Stannous fluoride (SnF_2)	1.23%,	2

124. How many milligrams of fluoride are contained in an 8.2 ounce tube of toothpaste?
A. 130 mg
B. 232 mg
C. 350 mg
D. 400 mg

125. High-gold alloys used for cast restorations are:
A. Greater than 20% gold or other noble metals
B. Greater than 30% gold or other noble metals
C. Greater than 50% gold or other noble metals
D. Greater than 75% gold or other noble metals

126. Which cavities below can involve any teeth, anterior or posterior?
A. Class I
B. Class II
C. Class III
D. Class IV
E. Class V
F. Class VI

127. The position of the gingival margin of a Class II amalgam restoration is dictated primarily by:
A. Aesthetics
B. The location of the gingival margin
C. The extent of the carious lesion
D. The thickness of the enamel

128. Delayed expansion of amalgam restorations is associated with which two factors listed below?
A. Insufficient trituration and condensation
B. High residual mercury
C. The contamination of the amalgam by moisture during trituration and condensation
D. The failure to use a cavity varnish

129. Triangularly shaped spaces located between the proximal surfaces of adjacent teeth are called?
A. Contact area
B. Heights of contour
C. Embrasures
D. Contact points

130. High copper dental amalgam alloys involve what ranges of copper in their composition?
A. 1 to 4%
B. 5 to 8%
C. 10 to 30%
D. 50 to 60%

131. The minimal reduction of working cusps for protection from the forces of mastication should be?
A. 2.5 to 3 mm for both amalgam and cast gold restorations
B. 1.5 to 2.0 mm for both amalgam and cast gold restorations
C. 2 mm for amalgam and 1 mm for cast gold restorations
D. 2.5 to 3 mm for amalgam and 1.5 mm for cast gold restorations

132. All of the following are true concerning dental caries except:
A. Dental caries is an infectious microbiological disease of the teeth that results in localized dissolution and destruction of the calcified tissues
B. The evidence for the role of bacteria in the genesis of dental caries is overwhelming
C. Streptococcus sanguis is considered to be a principal etiological agent in dental caries
D. Organisms which cause caries are called “cariogenic”
E. Lactic acid produced by acidogenic bacteria is the main cause of enamel decalcification

133. Pins should be inserted into:

A. Enamel only
B. Dentin only
C. Enamel and dentin (DEJ)
D. Any of the above

134. Chisels are used primarily to cut:

A. Cementum
B. Dentin
C. Enamel
D. Amalgam

Answer key to operative

1	C	2	C	3	B	4	B
5	C	6	D	7	C	8	C
9	B	10	B	11	C	12	B
13	E	14	D	15	C	16	C
17	C	18	C	19	C	20	A
21	B	22	C	23	D	24	C
25	D	26	E	27	C	28	B
29	E	30	D	31	C	32	C
33	C	34	C	35	A	36	E
37	B	38	B	39	E	40	C
41	C	42	B	43	A	44	B
45	C	46	A	47	D	48	D
49	D	50	B	51	A	52	D
53	A	54	D	55	C	56	D
57	B	58	A	59	D	60	F
61	D	62	B	63	C	64	C
65	B	66	C	67	E	68	C
69	C	70	B	71	C	72	B
73	C	74	B	75	A	76	B
77	B	78	A, B	79	F	80	F
81	A	82	C	83	B	84	B
85	A	86	C	87	C	88	A
89	A	90	C	91	C	92	C
93	D	94	C	95	E	96	B
97	C	98	E	99	—	100	C
101	D	102	C	103	B	104	D
105	C	106	B	107	C	108	B
109	B	110	G	111	C	112	C
113	C	114	A	115	E	116	A
117	B	118	B	119	C	120	E
121	B	122	C	123	—	124	B
125	D	126	A, E, F	127	C	128	C
129	C	130	C	131	D	132	C
133	B	134	C				

Reader's Notes

12

Oral Surgery

1. From the choices listed below, what are the two most important steps in the initial management of a laryngospasm?
A. Administering epinephrine
B. Applying oxygen under positive pressure
C. Administering succinylcholine
D. Placing the patient in the Trendelenburg position

2. The optimal bone grafting material should be of what origin?
A. Foreign
B. Synthetic
C. Autogenous
D. Mixed

3. Which of the following are requirements for successful implant placement?
A. Mucosal seal
B. Adequate transfer of force
C. Biocompatibility
D. All of the above

4. Which of the following can be used for removing bone?
A. Rongeur forceps
B. Chisel and mallet

C. Bone file
D. Bur and hand piece
E. All of the above

5. **Ultrashort-acting barbiturates produce loss of consciousness by depression of the:**
   A. Medulla oblongata
   B. Ascending portion of the reticular activating system
   C. Substantia nigra
   D. Descending portion of the reticular activating system

6. **The facial nerve, the retromandibular vein, and the external carotid artery lie within which salivary gland listed below?**
   A. Submandibular gland
   B. Parotid gland
   C. Sublingual gland
   D. None of the above

7. **All of the following may prevent a patient from developing a vasovagal syncopal reaction after the uses of a local anesthetic except:**
   A. Slowly injecting the anesthetic solution
   B. Watching the patient's color change during the injection
   C. Using a topical anesthetic prior to administration of the local anesthetic
   D. Injecting the anesthetic solution as quickly as possible
   E. Using a low concentration of vasoconstrictor
   F. Premedicating extremely anxious patients
   G. Sympathetic, but confident handling of the patient

8. **How will a larger than normal functional residual capacity affect nitrous oxide sedation?**
   A. Nitrous oxide sedation will happen much quicker
   B. Nitrous oxide sedation will take longer
   C. Functional residual capacity does not effect nitrous oxide sedation
   D. All of the above.

9. **A serious condition in which the quantity of blood pumped by the heart each minute (cardiac output) is insufficient to meet the body's normal requirements for oxygen and nutrients is called:**
   A. Heart block

B. Ventricular tachycardia
C. Congestive heart failure
D. Atrial fibrillation

10. All of the following are contraindication to implant placement except one. Which is the exception:
A. The presence of pathology within the bone
B. The presence of limiting anatomic structures such as the inferior alveolar nerve or maxillary sinus
C. Unrealistic expectations of the patient
D. The patient has a pronounced gag reflex
E. Acute illness or uncontrolled metabolic disease

11. A mandibular fracture that extends only through the cortical portion of the bone without complete fracture of the bone is called a:
A. Simple fracture
B. Greenstick fracture
C. Compound fracture
D. Comminuted fracture

12. Acetaminophen and propoxyphene are used together to treat moderate to severe pain due to:
A. Dental procedures
B. Headache
C. Arthralgias
D. Myalgias
E. All of the above

13. Major oral surgery includes all of the following procedures except:
A. The treatment of maxillary and mandibular fractures
B. Exodontia
C. Pre-prosthetic surgery
D. Reconstructive surgery
E. Traumatology

14. Which drug listed below is most commonly used to attain general anesthesia?
A. Valium
B. Chloral hydrate
C. Phenergan
D. Brevital

15. If the fracture line results in a muscle pull displacing the fractured segment, it is termed a (an):
A. Favorable fracture
B. Unfavorable fracture
C. Complex fracture
D. Complicated fracture

16. Which of the following is the process by which the total removal of a cystic lesion is achieved?
A. Marsupialization
B. Decompression
C. Enucleation
D. The Partsch operation

17. Which of the following is the primary direction of luxation for extracting maxillary deciduous molars?
A. Buccal
B. Palatal
C. Mesial
D. Distal

18. Which of the following are the most common causes of dehydration?
A. Fever
B. Vomiting
C. Diarrhoea
D. Heat exhaustion
E. All of the above

19. Which of the following can contribute to the non-healing (non- union) of a fracture?
A. Ischemia
B. Excessive mobility
C. Interposition of soft tissue
D. Infection
E. All of the above

20. Local anesthetics depress small, nonmyelinated nerve fibers:
A. First
B. Last
C. At the same time as large, myelinated nerve fibers
D. After the large, myelinated nerve fibers

21. Dead space in a wound usually fills with
A. Pus
B. Water
C. Blood
D. Tissue

22. All of the following are considered to be inhalational anaesthetics except?
A. Nitrous Oxide
B. Cyclopropane
C. Halothane
D. Isoflurane
E. Lidocaine

23. Which surgical approach listed below is the best to expose the TMJ?
A. Preauricular
B. Submandibular
C. Both are the same
D. None of the above

24. The internal jugular vein descends through the neck within the:
A. Arachnoid sheath
B. Carotid sheath
C. Spiral sheath
D. Dural sheath

25. All of the following statements concerning the articular eminence are true except:
A. It is also called the articular tubercle
B. It is convex
C. It is ridge that extends mediolaterally just in front of the mandibular fossa
D. It is considered to be the non-functioning portion of the temporomandibular joint
E. It is lined with a thick layer of fibrous connective tissue (fibrocartilage).

26. The universal sign of laryngeal obstruction is:
A. Mydriasis
B. Stridor (crowing sounds)

C. Sweating
D. Tachycardia

27. Squamous cell carcinoma is most easily managed when found where?
A. Floor of the mouth
B. Palate
C. Lower lip
D. Side of the tongue

28. What is the best way to palpate the posterior aspect of the mandibular condyle?
A. Intraorally
B. Lateral to the external auditory meatus
C. Through the external auditory meatus
D. Any of the above

29. Rheumatic fever is:
A. Inflammation of joints (arthritis) and the spleen (splenomegaly) resulting from a streptococcal infection, usually of the throat.
B. Inflammation of joints (arthritis) and the parotid glands (parotitis) resulting from a staphylococcal infection, usually of the middle ear.
C. Inflammation of the joints (arthritis) and the heart (carditis) resulting form a streptococcal infection, usually of the throat.
D. Inflammation of the joints (arthritis) and the thyroid gland (goiter) resulting from a staphylococcal infection, usually of the blood.

30. Which of the following is that phase of anesthesia that begins with the administration of anesthetic and continues until the desired level of patient unresponsiveness is reached?
A. Amnesia
B. Induction
C. Maintenance
D. Recovery

31. Which of the following is not an indication for excisional biopsy?
A. A small lesion (less than 1 cm in diameter)
B. A lesion that can be removed completely without traumatizing the tissue

C. When there is a suspicion of malignancy
D. A pigmented or small vascular lesion

32. Strong apical pressure with a small straight elevator may displace root tips of maxillary premolars and molars into the:
A. Submandibular space
B. Maxillary sinus
C. Mandibular canal
D. Infratemporal fossa

33. Which size suture listed below has the least strength and the smallest diameter?
A. 9-0
B. 3-0
C. 2
D. 5

34. All of the following drugs can potentiate a patient's bleeding following an extraction except:
A. Aspirin
B. Anticoagulants
C. Antianxiety drugs
D. Anticancer drugs

35. Which of the following delay healing process of an extraction site?
A. A patient that has a protein deficiency
B. A patient on glucocorticoid therapy
C. An older patient
D. Local infections
E. All of the above

36. All of the following statements concerning hemophilia are true, except:
A. Hemophilia A and B are inherited as a sex-linked recessive trait by which males are affected and females are carriers.
B. Bleeding time is abnormally prolonged.
C. The majority of people affected with manifestations include Type A and are under the age of 25.
D. The signs, symptoms and clinical manifestations include excessive bleeding from minor cuts, epistaxis, hematomas, and hemarthroses.

E. Chronic complications include impaired renal function and osteoarthritis.

37. What is the proper rate of rescue breathing in an adult?

A. 15 times per minute
B. 12 times per minute
C. 20 times per minute
D. 25 times per minute

38. Which vein listed below is the optimum site for I / V sedation for an outpatient?

A. Median basilic vein
B. Median cephalic vein
C. Median antebrachial vein
D. Angular vein

39. Which of the following is the most common pathognomonic sign of a mandibular fracture?

A. Nasal bleeding
B. Exophthalmos
C. Malocclusion
D. Numbness in the infraorbital nerve distribution

40. Which artery listed below supplies the mucosa of the hard palate posterior to the maxillary canine?

A. Sphenopalatine artery
B. Greater palatine artery
C. Posterior superior alveolar artery
D. Nasopalatine artery

41. Which of the following is the fixative of choice used for a routine biopsy specimen?

A. Hydrogen peroxide
B. Sodium hypochlorite
C. 10% formalin
D. Saline

42. The mandibular left second molar of a 14 year-old boy is unerupted. Radiographs show a small dentigerous cyst surrounding the crown. What is the treatment of choice?

A. Surgically extract the unerupted second molar
B. Uncover the crown and keep it exposed

C. Prescribe an anti-inflammatory medication and schedule a follow-up appointment in six months
D. No treatment is necessary at this time

43. All of the following drugs can reduce salivary flow during dental treatment. Which one, however, works by reducing anxiety and sensitivity during the procedure?
A. Scopolamine
B. Atropine
C. Local anesthesia
D. Benztropine

44. Therapeutic anticoagulation is administered to patients with all of the following except:
A. Post-myocardial infarction
B. Cerebrovascular thrombosis
C. Asthma
D. Pulmonary thrombosis

45. Body temperature can be measured in several different ways, which one is the least accurate?
A. Orally
B. Axillary
C. Rectally
D. Aurally

46. Serum calcium will be increased in all of the following conditions except:
A. Hyperparathyroidism
B. Chronic glomerulonephritis
C. Diabetes mellitus
D. Hypervitaminosis D
E. Malignant diseases of the skeleton (i.e., multiple myeloma)

47. Minor oral surgery includes all of the following procedures except:
A. Exodontia
B. The treatment of maxillary and mandibular fractures
C. The treatment of dental infections
D. The treatment of hard tissue pathologies
E. The treatment of soft tissue pathologies

48. Which of the following narcotics is contained in the analgesics Percodan and Percoset?

A. Codeine
B. Oxycodone
C. Hydrocodone
D. Morphine

49. Which form of the reduction listed below is best used to reduce a fracture when teeth are missing in one or more of the fractured segments?

A. Open reduction
B. Closed reduction

50. Which cranial nerve listed below provides motor innervation that allows for movements of the mandible?

A. Trigeminal (CN V)
B. Olfactory (CN I)
C. Facial (CN VII)
D. Vagus (CN X)

51. What is the only direction in which the TMJ can be dislocated?

A. Laterally
B. Medially
C. Anteriorly
D. Posteriorly

52. Which of the following are physiological symptoms of a patient taking barbiturates?

A. Slurred speech & Shallow breathing
B. Sluggishness & Fatigue
C. Disorientation & Lack of coordination
D. Dilated pupils (mydriasis)
E. All of the above

53. The mesioangular impaction is generally acknowledged as:

A. The most difficult impaction to remove
B. The least difficult impaction to remove
C. Neither of the above
D. Cannot be said.

54. The following signs i.e. a) Nausea b) Pallor and cold perspiration c) Widely dilated pupils d) Eyes rolled up e)

Brief convulsions are indicative of a patient having which type of reaction?
A. Somatogenic reaction
B. Psychogenic reaction

55. **Which of the following is considered to be the most common cause of TMJ pain?**
A. Internal derangement
B. Degenerative joint disease (DJD)
C. Myofascial pain dysfunction (MPD) syndrome
D. None of the above

56. **Which of the following statements are true concerning ecchymosis?**
A. Ecchymosis is an area of hemorrhage into the skin and subcutaneous tissue >1 cm in diameter.
B. An ecchymosis is often the result of injury; clotting and bleeding disorders can predispose to the formation of an ecchymosis
C. Grossly, an ecchymosis presents as a bluish lesion at the earliest stages of onset.
D. As the red blood cells in the lesion undergo progressive degeneration and the hemoglobin becomes converted through bilirubin into hemosiderin, the lesion progressively changes color from blue through green through purple to finally a brownish discoloration.
E. All of the above statements concerning ecchymosis are true

57. **Alloplastic grafts are:**
A. Those where the bone to be grafted to jaw is taken or harvested from one's own body
B. Taken from human donors
C. Inert, man made synthetic materials
D. Harvested from animals

58. **Which of the following is a peculiar thermal alteration that occurs during surgery in susceptible persons?**
A. Malignant hypothermia
B. Heat stroke
C. Malignant hyperthermia
D. Hyperreflexia

59. Ketamine is most commonly used to obtain:
A. Neurolept anaesthesia
B. Local anaesthesia
C. Dissociative anesthesia
D. Regional anesthesia

60. The American Society of Anesthesiologists would give what ASA classification to a healthy young patient with an unremarkable medical history and no systemic disease?
A. ASA-O
B. ASA-I
C. ASA-II
D. ASA-V

61. Which scalpel below is universally used for oral surgical procedures?
A. No. 2 blade
B. No. 6 blade
C. No. 10 blade
D. No. 15 blade

62. Chronic bronchitis is primarily a disease of:
A. Alcoholics
B. Cigarette smokers
C. Miners
D. Patients with a family history of allergy

63. What is the first step when initiating CPR?
A. Administer oxygen
B. Establish unresponsiveness
C. Administer epinephrine
D. Place a cool towel on the person's forehead

64. The most commonly used allogenic bone is:
A. Freeze-dried
B. Artificial
C. Both of the above
D. Neither of the above

65. Which of the following teeth could be removed without pain after administration of an inferior alveolar and lingual nerve block?
A. All anterior teeth on the side of the injection

B. Canine and first premolar on the side of the injection
C. Both premolars and first molar on the side of the injection
D. All the mandibular teeth

66. When a patient attempts protrusion, the mandible deviates markedly to the left which muscle listed below is unable to contract?
A. Buccinator muscle
B. Temporalis muscle
C. Right lateral pterygoid muscle
D. Left lateral pterygoid muscle

67. Incision for drainage (I&D) in an area of acute infection should only be performed after which of the following has occurred?
A. A culture for antibiotic sensitivity has been performed
B. Localization of the infection
C. A sinus tract is formed
D. All of the above

68. Which of the following is the maximum allowable dose for 2% lidocaine with 1:100,000 epinephrine?
A. 3.0 mg lidocaine/per lb.
B. 3.5 mg lidocaine/per lb.
C. 6.0 mg lidocaine/per lb.
D. 7.0 mg lidocaine/per lb.

69. The stylomandibular ligament of the TMJ is a band of cervical fascia that runs from the styloid process of the sphenoid bone to the:
A. Mandibular condyle
B. Ramus of the mandible
C. Angle of the mandible
D. Lingula of the mandible

70. The ideal time to remove impacted third molars is :
A. When the root is fully formed
B. When the root is approximately two-third formed
C. Makes no differences how much of the root is formed
D. When the root is approximately one-third formed

71. Which of the following will produce neurolept anesthesia?
A. Neuroleptic agent + narcotic analgesic

B. Neuroleptic agent + nitrous oxide
C. Neuroleptic agent + narcotic analgesic + nitrous oxide
D. Narcotic analgesic + nitrous oxide

72. When would you place a suture over a single extraction socket?
A. Routinely
B. Never
C. If the patient requests it
D. When there is severe bleeding form the gingiva or if the gingival cuff is torn or loose.

73. A patient with dry socket develops severe dull throbbing pain:
A. Two to three hours following a tooth extraction
B. One day following a tooth extraction
C. Two to four days following a tooth extraction
D. Immediately following a tooth extraction

74. A patient with a paralyzed left lateral pterygoid muscle is instructed to open his mouth wide. Which direction will the mandible take upon opening?
A. To the right
B. To the left
C. Straight
D. Is not able to open the mouth.

75. When performing CPR, if there is a pulse but the victim is not breathing, you should give rescue - breathing at a rate of:
A. 2 breaths every 20 seconds
B. 1 breath every 15 seconds
C. 1 breath every 5 seconds
D. 2 breaths every 30 seconds

76. Which suture pattern (or method) listed below is most commonly used in oral surgery?
A. Continuous pattern
B. Interrupted pattern
C. Mattress pattern
D. Sling suture pattern

77. Atelectasis can result from which of the following after a patient has undergone oral surgery?

A. Inactivity after surgery
B. Post operative narcotic analgesics
C. An endotracheal tube which has misplaced during the oral surgery procedure
D. All of the above

78. How long should one wait before obtaining a biopsy of an oral ulcer?

A. 4 days
B. 7 days
C. 14 days
D. 30 days

79. During an inferior alveolar nerve block injection, the needle passes through the mucous membrane and the buccinator muscle and lies lateral to the:

A. Masseter muscle
B. Temporalis muscle
C. Medial pterygoid muscle
D. Lateral pterygoid muscle

80. Nitrous oxide works on the:

A. Peripheral Nervous System (PNS)
B. Central Nervous System (CNS)
C. Autonomic Nervous System (ANS)
D. All of the above

81. Stage I of anesthesia describes which level of sedation?

A. Unconscious sedation
B. Conscious sedation
C. None of the above

82. Allogenic grafts (also called allografts) are composed of tissue taken from:

A. Another species
B. An individual of the same species who is not genetically related to the recipient
C. An individual of the same species who is genetically related to the recipient
D. The same individual

83. Which of the following is the most common indication for tooth transplantation?
A. Severe decay of a central incisor
B. Severe decay of a first molar
C. Severe decay of a third molar
D. Severe decay of a canine

84. All of the following are systemic contraindication to elective surgery except:
A. Blood dyscrasias (i.e., hemophilia, leukemia)
B. Controlled diabetes mellitus
C. Addison's disease or any steroid deficiency
D. Nephritis
E. Any debilitating disease
F. Cardiac disease

85. Management of an acute asthmatic episode occurring during oral surgery includes all of the following except:
A. Terminate all dental treatment
B. Position the patient in an erect or semierect position
C. Patient should administer their own bronchodilator using an inhaler
D. Administer nitroglycerin
E. Administer oxygen
F. Monitor vital signs

86. A 52-year-old woman requests removal of a painful mandibular second molar. She tells you that she has not rested for two days and nights because of the pain. Her medical history is unremarkable, except that she takes 20 mg of Prednisone daily for erythema multiforme. How do you treat this patient?
A. Have patient discontinue the Prednisone for two days prior to the extraction
B. Give steroid supplementation and remove the tooth with local anesthesia and sedation
C. Instruct the patient to take 3 grams of amoxicillin one hour prior to extraction
D. No special treatment is necessary prior to extraction

87. Wharton's duct is associated with the:
A. Parotid gland
B. Submandibular gland
C. Sublingual gland
D. von Ebner's glands

88. All of the following are reasons that vasoconstrictors are included in local anesthetics except:
A. They prolong the duration of action of the local anesthetic
B. They reduce the chance of an allergic reaction to the local anesthetic
C. They reduce the toxicity because less local anesthetic is necessary
D. They reduce the rate of vascular absorption by causing vasoconstriction
E. They help to make the anesthesia more profound by increasing the concentrations of the local anesthetic at the nerve membrane.

89. How many milligrams of epinephrine are in each cartridge (1.8 cc) of 2% lidocaine with 1:100,000 epinephrine?
A. 0.018 mg
B. 18 mg
C. 0.036 mg
D. 36 mg

90. The maxillary first molar is innervated by the:
A. Anterior superior alveolar and middle superior alveolar nerves
B. Middle superior alveolar and posterior superior alveolar nerves
C. Posterior superior alveolar and inferior alveolar nerves
D. Middle superior alveolar and palatine nerves

91. A surgical procedure for recontouring alveolar structures, usually in preparation for a prosthesis is called a (an):
A. Closed reduction
B. Operculectomy
C. Alveoloplasty
D. Gingivoplasty

92. Muscle fibers covered by a mucous membrane that attaches the cheek, lips and / or tongue to the associated dental mucosa is called:
A. Gingiva
B. Frenum
C. Operculum
D. Abutment

93. Cavernous sinus thrombosis can be caused by:
A. An infection of the central face or para-nasal sinuses
B. Bacteremia
C. Trauma
D. Infections of the ear or maxillary teeth
E. All of the above

94. Clinically scopolamine is used to:
A. Prevent nausea and vomiting associated with motion sickness
B. Reduce salivation and excess bronchial secretions prior to surgery
C. Reduce spastic states in parkinsonism
D. Produce sedation and as a preanesthetic medication
E. All of the above

95. In the head and neck, all the lymph ultimately drains into the:
A. Submental lymph nodes
B. Submandibular lymph nodes
C. Deep cervical lymph nodes
D. Retropharyngeal lymph nodes

96. Which local anesthetic listed below may possibly manifest its toxicity clinically by initial depression and drowsiness rather than stimulation and convulsion?
A. Lidocaine
B. Procaine
C. Benzocaine
D. Tetracaine

97. All of the following are contraindications to the use of nitrous oxide except:
A. Hypoxemia
B. Respiratory disease

C. Children
D. Emotional instability
E. Contagious diseases

98. All of the following are causes of metabolic alkalosis except:
A. Use of diuretics (thiazides, furosemide, ethacrynic acid)
B. Vomiting
C. Chronic renal failure
D. Overactive adrenal gland (Cushing's syndrome or use of corticosteroids)

99. Implants that are surgically inserted into the jawbone are called:
A. Endosseous implants
B. Subperiosteal implants
C. Transosscous implants
D. Supra-periosteal implants
E. None of the above

100. The treatment of a mandibular fracture using only intermaxillary fixation (IMF) is called:
A. Open reduction
B. Closed reduction
C. Fixation
D. Approximation

101. A complete blood count (CBC) includes:
A. Hematocrit
B. Hemoglobin
C. White blood cell count
D. Red blood cell count
E. All of the above

102. Zygomatic arch fractures can be nicely demonstrated by which radiograph?
A. Water's view
B. Lateral skull view
C. Posteroanterior skull view
D. Submento vertex view

103. Which artery listed below supplies the tongue?
A. Palatine artery
B. Inferior alveolar artery

C. Lingual artery
D. Vertebral artery

104. Which two of the following are useful for sedation and analgesia only?
A. Halothane
B. Methoxyflurane
C. Cyclopropane
D. Nitrous oxide
E. Ethylene

105. On physical examination, painless induration of soft tissue is suggestive of:
A. Normal tissue
B. Infection
C. Invasive malignant lesions
D. Benign lesions

106. Which division of the trigeminal nerve below passes through the foramen ovale and supplies motor innervation to the tensor veli palatini, tensor tympani, muscles of mastication (temporalis, masseter, lateral and medial pterygoids), and the anterior belly of digastric and mylohyoid muscles?
A. Ophthalmic division (V-1)
B. Maxillary division (V-2)
C. Mandibular division (V-3)
D. None of the above

107. All of the following drugs are anticholinergic except:
A. Atropine
B. Benztropine & Scopolamine
C. Fenfluramine
D. Trihexyphenidy
E. Ipratropium & Probanthine

108. By far and away the most commonly performed mandibular procedure for the correction of mandibular retrognathia is the:
A. Segmental osteotomy
B. Sagittal split osteotomy
C. Vertical ramus osteotomy
D. Body osteotomy

109. While attempting to remove a grossly decayed mandibular molar, the crown fractures. What is recommended next step in order to facilitate the removal of this tooth?

A. Use a larger forceps and luxate remaining portion of tooth to the lingual
B. Separate the roots
C. Irrigate the area and proceed to remove the rest of the tooth
D. Place a sedative filling and reschedule patient

110. All of the following are elements of general anesthesia except:

A. Analgesia
B. Relaxation
C. Hyperpyrexia
D. Hyporeflexia
E. Narcosis

111. Arrange the following five phases of healing of an extraction site in their correct order

1 Replacement of the connective tissue by fibrillar bone
2. Hemorrhage and clot formation
3. Replacement of granulation tissue by connective tissue and epithelialization of the site
4. Recontouring of the alveolar bone and maturation
5. Organization of the clot by granulation tissue

A. 4,1,3,5,2
B. 1,2,3,4,5
C. 3,4,2,1,5
D. 4,2,3,1,5

112. While extracting a mandibular third molar, you notice that the distal root tip is missing. Where is it most likely to be found?

A. In the infratemporal fossa
B. In the submandibular space
C. In the mandibular canal
D. In the pterygopalatine fossa

113. Which of the following is the most common error in recording blood pressure?

A. Applying the blood pressure cuff too tightly

B. Applying the blood pressure cuff too loosely
C. Overinflating the blood pressure cuff
D. Under-inflating the blood pressure cuff
E. Use of the wrong size cuff

114. A prothrombin time (PT) of:
A. 5-7 seconds is considered normal
B. 6-9 seconds is considered normal
C. 12-14 seconds is considered normal
D. 20-25 seconds is considered normal

115. All of following are weak points in the mandible where fractures are most common except:
A. The angle
B. The coronoid process
C. The condylar neck
D. The symphysis area

116. Which two diseases below cause more than 60% of all cases of end-stage renal disease in the United States?
A. Diabetes
B. Leukemia
C. High blood pressure (hypertension)
D. Pernicious anemia
E. Tuberculosis

117. All of the following local anesthetics are amides except:
A. Prilocaine
B. Bupivacaine
C. Lidocaine
D. Procaine

118. Which nerve below supplies motor function to the buccinator muscle?
A. Trigeminal nerve (CN V)
B. Facial nerve (CN VII)
C. Vagus nerve (CN X)
D. Glossopharyngeal nerve (CN IX)

119. Which of the following tests should be routinely performed in the preoperative work up for a patient that is being admitted to a hospital for surgery
A. A complete blood count (CBC)

B. A total white blood cell count
C. An assessment of the circulating platelets
D. A urinalysis
E. All of the above

120. Before dental treatment prophylactic antibiotic coverage is indicated for patient with each of the following conditions except:
A. Previous coronary artery bypass graft surgery
B. Rheumatic heart disease
C. Prosthetic aortic valve
D. Kidney damage needing hemodialysis
E. Total joint prosthesis

121. Inadvertent intravascular injection of a local anesthetic with a vasoconstrictor may cause which of the following clinical signs?
A. Nervousness
B. Dizziness
C. Blurred vision
D. Excitation and/or depression of the CNS
E. All of the above

122. Which of the following can result in masticator space infections?
A. Infections of the mandibular molar, especially the third molar
B. Non-aseptic technique in local anesthesia of the inferior alveolar nerve
C. Trauma to the mandibular (either external or fracture into the socket of a diseased third molar)
D. All of the above

123. Diazepam (Valium) can be used for
A. Candida albicans infections
B. Sedation induction
C. Hypothyroidism diagnosis
D. Myasthenia gravis

124. Which of the following are local contraindications for tooth extractions?
A. ANUG
B. Irradiated jaws

C. Malignant disease
D. All of the above

125. Chronic obstructive pulmonary disease (COPD) is a group of disorders characterized by airflow obstruction during respiration. Which one of those disorders listed below is marked by dyspnea and wheezing expiration caused by episodic narrowing of the airways?
A. Bronchial asthma
B. Chronic bronchitis
C. Emphysema
D. Bronchiectasis

126. Alloplastic materials used for augmentation genioplasty generally have a tendency to do what?
A. Produce an immunologic response
B. Be replaced by the host bone
C. Migrate from the position in which they were placed at the time of surgery
D. Be rejected

127. The most frequent location for a maxillary torus is:
A. The right sides of the hard palate
B. The left side of the hard palate
C. The midline of the hard palate
D. On the soft palate

128. Which teeth listed below are the most frequently impacted?
A. Maxillary canines
B. Maxillary third molars
C. Mandibular third molar
D. Mandibular premolars

129. Of the following drugs, which is most likely to cause seizures as an adverse reaction?
A. Aspirin
B. Morphine
C. Meperidine
D. Acetaminophen

130. The normal serum concentration of glucose is:
A. 20-40 mg/dl
B. 50-70 mg/dl
C. 80-120 mg/dl
D. 130-150 mg/dl

131. Which of the following are indications for biopsy?
A. A lesion that persists for more than two weeks with no apparent etiologic basis
B. Persistent hyperkeratotic changes in surface tissues
C. A lesion that has the characteristics of malignancy
D. An inflammatory lesion that does not respond to local treatment after 14 days (such as removing local irritant)
E. A persistent swelling, either visible or palpable, beneath relatively normal tissue
F. All of the above are indications for biopsy

132. A posterior superior alveolar nerve block (tuberosity injection) will provide anaesthesias for:
A. The second and third molar along with the mucoperiosteum of he palate
B. The first, second molars along with the mucoperiosteum of the palate
C. The first, second, and third molar but not the mucoperiosteum of the palate
D. The first, and third molars along with the mucoperiosteum of the palate

133. The unpleasant sensation of difficulty in breathing is called:
A. Hypercapnea
B. Dyspnoea
C. Hypocapnea
D. Apnea

134. Phlebitis of a vein after administration of IV valium is usually attributed to the presence of which of the following in the mixture?
A. Hydroquinone
B. Water
C. Alcohol
D. Propylene glycol

135. In preparing the edentulous mandible for dentures, each of the following may be safely excised except:

A. A labial frenum
B. A lingual frenum
C. The mylohyoid ridge
D. The genial tubercles
E. An exostosis

136. During extraction of a maxillary third molar, you realize the tuberosity has also been extracted. What is the proper treatment in this case?

A. Remove the tuberosity from the tooth and reimplant the tuberosity
B. Smooth the sharp edges of the remaining bone and replace and suture the remaining soft tissue
C. No special treatment is necessary
D. None of the above

137. Diabetes Mellitus Type 2 is associated with all of the following characteristic except:

A. Normal or increased insulin synthesis
B. Onset in adulthood
C. Autoimmune origin
D. Associated with obesity
E. Rare ketoacidosis

138. Which muscle below is responsible for the forward displacement of the condylar head when the neck of the condyle is fractured?

A. Masseter muscle
B. Mylohyoid muscle
C. Lateral pterygoid muscle
D. Medial pterygoid muscle

139. Which paranasal sinuses are the largest?

A. Frontal
B. Ethmoidal
C. Maxillary
D. Sphenoidal

140. How much hydrocortisone is secreted by the adrenal cortex daily?

A. About 1 mg
B. About 100 mg
C. About 20 mg
D. About 200 mg

141. Osteomyelitis is an infection of the bone and marrow. It is most often caused by:
A. Streptococcus pyogenes
B. Staphylococcus aureus
C. Mycobacterium tuberculosis
D. Neisseria meningitidis

142. Which of the following are important points to remember in the management of a diabetic patient?
A. Defer surgery until diabetes is well-controlled; consult physician
B. Schedule an early morning appointment and avoid lengthy appointments
C. Watch for signs of hypoglycemia
D. Treat infections aggressively
E. All of the above

143. The TMJ is the articulation between the condyle of the mandible and the squamous portion of the:
A. Sphenoid bone
B. Temporal bone
C. Ethmoid bone
D. Zygomatic bone

144. Which of the following arteries does not accompany the corresponding nerve throughout its course
A. Infraorbital artery
B. Inferior alveolar artery
C. Lingual artery
D. Posterior superior alveolar artery

145. The pterygopalatine fossa communicates laterally with the infratemporal fossa by way of:
A. The sphenopalatine foramen
B. The pterygoid canal
C. The foramen rotundum

D. The petrotympanic fissure
E. The pterygomaxillary fissure

146. The nerve to the mylohyoid muscle is a branch of the:
A. Ophthalmic nerve (CN V-1)
B. Maxillary nerve (CN V-2)
C. Mandibular nerve (CNV-3)
D. Facial nerve (CN VIII)

147. Which type of shock listed below is most often associated with severe trauma and reactive peripheral vasodilation?
A. Hypovolemic shock
B. Cardiogenic shock
C. Septic shock
D. Neurogenic shock
E. Anaphylactic shock

148. Which nerve listed below innervates the facial muscles with motor fibers, the lacrimal gland and salivary gland with parasympathetic fibers, and the anterior tongue with sensory fibers?
A. Trigeminal
B. Vagus
C. Facial
D. Glossopharyngeal

149. Which type of maxillary third molar impaction is most likely to be displaced into the antrum (maxillary sinus) and infratemporal space if correct extraction technique are not employed?
A. Vertical impaction
B. Distoangular impaction
C. Mesioangular impaction
D. Horizontal impaction

150. All of the following are advantages of using nitrous oxide analgesia except:
A. Rapid onset and recovery
B. Pleasant induction
C. It is a complete pain reliever
D. Nonirritating to the GI tract

151. Which of the following are likely signs and symptoms of a zygomatic fracture?
A. Nasal bleeding
B. Pain over zygomatic region
C. Numbness in the infratemporal nerve distribution
D. Exophthalmos
E. Diplopia
F. All of the above

152. When removing maxillary teeth, the upper jaw of the patient should be where in relation to the dentists's shoulder?
A. Below
B. Above
C. At the same height
D. It makes no difference where the patients's upper jaw is in relation to the dentist's shoulder

153. Local anesthetics are most effective in tissues that have what pH?
A. Below 7
B. Above 7
C. Below 4
D. Makes no difference what the pH of the tissue is.

154. What is usually the first clinical sign of mild lidocaine toxicity?
A. Itching
B. Nervousness
C. Vomiting
D. Sleepiness

155. Which type of bone healing involves both endosteal and periosteal proliferation?
A. Primary (bone- to bone)
B. Secondary (space fills in with callus)
C. Gap healing
D. None of the above

156. If a small communication is made with the maxillary sinus during extraction of a maxillary second molar, what treatment is recommended?
A. The sinus communication should be closed with a flap procedure

B. No additional surgical treatment is necessary
C. A figure- of - eight suture should be placed over the tooth socket
D. None of the above

157. Branches of which artery listed below supply the maxillary and mandibular teeth?
A. Vertebral
B. Occipital
C. Maxillary
D. Subclavian

158. Which of the following is a mandibular disorder caused by a chronic excess of glucocorticoids?
A. Cushing syndrome
B. Addison's disease
C. Cretinism
D. Grave's disease

159. How do local anesthetics affect the nerve membrane?
A. They increase potassium influx
B. They increase the membrane excitability by increasing the membrane's permeability to sodium ions
C. They decrease the membrane's permeability to sodium ions and reduce the membrane excitability
D. They increase the calcium and chloride flux

160. Which salivary gland listed below is the smallest and contains both serous and mucous acini?
A. Submandibular gland
B. Parotid gland
C. Subingual gland
D. Minor salivary glands

161. Which of the arteries listed below supply blood to the TMJ?
A. Facial artery
B. Lingual artery
C. Superficial temporal artery
D. Vertebral artery

162. The most common site of a pericoronal infection (pericoronitis) is
A. Around the site of a recent extraction

B. Around a newly erupted primary tooth
C. Around periodontally involved mandibular incisors
D. Around mandibular third molars

163. Which of the following is the most common cause of bleeding disorders?
A. Polycythemia vera
B. Thrombocytopenia
C. Myelofibrosis
D. Chronic myelocytic leukemia

164. Which of the following statement concerning the hypoglossal nerve are true?
A. It is a motor nerve supplying all of the intrinsic and extrinsic muscles of the tongue, except the palatoglossus, which is supplied by the vagus nerve.
B. It leaves the skull through the hypoglossal canal medial to the carotid canal and jugular foramen
C. It passes above the hyoid bone on the lateral surface of the hyoglossus muscle deep to mylohyoid muscle
D. It loops around the occipital artery and passes between the external carotid artery and internal jugular vein.
E. In the upper part of its course, it is joined by C1 fibers from the cervical plexus
F. All of the above statements are true concerning the hypoglossal nerve

165. Which nerve listed below is the largest of the 12 cranial nerves and is the principal general sensory nerve to the head, particularly the face?
A. Vagus (CN X)
B. Glossopharyngeal (CN IX)
C. Facial (CN VII)
D. Trigeminal (CN V)

166. Which of the following is the main reason to use water irrigation when cutting bone
A. It helps to wash away debris
B. Because heat generated by the drill affects bone vitality
C. To decrease the smell of freshly cut bone
D. It helps to flush out the high speed suction

167. The most severe tissue reaction is seen with which type of suture material?

A. Plain catgut
B. Chromic catgut
C. Polyglycolic acid
D. Polyglactin 910

168. Postoperative hypotension may be due to the effect of

A. Transfusion reaction
B. The anesthetic or analgesics on the myocardium
C. Liver failure
D. Anaphylaxis
E. All of the above

169. In patients having a Le Fort II fracture, a common finding is parasthesia over the distribution of the :

A. Infraorbital nerve
B. Inferior alveolar nerve
C. Mylohyoid nerve
D. Hypoglossal nerve

170. A person who has been on suppressive doses of steroid will

A. Never regain full adrenal cortical function
B. Take as much as a year to regain full adrenal cortical function
C. Take as little as a week to regain full adrenal cortical function
D. Take usually a couple of days to regain full adrenal cortical function

171. The initial event in a vasovagal syncope episode is the stress-induced release of increased amounts of catecholamines that cause all of the following except:

A. A decrease in peripheral vascular resistance
B. Tachycardia
C. Sweating
D. Bradycardia

Answer key to oral surgery

1	B, C	2	C	3	D	4	E
5	B	6	B	7	D	8	B
9	C	10	D	11	B	12	E
13	B	14	D	15	B	16	C
17	B	18	E	19	E	20	A
21	C	22	E	23	A	24	B
25	D	26	B	27	C	28	C
29	C	30	B	31	C	32	B
33	A	34	C	35	E	36	B
37	B	38	B	39	C	40	B
41	C	42	B	43	C	44	C
45	B	46	C	47	B	48	B
49	A	50	A	51	C	52	E
53	B	54	B	55	C	56	E
57	C	58	C	59	C	60	B
61	D	62	B	63	B	64	A
65	B	66	D	67	B	68	B
69	C	70	B	71	C	72	D
73	C	74	B	75	C	76	B
77	D	78	C	79	C	80	B
81	B	82	B	83	B	84	B
85	D	86	B	87	B	88	B
89	A	90	B	91	C	92	B
93	E	94	E	95	C	96	A
97	C	98	C	99	A	100	B
101	E	102	D	103	C	104	D, E
105	C	106	C	107	C	108	B
109	B	110	C	111	A	112	B
113	B	114	C	115	B	116	A, C
117	D	118	B	119	E	120	A
121	E	122	D	123	B	124	D
125	A	126	C	127	C	128	C
129	C	130	C	131	F	132	C
133	B	134	D	135	D	136	B
137	C	138	C	139	C	140	C
141	B	142	E	143	B	144	C
145	E	146	C	147	D	148	C

149	B	150	C	151	F	152	C
153	B	154	B	155	A	156	B
157	C	158	A	159	C	160	C
161	C	162	D	163	B	164	F
165	D	166	B	167	A	168	E
169	A	170	B	171	D		

Reader's Notes

13

Radiology

1. **Which of the following is not a disadvantage of the bisecting technique?**
   A. Image on x-ray film may be dimensionally distorted (amount may vary)
   B. Increased exposure time
   C. Due to the use of a short cone (which results in divergent ray), the image is not a true reproduction of the object
   D. May not be able to judge the correct alveolar bone height

2. **Your dental hygienist has a patient that says she needs bite - wing x-ray because it has been six months since the last films were taken. Your hygienist should respond in which manner listed below?**
   A. Agree with the patient
   B. Tell the patient that bite-wing x-ray should be taken once a year
   C. Tell the patient that dental x-ray are taken only when needed as judged by each patient's needs
   D. None of the above

3. **Which of the following positioning errors is the most likely cause of a reverse occlusal plane curve on a panorex (panoramic radiograph?**
   A. Chin tilted too far upward
   B. Chin tilted too far downward
   C. Head turned slightly
   D. None of the above

4. The period between radiation exposure and the onset of symptoms is called the:
A. Latent period
B. Period of cell injury
C. Recovery period
D. None of the above

5. All of the following are advantages of a panoramic radiograph except:
A. It shows areas that may not be visible on a full mouth series
B. It shows both arches on the same film
C. It gives better detail and definition than periapical radiographs
D. It is more comfortable for the patient (eliminates gagging)
E. It requires less time than a full mouth series

6. Which type of structure inhibits the passage of x-rays?
A. Radiopaque
B. Radiolucent
C. Translucent
D. All of the above

7. Kilovoltage controls the speed of:
A. Photons
B. Electrons
C. Anodes
D. Cathodes

8. The number of x-ray produced is controlled by:
A. Kilovoltage (kVp)
B. Milliamperage (mA)
C. Exposure time
D. All of the above

9. Which of the fallowing errors in radiographic technique is the most likely reason that an image on a radiograph would appear elongated?
A. Too much vertical angulation
B. Too little vertical angulation
C. Incorrect horizontal angulation
D. Beam not aimed at center of film

10. Which of the following is a major disadvantage of the paralleling technique?

A. The image formed in the film will not have dimensional accuracy
B. Due to the amount of distortion, periodontal bone height cannot be accurately diagnosed
C. An increase in exposure time is necessary due to the use of a long cone
D. An increase in exposure time is necessary due to the use of a short cone

11. One of the films in a full mouth series of dental radiographs has crescent shaped marks on it. What is the most likely cause of these marks?

A. Overbent films / cracked emulsions
B. Patient had glasses on
C. Exposure to secondary radiation
D. Cone cutting
E. X-ray arm drifted

12. Suppose that in a periapical examination of the mandibular incisor region, an exposure time of 1/4 second and focus- film distance of 8 inches were used. If you increase the focus-film distances to 16 inches, what would be the new exposure time required to produce the same density in the radiograph?

A. 1/2 second
B. 1 second
C. 2 second
D. 4 second

13. Which of the following is the name of the bony projection that arises from the sphenoid bone and extends downward and slightly posteriorly?

A. The lingula
B. The hamular process
C. Sella turcica
D. Pubic symphysis

14. Which x-ray is designed for diagnosis of basilar skull fractures?

A. Water's view
B. Submental-vertical / submento-vertex view

C. Towne's view
D. Panorex view

15. Image magnification may be minimized by :
A. Using a short cone
B. Placing the film as far from the tooth as possible
C. Using a long cone
D. Shortening the exposure time

16. X-ray fixer contains all of the following except:
A. A clearing agent
B. An antioxidant preservative
C. An accelerator
D. An acidifier
E. A hardener

17. The most effective means in reducing the time of exposure, the amount of radiation reaching the patient and the amount of radiation scattered to the dentist is:
A. A lead apron
B. Ultra-speed film
C. Lead diaphragms
D. Increasing target-film distance

18. It is recommended that the operator stand at least how many feet away from the patient when taking radiographs:
A. Two feet
B. Four feet
C. Six feet
D. Eight feet

19. Osteoradionecrosis is more common:
A. In the mandible
B. In the maxilla
C. Equally in both
D. Zygoma

20. Which of the following is a measure of the energy imparted by any type of ionizing radiation to a mass of any type of matter:
A. Absorbed dose
B. Exposure
C. Equivalent dose
D. Effective dose

21. The area from which x-rays emanate is called the:
A. Target
B. Focal spot
C. Intensifying screen
D. Cone

22. Which of the following is the best film for visualizing the condyles and neck of the mandible from an A-P projection?
A. Water's view
B. Caldwell's view
C. Towne's view
D. Panorex

23. Increasing the kilovoltage (kVp) causes the resultant x-ray to have
A. Decreased density
B. More latitude
C. A shorter scale of contrast
D. A longer scale of contrast

24. The image of the coronoid process of the mandible often appears in periapical x-ray of
A. The incisor region of the mandible
B. The molar region of the mandible
C. The incisor region of the maxilla
D. The molar region of the maxilla

25. All of the following are radioresistant cells except:
A. Muscle
B. Nerve
C. Mature bone
D. Lymphocytes

26. It is best to retain dental radiographs for how many years?
A. 2 years
B. 4 years
C. 6 years
D. Indefinitely

27. An assistant has taken three panoramic x-ray films today. During the day as she developed each film, she noticed the

films getting lighter and lighter. What needs to be done so that this problem can be corrected?

A. Decrease the temperature of the developing solution
B. Increase the temperature of the developing solution
C. Replenish the developing solution
D. Increase the mA setting
E. Increase the kVp setting

28. Which of the following are the uses of cephalometrics in orthodontics?

A. Diagnosis
B. Analysis of treatment results
C. Longitudinal study of growth
D. All of the above

29. Foreshortening and elongation are produced by:

A. Incorrect horizontal angulation
B. Incorrect vertical angulation
C. Either of the above
D. None of the above

30. The screening x-ray for pathology of the jaws is:

A. A panorex
B. A cephalogram
C. A periapical x-ray
D. An occlusal x-ray

31. All of the following are true concerning collimation except:

A. It prevents overexposure to patients
B. It increases the area of patient exposure
C. It reduces secondary radiation to the film
D. It reduces secondary radiation to the patient

32. Which of the following is the standard radiograph of choice for showing an anterior view of the paranasal sinuses and of the mid-face and orbits?

A. Panorex
B. Towne's view
C. Water's view
D. Cephalogram

33. Which of the following types of intraoral radiographs are most useful in detecting inter proximal caries?

A. Periapical radiograph
B. Bitewing radiographs
C. Occlusal radiographs
D. Cephalogram

34. The radiographs were taken with the buccal object rule in mind. In film # 2, the x-ray tube was directed from a mesial angulation. The object also moved mesially. What is the special position of the object in these radiograph?

A. The object lies lingual to the first molar
B. The object lies buccal to the first molar
C. The object lies between the second premolar and the first molar
D. The object lies directly apical to the first molar

35. After processing film, you notice that it appears brown in color. What is the most likely cause of this?

A. Solutions are too strong
B. Solutions are too weak
C. Fixing time was not long enough
D. Fixing time was too long
E. Film was under developed

36. X-ray developer contains all of the following except:

A. A developing agent
B. An antioxidant preservative
C. A clearing agent
D. An accelerator
E. A restrainer

Answer key to radiology

1	B	2	C	3	A	4	A
5	C	6	A	7	B	8	B
9	B	10	C	11	A	12	B
13	B	14	B	15	C	16	C
17	B	18	C	19	A	20	A
21	B	22	C	23	D	24	D
25	D	26	D	27	C	28	D
29	B	30	A	31	B	32	C
33	B	34	A	35	C	36	C

Reader's Notes

14

Preventive Medicine

Including Microbiology and Biochemistry

1. BCG vaccine should be used within how much time after preparation:
A. 1 day
B. 2 days
C. 3 days
D. 4 days

2. Drug resistance is produced most commonly by which of the following antituberculous drug ?
A. INH
B. Rifampicin
C. Ethionamide
D. Streptomycin

3. The metabolite which accumulates in blood, in epidemic dropsy, is :
A. Acetic acid
B. Pyruvic acid
C. Acetaldehyde
D. Formaldehyde

4. Hepatitis virus A can be killed by:
A. Ultraviolet light
B. Formalin 1 : 4000
C. Boiling at 1000° C for 5 minutes
D. Chlorination at 2 ppm

5. Which of the following statement is not true about sabin vaccine
A. 3 doses given
B. Given by intramuscular route
C. Given at monthly interval
D. Contain 3 viral strains

6. All of the following is/are true about measles vaccine except:
A. Not given if history of allergy to egg
B. Live attenuated vaccine
C. Given within one hour of reconstitution
D. Stored at 2°–10° C in a refrigerator

7. Most common method of detecting malnutrition by a health guide is:
A. Height
B. Weight
C. Mid-arm circumference
D. Skin fold thickness

8. Cereals lack which of the following amino acid:
A. Methionine
B. Lysine
C. Leucine
D. Phenylalanine

9. The protein content of cow's milk is
A. 1.2 gm%
B. 2.4 gm%
C. 3.5 gm%
D. 4.2 gm%

10. Vitamin A prophylaxis to be given 6 monthly is :
A. 6 μg
B. 66 μg
C. 6 mg
D. 66 mg

11. Which of the following is a dependent variable:
A. Cause
B. Effect
C. Association
D. Relative proportion

12. Disinfectants kill which of the following:
A. Microorganism
B. Pathogenic microorganism
C. Nonpathogenic microorganism
D. Viruses and fungi

13. Most common cause of neonatal deaths in India is :
A. Prematurity
B. Congenital malformation
C. Metabolic disease
D. Malnutrition

14. Incidence can be defined as :
A. Number of cases exiting at a given moment
B. Number of cases existing in a given population over a given period
C. Number new cases occurring during a specified period in a given population
D. Number of old cases present doing a specified period in a given population.

15. The community development programme is meant:
A. To bring about a Social and Economic change in village life through the effort of villagers themselves
B. To arrange welfare programme for women and children
C. To improve the agriculture product through better manure and seeds
D. To plan development programmers in about 100 villages with a population of about six to eight thousand.

16. The best method of health instruction is :
A. Providing reading assignment
B. Giving lectures
C. Setting example
D. Organizing film shows

17. The best teaching opportunity for a health worker in the community is while.
A. Giving health talk at home
B. Demonstrating to a group of mothers
C. Examining mother and children
D. Completing the records

18. Breast feeding is best for the baby:
A. But has no effect on the mother
B. But is likely to affect the mother's appearances adversely
C. But may cause Breast cancer in the mother
D. And is also good for the mother

19. Kwashiorkor is characterized by all of the following except
A. Apathy
B. Liver changes
C. Decreased body weight
D. Flag sign

20. Quarantine is the:
A. Minimum incubation period
B. Maximum incubation period
C. Period of infectivity
D. Serial interval

21. Cholera vaccine gives protection for:
A. 1-3 months
B. 3-6 months
C. 6-12 months
D. 12-18 months

22. Incubation period of mumps is:
A. 7 days
B. 7-14 days
C. 14-21 days
D. 21-30 days

23. Which of the following is a milk born disease:
A. Q-fever
B. Leptospirosis
C. Brucellosis
D. All of the above

24. Prevalence is calculated in a population by :
A. Finding the susceptible
B. Follow up
C. Studying cohorts
D. Studying the records

25. Correct nutritional status is best assessed by which of the following:
A. Weight for age
B. Height for age
C. Weight for height
D. Anthropometrics

26. Vi antigen of Salmonella is found to know the :
A. Carrier stage
B. Diseased stage
C. Infectivity
D. Immunity

27. For investigating an epidemic, all of the following are done except:
A. Confirmation of epidemic
B. Isolation of cases
C. Studying cofactors
D. Verification of case

28. What is the Role of Glucose in anti-diarrhoeal solution it:
A. Change taste
B. Increases absorption of sodium
C. Increases absorption of amino acids
D. Rapidly controls diarrhea by absorption of water

29. In a patient with burns more than 40%, average energy requirement in calories is:
A. 4000
B. 4500
C. 6000
D. 7000

30. Commonest cancer in males in India is of:
A. Bronchus
B. Stomach

C. Head and neck area
D. Urinary bladder

31. Appropriate fluoride levels in water in India is suggested to be:
A. 0.4 meq/L
B. 0.8 meq/L
C. 1.0 meq/L
D. 1.6 meq/L

32. Pellagra because of Jowar occurs due to:
A. High level of leucine
B. Low level of tryptophan
C. Increase in level of tryptophan
D. Low level of leonine

33. Chlorine available in fresh bleaching power is :
A. 20 %
B. 25 %
C. 33 %
D. 40 %

34. Man is intermediate host for:
A. Enterobiasis
B. Schistosomiasis haematobium
C. Taenia saginata
D. Echinococcus

35. Which of the following is a live vaccine
A. TAB
B. BCG
C. Diphtheria
D. DPT
E. Meningococcal

36. Newborn baby of a mother who had measles, is immune to this disease for
A. 4 to 6 months
B. 6 to 12 months
C. 1 to 3 years
D. 3 to 6 years
E. Life

37. Breast feeding is contraindicated if mother is receiving which of the following drugs?
A. Anti thyroid drugs
B. Broad spectrum antibiotics
C. Insulin
D. Saline
E. Streptomycin

38. Lepromin test is done to find out:
A. Indicative of delayed hypersensitivity
B. Indicative of infection
C. Negative in tubercular type
D. Positive in lepromatous type

39. The best method for sterilization of disposable items is:
A. Boiling heat
B. Dry heat
C. Gamma radiation
D. Incineration

40. Highest percentage of iron is present in which of the following:
A. Egg
B. Mutton .
C. Soybean
D. Spinach

41. In a standard normal curve, mean ± 2 standard deviation covers:
A. 60 %
B. 65 %
C. 95 %
D. 99 %

42. Ringer lactate solution contains which of the following electrolytes:
A. Na^+ and Cl^-
B. Na^+; K^+ and Cl^-
C. Na^+; K^+, Cl^- and Ca_2^+
D. Na^+; K^+ and HCO_3

43. Thiamine deficiency is best diagnosed by:
A. Erythrocyte transketolase assay
B. Blood free pyruvate levels

C. Acetyl –COA levels
D. Clinical severity of disease

44. Break point chlorination means:
A. Appearance of free chlorine in water
B. Appearance of residual chlorine in water
C. Point at which organic products are not oxidized
D. Twice the requisite amount of chlorine

45. Fiber optic instruments like endoscopes should be sterilized by:
A. Formaldehyde
B. Glutaraldehyde
C. Gamma radiation
D. Cetrimide

46. Vitamin A toxicity is manifested due to:
A. Mitochondrial damage
B. Glutaraldehyde
C. Microtubular damage
D. Endoplasmic reticulum damage

47. Ear-drum may rupture above which noise level:
A. 120 db
B. 160 db
C. 80 db
D. 90 db

48. MTP act permits termination of pregnancy up to which weeks of gestation:
A. 10
B. 12
C. 20
D. 28

49. Schick test is done to indicate:
A. Immunity to tetanus
B. Susceptibility to diphtheria
C. Immunity to diphtheria
D. Sensitivity of treatment

50. The freshly prepared ORS (Oral Rehydration Solution) should not be used for;
A. 2 hours

B. 8 hours
C. 12 hours
D. 24 hours

51. The daily extra calorie requirement in first trimester of pregnancy is:
A. 50
B. 150
C. 350
D. 450

52. Richest source of niacin is:
A. Egg
B. Meat
C. Liver
D. Milk

53. Screening of disease is what type of prevention:
A. Primary
B. Secondary
C. Tertiary
D. All of the above

54. Toxoid is prepared from:
A. Exotoxin
B. Endotoxin
C. Both
D. None of the above

55. Carcinoma more prevalent in persons working in dye industry of:
A. Bones
B. Skin
C. Lungs
D. Bladder

56. Dengue spreads by:
A. Anopheles
B. Culex
C. Aedes
D. Mansoides

57. Excessive crying is seen after vaccination of:
A. BCG
B. Polio
C. DPT
D. Measles

58. Strict vegetarians are deficient in:
A. B_1
B. Biotin
C. B_{12} / cyanocobalamine
D. Vitamin D

59. Most immediate treatment of night blindness is:
A. Topical Vitamin A
B. Vitamin A orally
C. Vitamin A parenterally
D. Any of the above

60. Treatment of choice for diphtheria carrier is:
A. Erythromycin
B. Tetracycline
C. Penicillin
D. DPT

61. Spread of dispersion means:
A. Mean
B. Mode
C. Median
D. Standard deviation

62. Constituents of 'Savlon' are:
A. Cetrimide +Chlorhexidine
B. Cetrimide + quarternary ammonium compound
C. Buffered glutaraldehyde
D. Certrimide only

63. Γ- globulins do not interact with immunity of:
A. Mumps
B. Measles
C. Rubella
D. Oral polio

64. Control of reservoir for presentation of disease is done with:
A. Tetanus
B. Rabies
C. Influenza
D. Diphtheria

65. Normal distribution of a curve depends upon:
A. Mean
B. Standard deviation
C. A + B
D. Mean + Range

66. 'Confidence + Limits' are:
A. Mean +Standard error
B. Median + Standard error
C. Mean + Range
D. Mean + Standard deviations

67. Which of the following immunoglobulins is found in saliva?
A. Ig M
B. Ig A
C. Ig E
D. Ig D
E. Ig G

68. Transplacental immunity is seen in all except:
A. Diphtheria
B. Pertusis
C. Polio
D. Measles

69. Primary prevention of diabetes mellitus includes all except:
A. Reduction of weight
B. Prevent hypertension
C. Exercise
D. Avoid-excessive sweets

70. Food poisoning is caused by all except:
A. Cl. septicum
B. Cl. welchii
C. Cl. Oedematicus
D. S. typhimururium

71. The fluid requirements per kilogram of body weight are highest:
- A. In the first week of the life
- B. Between ages of 1 to 6 months
- C. Between ages up to 24 months
- D. Above the age of 24 months.

72. Measles vaccine is not given below the age of:
- A. 9 months
- B. 12 months
- C. 15 months
- D. 18 months

73. Primary chemoprophylaxis belongs to which level of prevention:
- A. Ist
- B. 2nd
- C. 3rd
- D. 4th

74. All of the following are true vaccines except:
- A. Cholera
- B. BCG
- C. Typhoid
- D. DPT

75. Which of the following cereals is richest in calcium:
- A. Wheat
- B. Gram
- C. Rice
- D. Bajra

76. Hepatitis A virus is destroyed by all except:
- A. Chlorine 1 ppm
- B. Boiling at 100° C for 6 min
- C. UV rays
- D. Formalin 1:4000

77. Terms mild, moderate and severe are which type of variable:
- A. Interval
- B. Nominal.
- C. Ordinate
- D. Ratio

78. Man is an intermediate host for:
A. P.vivax
B. Strongyloides stercorales
C. Enterobius
D. Trichiuris trichura

79. Dally requirement of calcium in pregnancy is:
A. 50 mg
B. 100 mg
C. 500 mg
D. 1000 mg

80. Herd immunity is not useful in protection against:
A. Polio
B. Diphtheria
C. Measles
D. Tetanus

81. In a patient with AIDS, can not be given all of the following vaccines except:
A. BCG
B. DPT
C. OPV
D. Measles

82. The Best Epidemoilogical marker for the HBV:
A. HBc Ag
B. HBs Ag
C. Anti HBs Ag antibody
D. HBe Ag

83. Best indicator for Hepatitis – B infection of community:
A. Hepatitis B antigen
B. Core Antigen
C. Core Antibody
D. Hepatitis B Antibody

84. Best source of vitamin B_{12} is:
A. Milk
B. Liver
C. Soyabean
D. Leafy vegetables

85. Mosquito acts as intermediate vector in:
A. Filaria
B. Cholera
C. Typhoid
D. Malaria

86. Carcinoma least amenable to screening is of:
A. Lung
B. Breast
C. Cervix
D. Oral cavity

87. Variables are arranged in ascending or descending order to find:
A. Mean
B. Median
C. Mode
D. Standard deviation

88. Which of the following is an absolute contraindication for combined oral pills:
A. Diabetes mellitus
B. Hypertension
C. Previous history of thromboembolism
D. Heart disease

89. Incidence is calculated by:
A. Prospective study
B. Retrospective study
C. Cross-sectional study
D. Random study

90. Epidemiologic study of Hepatitis B:
A. HbsAg is used
B. IgG anti HBC
C. Hb C Ag
D. HBeAg

91. Student's t - test:
A. Is used to calculate attributable risk
B. Is used to calculate relative risk
C. To find out degree of significance
D. To calculate generation time of a disease

92. Vaccine not given to immuno-competent siblings of immuno deficient children:
A. Oral polio
B. MMR
C. Measles
D. DPT

93. Additional protein requirement per day during lactation is:
A. 14 g
B. 25 g
C. 35 g
D. 45 g

94. Benzathine penicillin given in RHD is which type of prevention:
A. Primordial
B. Primary
C. Secondary
D. Tertiary

95. Which of the following is a subcutaneous vaccine:
A. Measles
B. BCG
C. DPT
D. Polio

96. Quarantine is defined as:
A. Diseased individual isolated till symptoms subside
B. Healthy individual isolated after exposure to disease
C. Healthy individual isolated before exposure to disease
D. Diseased individual isolated till no secondary case occurs

97. Vaccine contraindicated in pregnancy is:
A. Tuberculin
B. Polio
C. Hepatitis B
D. Typhoid

98. In a patient with AIDS, you do not give which vaccine:
A. BCG
B. DPT
C. OPV
D. Measles

99. Most common cancer reported in India is:
A. Ca cervix
B. Ca lung
C. Ca breast
D. Ca oral cavity

100. 'DOTS' is:
A. Short term chemotherapy under direct observation
B. Long term chemotherapy under observation
C. Long term chemotherapy without supervision
D. Free drug distribution to patients

101. Quarantine is:
A. To keep the patient for longest incubation period
B. To keep the patient for shortest incubation period
C. To isolate for lag period
D. To isolate for generation time

102. Additional calories required during Lactation is:
A. 450
B. 550
C. 650
D. 750

103. Normal iron requirement during pregnancy is:
A. 2 mg
B. 40 mg
C. 80 mg
D. 100 mg

104. Active & Passive immunity is given simultaneously for the following except:
A. Hepatitis B
B. Tetanus
C. Measles
D. Rabies

105. Vitamin D is not present in:
A. Milk
B. Fish fat
C. Cod liver oil
D. Egg

106. Amount of weight gain per unit quantity protein is:
A. Protein efficiency ratio
B. Net protein utilization
C. Biological value
D. Digestibility coefficient

Answer key to microbiology including biochemistry and preventive medicine

1	A	2	A	3	B	4	C
5	C	6	D	7	C	8	B
9	C	10	D	11	B	12	B
13	A	14	C	15	A	16	C
17	C	18	D	19	C	20	B
21	B	22	C	23	D	24	B
25	C	26	A	27	B	28	B
29	C	30	C	31	C	32	A
33	C	34	D	35	B	36	B
37	A	38	A	39	C	40	B
41	C	42	C	43	B	44	A
45	B	46	A	47	A	48	C
49	B	50	D	51	B	52	B
53	B	54	A	55	D	56	C
57	C	58	C	59	B	60	A
61	D	62	A	63	D	64	B
65	C	66	A	67	B	68	B
69	A	70	C	71	B	72	A
73	A	74	D	75	D	76	A
77	A	78	A	79	D	80	D
81	B	82	A	83	B	84	B
85	A	86	A	87	B	88	C
89	A	90	B	91	C	92	A
93	B	94	C	95	A	96	B
97	A	98	D	99	D	100	A
101	A	102	B	103	B	104	C
105	A	106	A				

Reader's Notes

Reader's Notes

Reader's Notes